MICROBIOLOGICAL CLINICAL HYGIENE

MICROBIOLOGICAL HYGIENE

EINO ELIAS HAKALEHTO - SERIES EDITOR –

DEPARTMENT OF ENVIRONMENTAL SCIENCES, UNIVERSITY OF EASTERN FINLAND, KUOPIO, FINLAND

Microbiological Clinical Hygiene

Eino Elias Hakalehto (Editor)

2015. ISBN: 978-1-63463-428-1
(Hardcover)

MICROBIOLOGICAL HYGIENE

MICROBIOLOGICAL CLINICAL HYGIENE

EINO ELIAS HAKALEHTO
EDITOR

New York

Library of Congress Cataloging-in-Publication Data

ISBN: 978-1-63463-428-1

Library of Congress Control Number: 2014954519

Published by Nova Science Publishers, Inc. † New York

Contents

Preface

The idea of bringing together the different areas of microbiological hygiene in a book series came from the Publisher. In our modern times when microbial presence is perceived in more depth than before, it is an intriguing task to compile the research in the varied aspects of this unseen world of micro-organisms. The initial aim of this part, "Microbiological Clinical Hygiene", is to provide practical advice for those dealing with different aspects of health protection in the clinical environment. In addition, the book also aims at giving some cutting-edge information of the fascinating microscopic organisms which play a significant role in our life.

Dynamic balances are of utmost importance in the interactions between the human host and his microbiota. The interfaces between human cells and the ten time more numerous microbial cells can be seen as a protection against the hazards of the environment. It is, therefore, important to uphold the balances crucial to our health.

Our innovative PMEU technology (Portable Microbe Enrichment Unit) has proven useful in various fields of microbiological studies, producing novel information on microbial physiology and interactions as well as molecular communication during metabolic activity. However, more new methods and studies are needed before it is possible to satisfactorily simulate link between man and his microbiome.

If precautions on hygiene maintenance and control are properly managed in the hospital environment, the risks for not only direct microbiological contamination but also toxin and poisonous chemical load will diminish. Any combination of several malicious factors can multiply the risks of health hazards. Similarly, the positive effects accumulate. In fact, this is true also with respect to any internal factor contributing to the hygienic status within the body system of an individual. We may well consider the clinical hygiene as a concept much wider than the cleanliness in the patient proximity only. In this wider sense, the high standard of microbiological clinical hygiene could mean the combination of all the conditions, which best protect the patients and personnel, and the community, from any risks caused by microbial contamination or infection, or by their cohesive effect in the outer or bodily environment of the physiologically active host cells.

It has been an inspiring experience to see the accumulated scientific conception and confirmation of the work tradition of many pioneers, such as Ignaz Semmelweis, Louis Pasteur, A. J. Kluyver, C. B. Van Niel, William Firth Wells, Helge Gyllenberg and many others, during the era of microbiological research.

Microbiological Clinical Hygiene can be understood to play an important role in maintaining or achieving health. As a field of study, it combines scientific theory with practical work in hospitals, clinics, and in the field. Microbiological Clinical Hygiene refers to cleanliness of the human environment in situations and facilities, where the risk of invasive infection or physiological malfunction exists. Its main purpose is to protect individuals from pathogenic or otherwise harmful microbes. However, it can also mean a healthy balance of the microbiota on different surfaces of the body, i.e., the mucosal membranes and the skin, which protect the body from harmful microbes.

This volume, "Microbiological Clinical Hygiene" is the first book in a series of four. The following three volumes will be "Microbiological Food Hygiene", "Microbiological Industrial Hygiene" and "Microbiological Environmental Hygiene".

I wish to thank all the contributors of this book for fruitful cooperation, as well as those who took part in various phases of the technical edition. Most of you were conscious of the serious microbial illness of our son, supporting in many ways during the hard times and shared the joy of his recovery with us. My sincere and warmest thanks to all of you.

My thanks are also due to the Publisher, Nova Scientific Publishers Inc., for taking up this important field of Microbiological Hygiene.

In Kuopio, Finland, 21st of July, 2014.

Elias Hakalehto, Editor
Department of Environmental Sciences
University of Eastern Finland
P.O.B. 1627, FI-70211
Kuopio, Finland

Introduction

Elias Hakalehto

Department of Environmental Sciences,
University of Eastern Finland, Kuopio, Finland

Although various microbiological strains are more or less omnivalent in the environment or even within the human body system, there are some areas in the latter where they are basically kept out. Such tissues include several organs and cavities: the bladder, the neural network, the peritoneum, and some other areas of the body. In turn, our body is tightly connected with its environment via its microbiome. Therefore, many principles of ecology apply to human microbial communities.

With respect to the the stomach it was long believed that hardly any bacteria reside there permanently. However, this picture has changed after the finding that helicobacteria are embedded into the epithelia inside the polysaccharide capsules which protect the bacteria against the acidic environment (Marshall 1995). More recently, the presence of lactic acid bacteria (LAB) in the gastric areas has been established (Hakalehto et al., 2011, Hakalehto, 2012). In the duodenum, bile acids, immunoglobulins, defensins and other protective mechanisms prevent most microbe populations from growing too much (Hakalehto, 2012). Correspondingly, "aerial protection" is found elsewhere in the Nature, for example, in the antibacterial peptides of frogs' skin (Samgina et al., 2012).

In hospitals and within all the healthcare systems, we should recognize the importance of maintaining sterile and almost sterile sites. Protection is needed against diseases and hygienic risks that the patients and personnel encounter in man-to-man contacts and environmental contamination. In order to achieve this, more information on pathogenic and harmful organisms is required, as well as knowledge on their dissemination and distribution inside the healthcare environment (Hakalehto, 2006). A prevalent trend is towards point-of-care applications in the microbiological verification. Understanding the biofilm formation is of crucial importance in the understanding of microbial communities on surfaces (Costerton et al., 1999). We should also block "the routes of contamination" into the body system and inside hospitals (Tran et al., 2006).

This is simply what this book is about. Hopefully we will be able to elucidate some ways in which the results from scientific explorations can be useful in the practical situations in healthcare. Actually, It is not only a matter of verifying the microbial presence, but of characterizing the microbes and assessing their relevance and potential risks also. With genetic techniques, such as Polymerase Chain Reaction (PCR), it has been found that human intestines contain far more bacterial species than it is possible to cultivate in the laboratory (Ott et al., 2004). Consequently, in hygienic studies, it is important – after finding out the key organisms – to study the action or activities of the microbial population as a whole as well as the physiological functions of individual strains. In variable conditions, these strains choose variable modes of metabolic behavior and interaction.

Molecular communication between the human body system and the microbes determine the consequences of microbial presence. For example, *Klebsiella pneumonia* can colonize the intestines of a small child and become an integrated member of the normal flora. But in some conditions later in life, it can develop detrimental pathogenesis in the lungs (Hakalehto, 2012, 2013). The basic characteristics of various strains also explain why some klebsiellas are pathogenic, while the majority of the strains are harmless members of microbiota.

In order to understand better the roles of bacteria and other microbes in our health and sickness, new methods are warranted. There is an increasing need to understand the relations between the neogenesis of bacterial strains and the altered mode of pathogens. As an example we can consider the case the El Tor variant of *Vibrio cholera*e, which in the 1960's was found to possess new metabolic traits and cause an entirely new dominant El Tor pathotype (Watrick and Kolter, 1999). It is likely that this "metamorphosis" occurred in the water environment into which the disease causing agent had disseminated. Its biofilm formation includes a mannose-sensitive step which indicates the involvement of type-1 fimbriae. Therefore, aspects of environmental health need to be investigated behind the outcome of new, emerging epidemics (Hakalehto, 2014). They need to be studied in the light of structural and physiological knowledge on the particular strains. The epidemiological survey on the *Mycobacterium tuberculosis* genotypes reveals the main routes of contaminations of various subtypes of this devastating disease, which has killed perhaps more people than other contagious diseases together (Bisen and Raghuvanshi, 2013) in the history of mankind.

In the close proximity of the patient and the personnel, we have to take into account the simple basic laws of transmission. Some of the most important contributions on safeguarding human health have risen from the understanding of the mechanisms of dissemination and the routes of contamination. For example, the Hungarian doctor Ignaz Semmelweis, introduced the principles of hand hygiene into hospital hygiene more than 150 years ago (Hakalehto, 2006).

Many parts of the current book are based on the PMEU technology (Portable Microbe Enrichment Unit) which has proven useful in various fields of microbiological studies, producing novel information on microbial physiology and interactions as well as molecular communication during metabolic activity. However, more methods and studies are needed before it is possible to satisfactorily simulate link between man and his microbiome.

In modern microbiology, reservoirs of microbial pathogens need to be carefully researched, and eradicated as a source of infection, consequently. Some disease-causing bacteria such as borrelias can remain hideous for long periods of time. They stay latent in tissues or overall inside host cells. On the gut epithelia, such pathogens as the salmonellas, may often take part in the metabolism and molecular communication of the microbiota without inducing any illnesses. The immunodefenses and other individual traits of the host body and its microflora often determine the potential of a pathogen to develop a contagious sickness. On the other hand, common members of the normal flora can be disastrous for some people in hazardous conditions, such as in the case of lowered immunoresponse. The absence or presence of pathological influence on the host can often be seen as alterations in the immediate physiological condition of the patient. His or her condition as well as the composition of the microflora and its activity are in a continuously changing process. In the forthcoming era of personalized medicine, it will be more and more important to gather information directly from the microflora.

The sources and routes of microbial contamination, as well as the dominant infectious behavior of the contagious microbes, need to be evaluated carefully. For example, the human skin offers niches for the more numerous anaerobic flora underneath the aerobic flora. In fact, many bacterial parasites of man are typically facultative anaerobes. In their "shadow", a population of tediously detectable obligate anaerobes often causes less recognized but serious health problems. In order to prevent microbial diseases, it is necessary to take into account all members of the flora, and their interactions with each other and with the host.

One aspect of our microbes that is often neglected is their ability to "maneuver" in a metabolic context. Their interactions between each other and with the host form a matrix and an additional feature of the intestinal or other symbiotic ecosystems, whose importance to our health is increasingly more widely confirmed in scientific research and also more commonly recognized (Hakalehto, 2012). The concept of "molecular communication" gets a true meaning, when we achieve understanding on the routes of contamination and the mechanisms of the distribution of the diseases, as well as when we accomplish in elucidating their dependences on the host and microbial metabolism.

In this book, our aim has been to build a bridge between, on the one hand, the knowledge on microbial cells in mixed populations, and on the other, their contribution to the practical clinical hygiene. This includes giving a justification to practical solutions in clinical microbiological hygiene on the basis of scientific research and intuition, which have to be continuously tested and re-evaluated. This ultimately leads to the best result for the patient and for the entire healthcare system. We have also tried to include also ideas of the "hypothesis" level into this book. Some reasoning and experimentation behind these ideas is presented.

References

Bisen, PS; Raghuvanshi, R. Emerging Epidemics. Management and control. New Jersey, USA: John Wiley & Sons; 2013.

Costerton, JW; Stewart, P-S; Greenberg, EP. Bacterial biofilms: a common cause for persistent infections. *Science*, 1999; 21, 1318-1322.

Hakalehto, E. Semmelweis' present day follow-up: Updating bacterial sampling and enrichment in clinical hygiene. *Pathophysiology,* 2006; 13, 257-267.

Hakalehto, E, editor. Alimentary microbiome - a PMEU approach. New York, NY, USA: *Nova Science Publishers Inc.*; 2012.

Hakalehto, E. Interactions of *Klebsiella* sp. with other intestinal flora. In: Pereira, LA, Santos, A, editors. *Klebsiella Infections: Epidemiology, Pathogenesis and Clinical Outcomes.* New York, USA: Nova Science Publishers, Inc.; 2013; pp. 1-33.

Hakalehto, E. Bacteriological indications of human activities in the ecosystems. In: Armon, R; Hänninen, O editors. *Environmental indicators*. Germany: Springer Verlag; 2014. In Print.

Hakalehto, E; Vilpponen-Salmela, T; Kinnunen, K; von Wright, A. Lactic Acid bacteria enriched from human gastric biopsies. *ISRN Gastroenterol.* 2011; 2011, 109183.

Marshall, BJ. Helicobacter pylori. The etiologic agent for peptic ulcer. *JAMA*, 1995; 274, 1064-1066.

Ott, SJ; Musfeldt, M; Ullman, U; Hampe, J; Schreiber, S. Quantification of intestinal bacterial populations by real-time PCR with a universal primer set and minor groove binder probes: a global approach to enteric flora. *J. Clin. Microbiol.*, 2004; 42, 2566-2572.

Samgina, TY; Vorontsov, EA; Gorshkov, VA; Hakalehto, E; Hanninen, O; Zubarev, RA; Lebedev, AT. Composition and antimicrobial activity of the skin peptidome of Russian brown frog Rana temporaria. *J Proteome Res*. 2012; Dec 7;11(12), 6213-22.

Tran, NK; Kost, GJ. Worldwide point-of-care testing: compendiums of POCT for mobile, emergency, critical, and primary care and of infectious diseases tests. *Point of care: the Journal of Near-Patient Testing & Technology*, 2006; 5, 84-92.

Watnick, PI; Kolter, R. Steps in the development of a Vibrio cholerae El Tor biofilm. *Mol Microbiol.* 1999; Nov;34(3), 586-595.

In: Microbiological Clinical Hygiene
Editor: Eino Elias Hakalehto

ISBN: 978-1-63463-428-1

Chapter 1

Trends in Clinical Microbiology toward Point-of-Care Diagnostics

***Elias Hakalehto*[1], *Jouni Pesola*[2] *and Eino Puhakainen*[31]**
[1]Department of Environmental Sciences,
University of Eastern Finland, Kuopio, Finland
[2]Department of Pediatrics, Kuopio University Hospital, Kuopio, Finland
[3]HUSLAB, Helsinki University Hospital, Helsinki, Finland

Abstract

Laboratory diagnostics in hospitals is no longer defined into lab units only. Bed-side sampling protocols and analysis and on-site hygienic surveying have become part of everyday clinical action. For the patients, the increased point-of-care (POC) adds to speed in diagnostics and safety. For the entire hospital system, improved linking of diagnostics into actual treatments results in better cure outcome. This is assisted with modern technologies (POC-IT). The current trends and advancements are discussed basedon the situation in Finland, especially in the Helsinki area, but these experiences and developmental thoughts could be adapted also elsewhere.

1. Introduction

Because various micro-organisms play important roles in human health and disease, adequate microbiological testing resources should be readily available in all parts of the healthcare chain. This "continuous emergency status" gives us the benefits of instantaneous processing of the samples, as well as quicker further testing option and viable real-time information transfer. Consequently, no losses of time or sample quality are caused in the analysis process (Hakalehto, 2006). This is especially significant in case of analysis on emerging infections and other urgent microbiological samples.

[1] Chief Chemist (retired)

The normal flora contributes to the body's defensive actions. It forms the matrix where aggressive pathogens may come up and conquer the space, produce toxins, or otherwise rapidly harm the body system.

Thus, the surveillance of both hazardous microbes and follow up of the alongside normal microbiota have to be active inside the hospitals and clinics. Consequently, the laboratory functions need to be available anywhere in case of sudden need for microbiological sampling and analysis, not only in the centralized laboratory. Equally important, any patient in need or in danger should be subjected to continuous monitoring of his or her microbiological condition. The microbiological labs should be innovatively designed in such a way that they are accessible from everywhere via remote connections, and the samples are to be taken to them without delays. The laboratory concept should thus include the point-of-care concept. In the other words, the concept itself has and needs to be reformed into such an arrangement, or series of arrangements that offer major increases in the effectiveness of the hospital care producing also remarkable economical savings. For example by:

- Bedside monitoring
- Monitoring at the ward close to the patient
- Close co-operation between clinicians and clinical microbiology laboratory personnel
- Involvement of clinical personnel in the microbial monitoring

Besides the distinction between regular or standard lab operations on the other hand, and point-of-care or bedside diagnostics on the other, also the division into lab and field methods has become an increasingly ambivalent one. This is a direct consequence of widening or opening up of the concept of microbiological laboratory work or clinical microbiology in general. An analogue could be searched from the water hygiene sector where the PMEU techniques have been used for the monitoring of a water distribution systems in Finnish Polaris study (Hakalehto et al., 2011), or in source-tracking of the origins of the contaminating strains in the waterways (Heitto et al., 2006, Heitto et al., 2009), in sensitive detection of pathogenic, hazardous or otherwise harmful strains (Hakalehto, 2013, Mentu et al., 2009, Pitkänen et al., 2009), or in the ASCS (Automated Sample Collection System) type of monitoring of clean water production (Hakalehto et al., 2013, Heitto et al., 2012). In this context it is possible to also screen up the antibiotic susceptibilities of different strains (Hakalehto, 2011). All these examples could be related to the hygiene control of fluids and clinical specimens as well as that of the equipment and surroundings in hospital premises.

In practice, the point-of-care testing means usually bedside monitoring. The equipment is close to patient and continuously operable. In any case if it is not continuously monitoring his or her body functions or taking samples automatically, and this it can still be considered to perfectly match with the idea of *in vitro* diagnostics. Nevertheless, the sampling can usually start directly on sampling sites, and the testing or sample processing system is beneficially situated close to patient at the ward, for example. Hence, it is not taking place in a separate laboratory. Therefore, the training of the personnel at the wards is of utmost importance for the entire implementation of the point-of-care approach. This comprises of the inparts of the nurses on site, responsible for the patient treatments, who have to take the samples and to use the equipment.

Equally well, the responsible physicians have to learn to exploit this novel source of information, and specific tools, for decision making in the patient care.

The point-of-care functions could then be an expansion to the evidence-based medical treatments. Similarly, the laboratory could be extended beyond its physical walls, into carrying out an increasing amount of point-of-care duties.

2. Experiences from Clinical Field

Point of Care Testing (POCT) in general has increased greatly during last years in healthcare in western countries. For instance in Finland the costs of POCT have presently increased to an amount corresponding to about ¾ of that of basic routine laboratory tests because of the low cost of automated analytics. The biggest portion of the POCT costs, about 50%, is caused by common blood glucose testing among the diabetic population. There are many other diseases besides diabetes which are increasingly tested by POCT especially in clinical chemistry and hematology practices, but POCT is increasingly implemented into also clinical microbiology applications. One big advantage in POCT is that it will shorten the turnaround time in many clinical decisions. Many microbes also lose their vitality during transportation to the analyzing laboratory after sample collection, if this time period is prolonged.

It is essential for successful POCT activities that certified and verified methods are used, and that whole personnel performing the analyses is well trained. In organized healthcare there must be qualified training and quality assurance system in routine use.

In many clinical laboratory organizations this kind of processes are already belonging to everyday practices and also POC-IT is used in data transfer and quality assurance. Some big POCT selling companies offer this kind of services, too.

However, it is important to take into account that adequate levels of flexibility are maintained in the POCT. In practice, this means that healthcare units could have specific departments for evaluating novel procedures or practices for the diagnostics, and for analytical purposes. Also the small companies which carry out important basic work in researching and developing innovations should have their say in the overall development. In BIOtech 2014 Conference in Tokyo, Japan, Chia Feng Lu, a US lawyer with his academic background in pharmacy and economics, from Baker and McKenzie, underlined the importance of getting new inventive medical devices rapidly under validation and official acceptance procedures (Feng Lu, 2014). In Japan this had been identified as one of the key elements of the development in the clinical field.

There is an action program for enhanced application of medical devices pursued in Japan for shortening the period of time required for new devices to reach the patients. The number of approval devices had increased from 13 in 2009 to 104 in 2013. New legislation is also to be implemented with the aim of lowering the validation and acceptance period from three years to one year only.

Remote Control Programs in Controlling the POCT

Remote control programs in controlling the POCT is referring to a system which enables the simultaneous control of several similar or different type of POCT equipment. They should also be linked with HIS/LIS (Hospital Information System / Laboratory Information System) systems for safe and traceable patient result information flow.

For background, in Finland the total healthcare costs were 14.7 billion euros (year 2008). From this input the division into different sectors was:

- basic health care 3,1 billion €
- special health care 4,9 billion €
- outpatient care, medicines and medical consumables 2,1 billion €
- clinical laboratory expenses 588 million € (corresponding to 4 % of all healthcare costs)
- POCT turnover in Finland was 65 million €, equivalent to an amount corresponding to 70 % of the total reagent costs of the actual clinical laboratories
- POCT total costs thus comprise 42 % of all the reagent expenses of Finnish clinical laboratories
- 30 million € of the POCT costs is caused by the glucose blood tests which however constitutes only for 2 % of the entire costs caused by diabetes (1.35 billion €/y)

(Approximately 60-80 %) Must of the clinical decisions approximately 60-80 % are based at least partially on clinical laboratory results. The device, equipment and reagent costs of the laboratories were 90 million €.

The entire amount of laboratory testing in Finland 2009:

- Registered lab tests 55-60 million €
- HUSLAB (Helsinki area) share of this about 17 million € (25-30 %)
- Private laboratories performed about 8 million tests (614 test producers)

Point of Care Information Technology (POC-IT)

Centralized maintenance of the POC-IT is based on the following principles:

1 Device control and configuration
2 Quality assurance
3 Patient data handling (POC, Telemedicine)
4 Rights to use
5 Reagents and control
6 Automated validation
7 Maintenance services

Further on POC-IT-systems can be divided into three main types:

1 Closed equipment-centered systems, no outside equipment attachable, in some options for remote control
2 Half-open systems, where equipment of several manufacturers can be linked, although in limited fashion, often with mediator
3 Open system, which can comprise of devices from numerous manufacturers

Properties of POC-IT systems:

1 Portable or desktop POC device, which can be connected to HIS/LIS
   - connection via docking station and/or IP-address to server either straight or via mediator → LIS/HIS:
     * Software
     * Serial RS232
     * Bluetooth, USB, WLAN
     * Ethernet (LAN/IP-address)
     * Different combinations of the above
2 Verification of the user ID, and the level set up by POC coordinator or main user
3 Password alternatives for the ID
4 Result saving on the basis of patient or sample identification code or tag
5 Bar code reader in feeding input data (e.g., control data)
   - POC-IT system characteristics
6 Option for result commentary
7 Acceptance, rejection, result transfer via server
8 QC data / acceptance, lock out, automatic validation
9 Lot numbers

Analytics adjoined with POC-IT-systems

1 Glucose, microalbuminuria
2 Urea analysis
3 Blood clotting analysis
4 Heart function markers
5 Inflammatory markers
6 Blood gas analytics
7 Clinical chemistry
8 Basic hematology
9 Microbiological parameters

Examples of available POC-IT systems are listed in Table 1. The integration of POC into a network of devices with adequate and appropriate protocols is producing remarkable benefits, which will be replacing the old-fashioned concept of a laboratory distinct from other hospital functions:

POC-IT advantages

1 Point-of-care is rationalized, cost savings
2 Equipment connections, registers
3 QA of the analysis
4 Patient safety, avoidance of mistakes
5 Result transmission and saving (in real-time, traceability)
6 Supports intensive care and active care units in maintaining blood gas analytics and bedside microbiological monitoring
7 Aerial action map, harmonization of POC devices

One example of the above-mentioned solutions:

- Integration of 350 Accu-Chek Inform II instruments
  * Central monitoring of instrument status
  * Centralized update of instrument software
- Central training and certification of 3000 operators
- Central registration of controls
  * Possible to ensure controls are run on all instruments both in the morning and in the evening
- Auto-validation of test results
  * Validated results are delivered direct to the patient journal within minutes while patient is still there
- Special features
  * Elegant handling of tolerance tests
  * Possibility to work both with or without advance orders in LIS (sample ID vs. Patient ID scanned)

Some potential limitations of the POC-IT have been identified. They include the attachment to particular equipment suppliers, increased need for coordination on all levels, and increased maintenance and service efforts required. This could cause extra work for the laboratory, which should be rearranged for integrating the increasing POC activities into its protocols. In microbiology, openness of system is comprising of other factors besides the actual device, namely e.g., media and detection protocols that need to be evaluated together.

Maintenance responsibilities may cause extra work for the laboratory in the beginning, during the setup of the system, but once POC-IT has been kicked off, the benefits accumulate. Special points to be taken into account in practical laboratory action:

1 Cooperative teams for data handling headed
2 Result data transmission to be secured, fire walls
3 Net topology design together with central data management
4 POC device life time surveillance, maintenance contracts
5 Future compatibilities in growing markets
6 Increase of POC testing
7 Automatic verification of the results/QC interface

8 Transferability of the control data
9 Administration of the user rights and ID's

Table 1. Some available POC-IT systems

Manufacturer	System	Type
Abbott	Central Data System, CDS	Closed
Alere	Aegis POC™	Open
Conworx	POCCelerator™	Open
HemoCue	HemoCue® Data Management	Closed
MCS AG	POCTExpert	Open
Orion Diagnostica	QuickRead® QuickLink®	Closed
Radiometer	Radiance	Closed/Half open
Roche	Cobas® IT 1000	Half open
Siemens	Siemens Link	Closed

Future views have to be formed according to the user experience and chemical and microbiological, scientific advancement of methods and devices. POC-IT systems have to be integrated into practical methods for conceivable entities.

The importance of education is increasing. This requires more cooperation between POC device manufacturers and POC-IT firms. At best, these systems will shorten the data acquisition, prevent sample spoilage, and diminish the need for moving the patients.

Data IT transfer is improving the usability and acuteness of the patient analysis information. Work time of the caretaking personnel is directed into unit task related with the guidance and treatment of the most diseased patients.

A validation project aiming at the development of blood culture analysis method has been pursued at Neonatal Intensive Care Unit and Pediatric Hematology and Oncology ward in Kuopio University Hospital, Finland. The blood culture samples are enriched at the ward in PMEU Scentrion® (Finnoflag Oy and Samplion Oy, Finland; Figures 1-3) detecting the microbial growth by sensing volatiles originating from enriched samples.

This concept can be used bedside. Both enrichment cultivation for the identification of the pathogen and antibiotic susceptibility testing could be performed at the same time during sepsis diagnostics, for example.

As a matter of fact this kind of analysis structure of multiple tests from single samples is the basis of modern clinical laboratory automation. It could be combined with the POC-IT system.

3. Concept of Continuous Monitoring

Based on our earlier discussions, a checklist has been proposed (Hakalehto, 2011):

1. Identifying the disease as accurately as possible.
2. Finding the causes for the disease and the course of it (patient history).
3. Deciding upon the correct treatment including the medication.
4. Evaluating the overall health and condition of the patient.
5. Deciding about consulting with specialists of other fields.

(Continued)

6. Taking into account the potential complications.
7. Carrying out risk assessment with respect to the chosen methods of care.
8. Modifying a plan for the patient follow up and further analysis.
9. Giving a prognosis and establishing milestones for the recovery.
10. Deciding where to locate the patient in the hospital / in the healthcare system.

The individual steps in the list above need to be carefully evaluated. This process requires continuous monitoring of the patient's condition, and his or her microflora.

Bedside Monitoring of Microbiota

Monitoring of the microbiota of patients from samples collected repeatedly at different phases of treatment would offer new possibilities for monitoring characteristics of microbiota and also for following up the development prevelance in antibiotic resistance of the strains belonging to the this flora.

This approach would also guide the decision making physician regarding the selection of antibiotic drugs e.g., in cases of neonatal sepsis or neutropenic fever leading to more individualized treatment. It would also broaden the understanding on the routes of spreading of antibiotic resistant microbes and other contagious microbes of special interest with respect to hospital environmental microbiology.

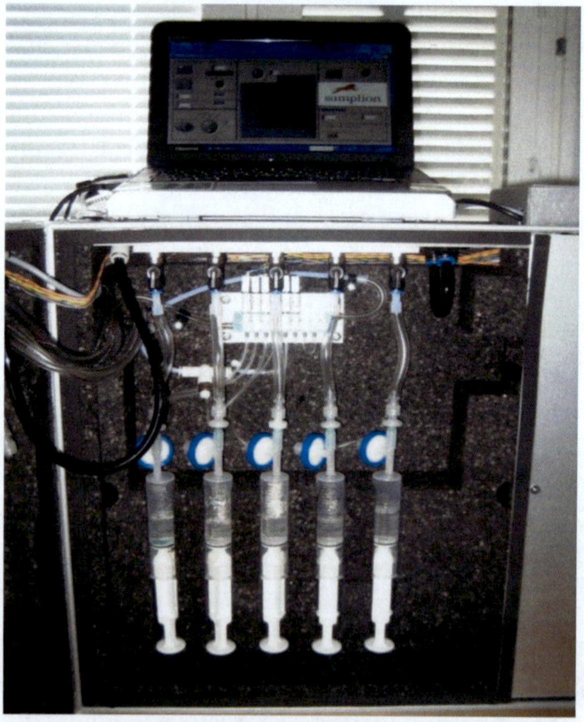

Figure 1. Bedside monitoring of microbiological samples in PMEU Scentrion® enrichment syringes (Finnoflag Oy and Samplion Oy).

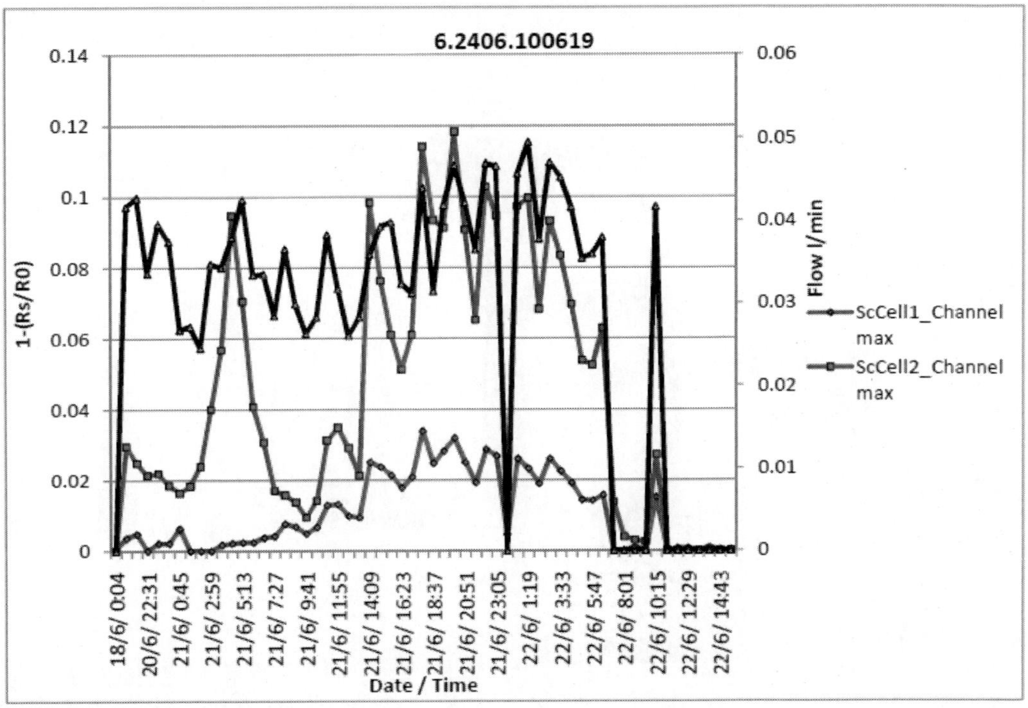

Figure 2. Microbial growth detected on the basis of clear increase of vapours or volatiles emitted from blood culture sample taken at Kuopio University Hospital Neonatal Intensive Care Unit by PMEU Scentrion® (Finnoflag Oy and Samplion Oy, Finland). The bacterium was identified as *Staphylococcus capitis*. Evaluated emissions indicate blood contamination rapidly.

By continuous monitoring of microbiota the changes could be detected timely. Ideally, the corrective treatments by e.g., pro- and/or prebiotics could be used.

This would also provide data on the impact of the microbiota on human health in different situations. This type of personalized medicine combined with research on individual patient microflora could hopefully give direction to the successful treatments in the future.

Bedside Monitoring of Blood Cultures

Monitoring blood culture samples at the ward bedside would offer clinicians a new possibility to evaluate the response of patients to the antibiotic treatments introduced at on-line basis. This would also allow timely modification of antibiotic treatments, when needed. Ideally this concept would be performed in close collaboration between clinicians and microbiology laboratory personnel and in order to interpret the results and confirm them by other methods, when needed.

Monitoring the samples at the ward close to the patient requires involvement of clinical personnel to the microbial monitoring. Moreover, close co-operation between clinicians and clinical microbiology laboratory personnel is usually a necessity, because the resulting data has to be stored and combined with other laboratory data.

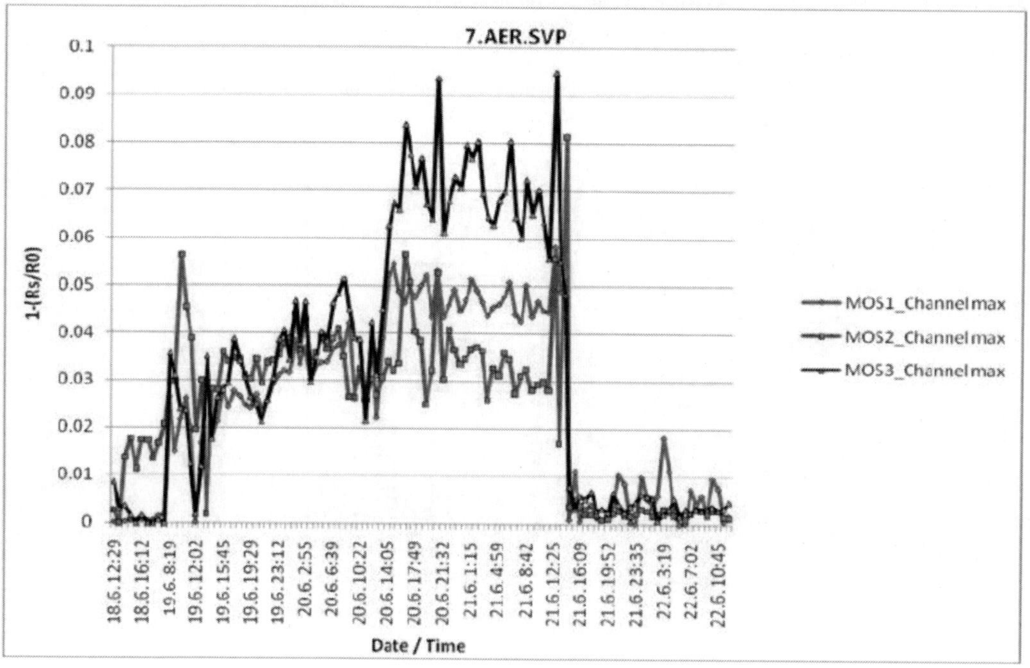

Figure 3. Blood culture sample enriched in PMEU Scentrion®. The sample was drawn from central venous catheter of a patient at a diagnosis phase of neutropenic sepsis before starting empiric antibiotics. The appearance of microbial growth is visualized by the raise of the curves indicating emitted volatiles originating from microbial metabolism, as detected by three Metal Oxide Sensors (MOS).

Methods for Continuous Monitoring

There are new, effective methods for microbe detection and identification like mass spectrometry based matrix-assisted laser desorption ionization time of flight mass spectrometry (MALDI-TOF MS).

However, there remains a need for studying living and metabolizird organisms e.g., for antibiotic susceptibility testing emphasizing the importance of development of cultivation-based methods (van Belkum et al., 2013).

"Culture has been the mainstay of clinical microbiology for the past century and will likely remain so for decades to come despite accelerating technological development and the introduction of novel diagnostic procedures.

However, there remains an absolute need for significant quantities of living organisms - not as much for detection and identification of microbial species, since strong alternative technologies are being introduced including MALDI-TOF MS, but more specifically for antibiotic susceptibility testing." (van Belkum et al., 2013).

It has been stated that the antibiotic susceptibility testing in liquid phase could be easily automated. There are already a number of systems available for the clinical microbiology laboratory including the Becton Dickinson Phoenix, the Siemens MicroScan WalkAway or the bioMérieux VITEK2™ systems (Jin et al., 2011). However, in the future also a growing need for investigating or simulating bacterial interactions in pathogenic situation will arise.

Gas Phase Provides an Interesting Option

The gas phase of the individual patient and his microbes is being continuously reshaped as the microflora goes through alterations in the metabolism regulation, nutrition, hormonal or neuronal signaling, or pathogenic developments.

Also, the effects of the uptake of various medications could essentially formulate the emitted gases (Hakalehto et al., 2012). The complete or big-scale changes in the gas formation patterns could also occur when the microflora, or its major component, is switching itself to a secondary metabolism (Khetan et al., 1999, Price-Whelan et al., 2006, Bernal et al., 2007) or into the mode of the overflow metabolism (Hakalehto et al., 2014b).

As such, these comprehensive alterations could be associated with the nutrient uptake of the body, or the body system and its microbes together.

Interestingly, there is not always a distinction between the speed of the aerobic and anaerobic metabolism in bacterial growth (Hakalehto et al., 2007).

By the use of continuous monitoring continuous accumulation of data is obtained instead of single results. Enrichment based methods would be preferable, because enhanced survival of microbes suffering from environmental stresses can be made detectable by them . As a result of enrichment living microbes could be isolated offering possibilities for further studies for e.g., antibiotic resistance monitoring or investigations of host-bacterial and bacterial-bacterial interactions.

The results obtained by enrichment provide material for further studies. This can be seen as a methodological link to the branching tree of analysis. This produces hierarchic information; possible early warnings, preliminary data to be confirmed or assessed by further studies. It could also give information on important variables, such as development of microbial virulence. When growth is detected during the PMEU cultivation, subsamples could automatically lead to other containers or syringes containing antibiotics relevant for the clinical purpose. By this means clinically important data could be achieved in an efficient manner.

4. Personnel Training As a Bottle Neck at the Bedside

We have noticed in our studies at Kuopio University Hospital and elsewhere that health care personnel should be carefully and repeatedly informed and advised for the concept of continuous microbiological monitoring. This concept should be introduced both to the physicians and nurses. The local modification of this concept should be worked out together with the clinical microbiology laboratory personnel in order to provide unlimited collaboration. Personalized investigation of patients as well as hospital epidemiology data collection have to be taken into account.

Usually, as anything new is taking place in the laboratory world, there is a special need for personnel training emerging. It would be important to find out enthusiastic individuals and medical units for testing purposes, which are ready to adopt this kind of new concepts within the field of clinical microbiology. They will be important key individuals later delivering their experience and knowledge to their colleagues worldwide.

Because the principles described above have to be transferred bedside developing a basis for new world of point-of care diagnostics in microbiology, the health care personnel should be well trained in order to get all the benefits out of it.

5. Microbiological Control in the Field

The microbiological operations in field conditions require specific applications. The PMEU units have been used for monitoring *Campylobacteria* in waters (Pitkänen et al., 2009). However, in Burkina Faso, in the studies for determining pathogenic *Campylobacter*, *Yersinia* or *Salmonella* species disseminating with water or food no reasonable source of bottled microaerobic gas was available. (Hakalehto et.al. 2014a).

Therefore, we developed a field capable system for arranging the appropriate gas supply. In this procedure a strong fiber plastic sac (with a full volume of 200l) was filled with a gas mixture generated by commercial sachets into sterile filtered air. This mixture was then directed throughout a sterile filter and valve into the PMEU Scentrion® unit equipped with standard sterile filtered gas outlets.

For a review of the use of PMEU technology in monitoring hazardous microbes see also Hakalehto (2006, 2010, 2011, 2014). In water hygiene the PMEU system has been applied for the fast microbiological screening of a water distribution system (Hakalehto et al., 2011), as well as for the source-tracking of water contaminants (Heitto et al., 2009).

A review of using the PMEU method for water microbiology is included in the book "Alimentary Microbiome – A PMEU Approach" in a chapter by Heitto et al.(2012).

6. Future Views Healthcare in Microbiology

The sample and subsample logistics will offer an avenue to the adequate information for optimal patient treatment. This will increase the effectiveness in hospital microbiology leading to improved patient care and overall economics of the hospital.

Extension of diagnostics and patient monitoring into homes and care centers will eventually lead to maximal transfer of information instead of patient movements, or even sample transportation.

The latter is, in case of microbiological studies causing unnecessary ageing and lessening of quality of the samples as well as information content of the unit samples.

Eventually the "spreading out" of the laboratory concept into clinical POC will lead to the implementation of the microbiological diagnostics in some safe form into homes, offices, nursing homes, and elsewhere.

Conclusion

As a producer of analysis data, POC field is reaching the levels of the "old-fashioned" laboratories. In microbiology, this produces better maintenance of the samples and elevated speed for their analysis.

Consequently, the entire treatment operation could be enhanced positively. Automated data transfer (POC-IT) improves the economics and traceability and other parameters of the diagnosis functions. Overall costs for the hospital system, and for the entire society can be better controlled with obvious savings in the lab sector.

Therefore, the laboratories should extend their functions into the direction of spreading out into the entire hospital system and healthcare in an omnipresent fashion.

References

Bernal, V., Sevilla, A., Cánovas, M., Iborra, J. L. Production of L-carnitine by secondary metabolism of bacteria. *Microb. Cell Fact.*, 2007; 6, 31-47.

Feng Lu, C. Critical issues ahead on our way to personalized medicine. *Lecture in: BIOtech 2014 Conference,* Tokyo, Japan, 2014.

Hakalehto, E. Antibiotic resistant traits of facultative *Enterobacter cloacae* strain studied with the PMEU (Portable Microbe Enrichment Unit). In: Méndez-Vilas, A., editor. *Science against microbial pathogens: communicating current research and technological advances.* Microbiology book series Nr. 3, Vol. 2. Badajoz, Spain: Formatex Research Center; 2011; 786-796.

Hakalehto, E. Bacteriological indications of human activities in the ecosystems. In: Armon, R., Hänninen, O., editors. *Environmental indicators*. Germany: Springer Verlag; 2014. In Print.

Hakalehto, E. Enhanced mycobacterial diagnostics in liquid medium by microaerobic bubble flow in Portable Microbe Enrichment Unit. *Pathophysiology*, 2013; 20, 177-180.

Hakalehto, E. Hygiene monitoring with the Portable Microbe Enrichment Unit (PMEU). *41st R3 -Nordic Symposium. Cleanroom technology, contamination control and cleaning. VTT Publications 266.* Espoo, Finland: VTT (State Research Centre of Finland); 2010; 164-176.

Hakalehto, E. Semmelweis' present day follow-up: Updating bacterial sampling and enrichment in clinical hygiene. *Pathophysiology,* 2006; 13, 257-267.

Hakalehto, E., Heitto, A., Heitto, L. Fast coliform detection in portable microbe enrichment unit (PMEU) with Colilert® medium and bubbling. *Pathophysiology*, 2013; 20, 257-262.

Hakalehto, E., Heitto, A., Heitto, L., Humppi, T., Rissanen, K., Jääskeläinen, A., Hänninen, O. Fast monitoring of water distribution system with portable enrichment unit – Measurement of volatile compounds of coliforms and *Salmonella* sp. in tap water. *J. Toxicol. Environ. Health Sci.,* 2011; 3, 223-233.

Hakalehto, E., Nyholm, O., Bonkoungou, I. J., Kagambega, A., Rissanen, K., Heitto, A., Barro, N., Haukka, K. Development of microbiological field methodology for water and food-chain hygiene analysis of *Campylobacter* spp. and *Yersinia* spp. in Burkina Faso, West Africa. *Pathophysiology*, 2014 Aug 4. pii: S0928-4680(14)00043-1. doi: 10.1016/j.pathophys.2014.07.004. [Epub ahead of print]

Hakalehto, E., Pesola, J., del Amo Paez, E., Hänninen, O. Bacterial interactions in the small intestine and their contribution to host nutrient uptake. In: Hakalehto, E., editor. *Alimentary microbiome: a PMEU approach*. New York, US: Nova Science Publishers, Inc.; 2012; 61-94.

Hakalehto, E., Pesola, J., Heitto, L., Närvänen, A., Heitto, A. Aerobic and anaerobic growth modes and expression of type 1 fimbriae in *Salmonella*. *Pathophysiology,* 2007; 14, 61-69.

Hakalehto, E., Tiainen, M., Laatikainen, R., Paakkanen, H., Humppi, T., Hänninen, O. *Klebsiella* sp. ferments hydrolysed cellulose and other carbohydrates by overflow metabolism to 2,3-butanediol and ethanol balancing pH and osmotic stress without population growth. *Manuscript in preparation, 2014b.*

Heitto, L., Heitto, A., Hakalehto, E. Environmental monitoring using the enrichment of hygienic indicators. In: Hakalehto, E., editor. *Alimentary microbiome - a PMEU approach.* New York, NY, US: Nova Science Publishers, Inc.; 2012; 213-231.

Heitto, L., Heitto, A., Hakalehto, E. Tracing waste waters with faecal enterococci. *Poster in European Large Lakes Symposium*, Norrtälje, Sweden; 2009.

Heitto, L., Heitto, A., Hakalehto, E. Tracing wastewaters with faecal coliforms and enterococci. In: Simola, H., editor. *Seminar on Large Lakes 2006*. Joensuu, Finland; 2006; 101-106.

Jin, W. Y., Jang, S. J., Lee, M. J., Park, G., Kim, M. J., Kook, J. K., Kim, D. M., Moon, D. S., Park, Y. J. Evaluation of VITEK2, MicroScan, and Phoenix for identification of clinical isolates and reference strains. *Diagn. Microbiol. Infect. Dis.*, 2011; 70, 442-447.

Khetan, A., Malmberg, K. H., Kyung, Y. S., Sherman, D. S., Hu, W. S. Precursor and cofactor as a check valve for cephamycin biosynthesis in *Streptomyces clavuligerus. Biotechnol. Prog*., 1999; 15, 1020-1027.

Mentu, J. V., Heitto, L., Keitel, H. V., Hakalehto, E. Rapid microbiological control of paper machines with PMEU method. *Paperi ja Puu / Paper and Timber* (90th Anniversary issue), 2009; 91, 7-8.

Pitkänen, T., Bräcker, J., Miettinen, I. T., Heitto, A., Pesola, J., Hakalehto, E. Enhanced enrichment and detection of thermotolerant *Campylobacter* species from water using the Portable Microbe Enrichment Unit (PMEU) and realtime PCR. *Can. J. Microbiol.*, 2009; 55, 849-858.

Price-Whelan, A., Dietrich, L. E., Newman, D. K. Rethinking 'secondary' metabolism: physiological roles for phenazine antibiotics. *Nat. Chem. Biol.*, 2006; 2, 71-78.

Van Belkum, A., Durand, G., Peyret, M., Chatellier, S., Zambardi, G., Schrenzel, J., Shortridge, D., Engelhardt, A., Dunne Jr, W. M. Rapid clinical bacteriology and its future impact. *Ann. Lab. Med.,* 2013; 33, 14-27.

In: Microbiological Clinical Hygiene
Editor: Eino Elias Hakalehto

ISBN: 978-1-63463-428-1

Chapter 2

Structure and Function of Bacteria in Contact with Host

Elias Hakalehto
Department of Environmental Sciences,
University of Eastern Finland, Kuopio, Finland

Abstract

Microbes metabolize and communicate with their surroundings through their surface structures. The role of these layers and appendiges depends on the kind of microbe, and the prevailing conditions. Several fundamental differences between various micro-organisms can be found, such as Gram-reaction in case of eubacteria. The Gram-positive genera usually have a thicker peptidoglycan layer (murein, PG) as cell skeleton, whereas Gram-negative bacteria possess two distinct membranes on their surface, surrounding the peptidoglycan from both sides. Between the cytoplasmic or cell membrane (CM) and the outer membrane (OM) they have, besides the peptidoclycan, also the periplasmic space (PS). The Gram-negative structures offer means for immunological variation of outer cell surfaces, as well as a limited space to carry out some extra-cytoplasmic reactions in an energetically feasible way in the periplasm. Some crucial practical questions in the hospital hygiene are:

- What characteristics are required from bacteria that can cause hospital infections?
  - structure
  - function
  - interactions with host body
- Which bacteria can be transmitted from surfaces to the patients?
- What should be done to avoid it?
  - cleaning
  - protective clothing
  - monitoring of preventive measures

All these questions relate to the actual basic traits of a particular microbe and the general features of microbial life. The borderlines or interfaces within our tissues are important links both for the microbes and for us as host.

Also the "microbiological characteristics" of any material, liquid, devices, textiles etc. in the hospital milieu are not meaningless from the point of view of achieving or maintaining an adequate level of hygiene. In dealing with the basic factors influencing the cleanliness, we need to know our microbes, both by their structure and function, not only by name.

Some key structural and functional characteristics of different microbes, and their contribution to the molecular communication phenomena such as attachment and metabolic capabilities and interactions, are outlined.

1. Introduction

In order to understand the behavior of microbial cells, strains and communities it is crucial to study the individual cells, and their interactions with other entities. Any result of the assessment on this basis is an estimate on the "microbiological reality". This reflects the actual presence of microbes in and around a particular object, and it constitutes a rather challenging task for any investigations. Cell surface contributes to the characteristics of the microbial contaminant, because it mediates both physiological results of microbial metabolism, as well as contacts of the microbes on human tissues and other surfaces. It plays therefore an important role in structure and function relations of various bacteria with respect to infections and interactions with hosts or hospital surfaces.

Interactions with epithelial and other solid surfaces are essential microscale phenomena determining the behavior of particular strains in human body system and in the healthcare environment. Different categories of sorption are listed below (according to Florence and Attwood, 2006):

1 absorbing onto larger solid particles
2 free cells in suspension
   a. motile
   b. non-motile
3 small particles absorbed onto larger microbial cells
4 cells absorbing onto flocculating particles
5 cells absorbing onto solid surfaces
   a. attachment by capsule
   b. attachment mediated by fimbriae or adhesions
   c. attachment of the flagellated cells using the flagellae
   d. attachment of the flagellated cells using the non-flagellated cell surface areas

The adsorbed microbes tend to form structural layers, often called as biofilms (Costerton et al., 1999). These complex "microbial states" are a consequence of multi-strain growth on the surfaces. Microbes live in such a many "dimensions". Micrographs illustrating the biofilm formation can be found in the Chapter 2.

In other words, microbial presence and activity is dependent on numerous parameters enough, that their future behaviour is difficult to foresee. – On the other hand, by series of sampling and enrichment experiments with the PMEU, it is made possible to obtain data on the tendencies and successions within any microbial ecosystems (Hakalehto, 2012).

In the cell surface research, it is important to take into account that the cells in active phase are going through continuous changes which influence the surface composition.

In one attempt to describe the microbiological reality, the many-sided environment in the human gastrointestinal tract has been described with the aid of the PMEU. The experiments involved in the book describe the case of the PMEU for cutting of the specific moments (time units) in order to evaluate their microflora on the basis of the enrichment results from samples thereof. Single cultivation syringes simulate the behaviour of single cells or populations.

According to the principles of laboratory microbiology, the homogenous cultures reflect the status of any individual cells. Because of the special gas conditions in the PMEU syringes, it is possible to obtain information on the behaviour of single cells in nearly real-life conditions. This is in line with the general trend in the rapid clinical microbiology for developing the gas detection applications (van Belkum et al., 2013).

When the syringes are connected in series with respect to gas flow, it is made possible to investigate various gaseous gradients in a population of microbial cells (Hakalehto, 2011, 2013). These gradients occur in many situations, such as layers of cells, biofilms, sediments, alimentary tract, degradative successions in soil, industrial processes etc. The flow of gases carries also the volatile compounds liberated by the cells. These could have a big influence on the microbial ecology as well as on the development of metabolic interactions.

Gases also act as signal molecules between microbes. For example, lactobacilli and other benign normal flora are boosting the growth of *Clostridium* sp. in the human gut. This accelerated growth makes the clostridial cells as swarmer cells which help in maintaining the BIB (Bacterial Intestinal Balance) for their part (Hakalehto and Hänninen, 2012). If gas flow slows down, it could cause the ceasing of active growth phase, which leads to increased attachment of *Clostridium* sp. onto the epithelial walls, and to their rooting in there.

Therefore, the liquid extracellular products are not the only ones to regulate the metabolic action of a microbial population, but the gas-liquid interface phenomena contribute essentially to the outcome of the joint activities of a microbial community.

2. Cell Surface Determinants in Cell-To-Cell Contacts and in Biological Activities Thereof

In case of many microbes, the cell surface characteristics are the determining factor in the attachment. One additional category to the list above could be the cell to cell adhesion in its many forms. In here, an example related to some food contaminants is highlighted in order to demonstrate the links between structure and function in bacterial cells. There the surface characteristics are decisive in case of attachment (or aggregation, flocculation) between homogenous cells, as like in the case of *Pectinatus* strain DSM 20465 (Back et al., 1979). Besides having slightly different cell surface mild acid extractable protein patterns (Hakalehto et al., 1984), this strain possessed a shorter or almost non-existent O-specific side chain of the lipopolysaccharide molecules (LPS) on the outer cell surfaces (unpublished results).

This strain was also the only one of five strains of these strictly anaerobic Gram-negative bacteria containing heptoses in their core oligosaccharides of the LPS (Helander et al., 1983).

All these attributes could possibly influence the aggregation of this strain, by the following mechanisms:

1 less coverage by the LPS O - specific side chain
2 specific surface proteins with revealed cystine moieties
3 heptose-mediated attachment to the cystine amino acids on the surface proteins

Moreover, when lethal toxicities of the various *Pectinatus* strains were determined, the strain DSM20465 turned out to be remarkably less toxic, together with strain ATCC29359 on galactosamine-sensitized mice (Helander et al., 1984). These two strains were later on identified to belong to the species *P. cerevisiiphilus*, whereas the other tested ones were designated as members of *P. frisingiensis* (Haikara, 1991). The strains of *P. cerevisiiphilus* (surface-protein type II) were later on shown to possess an immunodeterminant protein (22-25 kilodaltons in molecular size) (Hakalehto and Finne, 1990, 1992). The cytotoxicity variations on the basis of the LPS solubility were assumed by Helander et al. (1984). It was also found out that the genus *Pectinatus*, whose actual source or natural habitat is unknown, was resembling the coccoid rumen anaerobes of the genus *Veillonella* with respect to the LPS fatty acid composition (Hewett et al., 1971, Helander et al., 1983). In fact, another species belonging to the family *Veillonellaceae*, namely *Megasphaera*, has been repeatedly isolated from packaged beer (Weiss et al., 1979; Helander et al., 1984; Haikara, 1991). The *Megasphaera* antisera even cross-reacted with *Pectinatus* brewery isolates (Hakalehto, 2000). Later on, the relatedness of *Pectinatus*, *Megasphaera*, *Veillonella*, *Selenomonas* and other rumen bacteria was confirmed by rRNA analysis (van Gylswyk et al., 1997). Most of them were also isolated from the turbid beer. It has also been documented in several studies that the peptidoglycan layer of *Pectinatus* sp. is exceptionally thick for a gram-negative bacterium thus resembling these relatives isolated from rumen conditions (about 30 nm) (Hakalehto, 2000).

It could be presumed that this kind of cell surface skeleton layer increases rigidity and protects the cells in high pressures, such as in the digestive system or in the respiratory tract where gases are exchanged but their flow could be obstructed. See also the Chapters 4 and 14. Moreover, the osmotic pressure can be better withstood by bacterial cell with a strong and solid peptidoglycan envelope. Also for the bacteria, some protection against dehydration could be then achieved.

3. Airborne Transmission

With respect to the transmission of bacterial contaminants in air, it was demonstated that strictly anaerobic *Pectinatus* strains were distributed via aerosols close to the bottling line in a brewery (Hakalehto, 2000). This data fits together with the supposed distribution of the anaerobes as airborne contaminations in the product filling areas (Henriksson and Haikara, 1991). This is an indication of the relevance of microenvironments or niches for the survival of different bacterial species. Obligately anerobic *Clostridium difficile* was detected in less than 19 hours by the PMEU in a patient room (Hell et al., 2010). In the light of the above-mentioned case of the spread of anaerobic industrial contamination, it could be assumed that even vegetative cells, not only the endospores, of e.g., *C. difficile* hospital infections could be disseminated by air movements in aerosols.

If these mechanisms of airborne transmission are functionable, they could significantly increase the risk of contagion. The attachment and particle forming characteristics of different strains related to cell surfaces could then play an important role in aerosol protection of the contaminants. A list of postulates related to the air transmission of pathogens presented by Wells (1955). See Appendix 1.

The behavior of the aerosol (or dust) droplet (or particle) in the respiratory tract is essential for the development of disease. The curvature in the pharynx is acting as an "anatomical sieve" in preventing most of the small particles from achieving the lower pulmonary airways. Instead, the particles attach to the neckside surface of the pharynx. In this area, it is believed that a prior viral infection is damaging the ciliary structures, thus allowing easier "landing", i.e., attachment and colony formation, of bacterial agents. For example, Wells (1955) is stating: "While it is quite impossible to say which inhaled bacilli will induce tubercles, under a given set of conditions the fraction may be predicted with a sufficient degree of probability to correlate infection with dosage." According to our conception, also the form and function of the individual cells in the distributed population influence the infective properties. Wells also emphasizes the route of infection in the ecology of communicable diseases. As an example he points out the more severe consequences of peritoneal infection (as measured in relation with bacterial cell numbers) than that of pulmonary origin. Moreover, he concluded that even though this is true for both group C streptococci and type 1 pneumococci, the latter had still far more damaging effect in peritoneal injections into experimental mice. The seriousness of the infection is thus related to the particular cell surface traits, toxins, immunoreactivity, and other characteristics of the strain, as well as the local preparedness or defenses of the host tissues to resist the infections.

4. Bacterial Cell Appendages

Another type of cell to cell aggregation is related to the interactions of heterogeneous cells, such as bacterial cells and red blood cells, for example. The mannose-sensitive binding of type 1 fimbriae is an example of this binding (Korhonen *et al.*, 1982). Then the properties of individual molecules play also a role in the attachment (Kim and Baldwin, 1990). With respect to type 1 fimbriae, it was shown that this structure is taking part to primary attachment to the epithelia or to the miscellaneous surfaces in the hospital milieu. In all studied eubacteria possibly an universal asparagine amino acid in the position No 7 in the N-terminal end of the peptide chain of flagellar filament structural proteins was detected (Hakalehto et al., 1997).

In case of studying the immunological cross-reactions between the closely related *Salmonella* and *Citrobacter* genera it turned out that some fimbrial sequences of *Salmonella* were provoking the production of more interactive antibodies than the others (Hakalehto, 2000). In our laboratory in the experiments using RVS (Rappaport Vassiliadis Soya peptone) broth it turned out that *Citrobacter* sp. strains were more readily eliminated at higher temperatures (42-43 °C in comparison to 37 °C) when the selective medium for salmonellas was used. It is also noteworthy that in low growth temperatures (e.g., 20 °C) type-1-fimbriae are not expressed, and not even a shift into the high temperature (42 °C) did alone facilitate their expression implying to other underlying mechanisms for fimbrial surface protrudement (Hakalehto et al., 2000).

In physiological or higher temperatures the type-1 fimbriae were expressed, as seen by micrographs, in 3-5 hours, whereas in 7 hours almost no surface appendages were found (Hakalehto et al., 2000). These appendages are produced quickly in a few seconds after the bacteria pass the acidic stomach and enter the more permissive duodenal areas (Hakalehto et al., 2000; Hakalehto et al., 2007). In the acidic conditions of the stomach (pH 1-2) the fimbriae and flagellae would dissociate (Hakalehto et al., 1984; Hakalehto, 2000). It could also be deduced that the protein-rich nutrition is favouring these rapidly attaching strains. This has proven to be the case, as would human population was recently divided into three main types according to the microbiota (Wu et al. 2011). The basic distinction in the development of intestinal microbiome with the protein nutrition and in the carbohydrate diet was noticed already a long time ago. This fundamental distinction in diet also has important contributions on our well-being and the etiology of various common diseases.

The PMEU technology has been successfully used for investigating the intestinal microbial ecosystems and host – microbe interactions (Hakalehto, 2012).

The salmonellas were shown to grow equally well both in aerobic and anaerobic conditions in the PMEU, whereas the type 1 fimbriae were more abundant in the aerobiosis (Hakalehto et al., 2007). This clear difference in antigenic expression could reflect the tendency of invading salmonellas to strive for blood oxygen in the human body system. As a consequence, the tissue penetrating bacterial cells root into areas with fresh blood contents. Otherwise it has been documented that in the anaerobic conditions the salmonella cells are increasingly uptaken by epithelial and peritoneal cells due to the synthesis of additional proteins (Lee and Falkow, 1990). Consequently, also the use of PMEU for creating cultures with homogenous bacterial cells in identical growth phase is a tool for researching infectivity (Hakalehto et al., 2007). In fact, as stated above, it was shown the type-1 fimbriae of facultative salmonellas were expressed more readily in the presence of some oxygen.

The adhesions and invasing strains of e.g., *E. coli* can form adhesive organelles as well as reservoirs of pathogenic bacteria into the host and host cells (Le Bouguénec, 2005). After adhesive sheath structures mediate the mannose resistant adhesion, the entry of organisms such as enteropathogenic *E. coli* and *Yersinia* is facilitated. Anti-adhesion therapies of bacterial diseases have been reviewed (Ofek et al., 2003).

Also therapeutic antibodies from outside the body system such as the egg yolk antibodies (IgY) can be used for passive immunization (Hakalehto and Kuronen, 1998).

5. Gas Emissions in Cell-to-Cell Interactions

By the PMEU it is also possible to investigate the influence of gas flow emitted from adjacent cells on the basis of observing the growth speed and the onset of growth (Hakalehto, 2011; Hakalehto and Hänninen, 2012; Hakalehto, 2013). This kind of interaction is mediated by gaseous signals form cell to cell. Lactobacilli were found to boost the growth of butyric acid bacteria. Then the carbon dioxide produced by the former ones was provoking the active growth of the others (Hakalehto and Hänninen, 2012). It was also supposed that by this mechanism the lactobacilli could actually compete for space with clostridia and prevent them from rooting onto the gut epithelia.

This could take place by keeping the *Clostridium* sp. strains in an active state, and by preventing them from producing S-layers or other structures for attachment, or spores.

The above-mentioned example illustrates the ways bacterial strains maintain the balance in the anaerobic colon and other areas of lower intestines. It was also found that the clostridia could grow well in 100% CO_2 (Hell et al., 2010). In the duodenum, the lactobacilli and clostridia are not present in high numbers due to e.g., bile substances (Hakalehto et al., 2010). In the areas of upper intestines e.g., coliforms and salmonellas could dominate by attaching quickly with the aid of fimbriae and flagellae produced by the young cultures (Hakalehto 2000; Hakalehto et al., 2007).

6. Cell Surface Layers of Bacteria

Since microbial cells are compartments surrounded by cell walls and membranes, their metabolic activities could be divided into the following categories:

1 Intracellular
2 Membrane-bound
3 Extracellular

In case of the Gram-negative bacteria also periplasmic (4.) metabolism could occur. The structures of bacterial outer surfaces are illustrated in Figure 1 (modified from Hakalehto 2000). This is a fascinating issue, because in the periplasm between the cell membrane (CM) and outer membrane (OM) many transport enzymes and also hydrolyzing and other functional enzymes are actively operating. The periplasm offers the Gram-negative bacteria a limited space where the need of particular enzymes is lower, and they can be more "economically" produced and easily regulated than in the potentially vast extracellular area. Active transport inside the cells of all substrate compounds is not necessarily required when some of them can be processed in the periplasm. The cells can also adjust themselves into changes in osmotic pressures. We have hypothesized that in the small intestines the periplasm could play an important role in buffering hydrostatic pressure (Hakalehto et al., 2014). It is growing in volume if the outside pressure is increasing.

7. Periplasmic Space Function

Periplasmic enzymes are involved in transport, degradation and synthesis of molecules. In pathogenic Gram-negative species many lytic virulence factors locate in the periplasm:

- collagenases
- hyaluronidases
- proteases
- β-lactamases

- phosphatases
- lipases
- nucleases
- carbohydrate-degrading enzymes

Some periplasmic proteins are components of the chemotaxis system, which senses the external environment of the cell.

In case of glucose dehydrogenase enzyme (GDH), catalysis of an oxidation-reduction (redox) reaction in which a CH-OH group act as a hydrogen or electron donor and reduces a hydrogen or electron acceptor.

In case of *Klebsiella* ketogluconate addition of $CaCl_2$ to the medium of magnesium-limited cultures increased GDH activity but simultaneously decreased the specific CO_2 production rate (Buurman et al., 1990, 1994). The CO_2 production was coupled with acetate production with the molar ratio of 1:1, whereas the corresponding ratio of CO_2 to 2,3 – butanediol and acetoin was 2:1. Net production of succinate and 2-oxoglutarate from glucose via phosphoenolpyruvate carboxylase involves fixation of CO_2 (1:1) that has been formed by the culture ccording to the equation: $qCo_{2\,(TCA)} = qCO_2$ (measured) + q2-oxyglutarate + q-succinate – q-acetate – 2q-acetoin - 2q-2,3-butanediol.

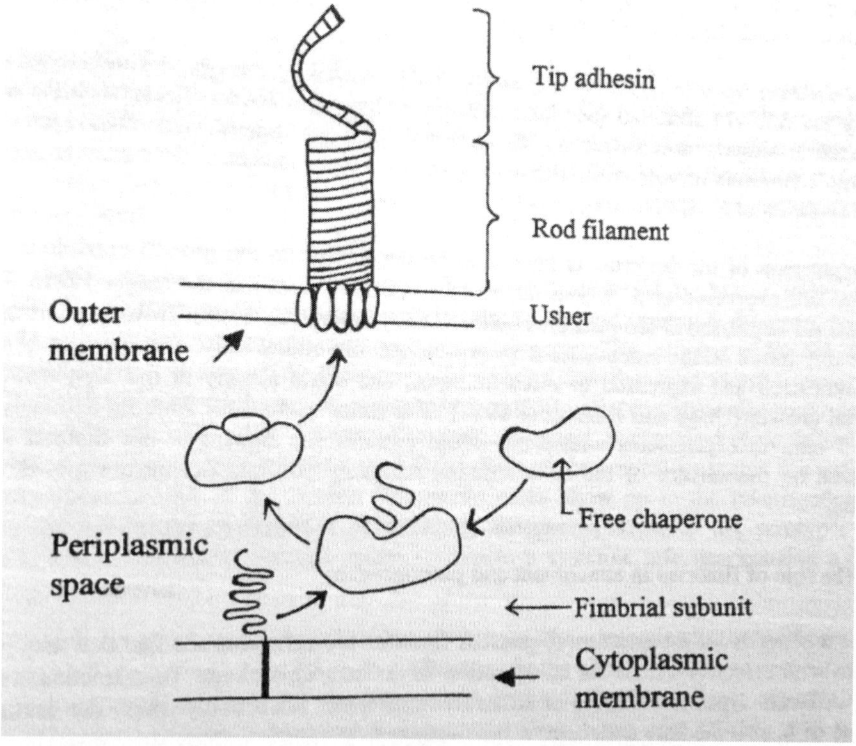

Figure 1. A scheme of the assembly of fimbrial subunits assisted by periplasmic chaperones via the chaperone-usher pathway. Modified from Hakalehto 2000.

"Under phosphate-limited conditions activation of periplasmic oxidation of glucose in *K. pneumoniae* can provide a competitive advantage to the organism without resulting in a net increase in production rate of ATP equivalents."

Catalytic site of GDH is available for periplasmic glucose oxidation (Midglay and Dawes, 1973). This enzyme oxidases glucose in *Klebsiella aerogenes* (Neijssel et al., 1983). It has been found that *K. aerogenes* possess the potential to produce carbon substrate (glycerol) at a vastly enhanced rate, without an increase in growth rate (Streekstra et al., 1987). This is in line with our assumption that also 2,3-butanediol could be produced by a periplasmic mechanism with the klebsiellas during a no-growth situation (Hakalehto et al., 2014). It has been suggested that the β-galactosidase of *Fibrobacter succinogenes* strain L2 cleaves lactose outside the cell and that the glucose released is catabolized while the galactose accumulates in the extracellular culture fluid (Javersky et al., 1990). This activity was on the highest level in the periplasmic space.

Interacting selectively and noncovalently with a quinone, any member of a class of diketones derivable from aromatic compounds is obtained by conversion of two CH groups into CO groups with necessary rearrangement of double bonds.

8. Origins of Bacterial Strains and Their "Molecular Heritage"

As members of the alimentary microbiome bacterial strains act in distinct ways from individual, separated or swarming cells. In the microbial communities they belong to some definable ecosystems (Hakalehto, 2012). As interactive members they carry molecular traits of these multiorganismal partnerships and joint actions within their molecular structures, and reflect the laws of the microbiome constitution. In a somewhat similar way, our own blood cells could carry signs of infectious development well before any symptoms are observable (as hidden information in circulating leucocytes) (Knight et al., 2013).

Consequently, we could well make a philosophical question, whether they never entirely cease to belong to the microbial communities where they originate from. This question, although being a rather theoretical one, is having some practical relevance e.g., in the hospital surroundings.

Are the hospital strains and other microbes in this setting bearing any associations to the host-microbe ecosystems where they possible derive from? If delivered to a human body again, are their patterns of action unchanged, also carrying detectable traces of their earlier "environmental fate" or "strain history"? – The PMEU technology could be used for studying any individual microbial strain in conditions simulating the real-life challenges which these microbes face in natural environments.

In a normal laboratory culture these aspects usually remain unsolved since the main purpose is then to measure the growth of a micro-organism. In the PMEU, for example, the small dose of defensin proteins (HBD-2) required for limiting the microbe growth in human body, could be effectively tested and verified (Hakalehto, 2011).

These kinds of sensitive interactions of "molecular communication" mechanisms need to be evaluated for better views on pathogenesis and host defence.

9. Generation and Verification of Volatiles Inside and Out from the Body System

As indicated before, the gas conditions required by various microbes in the hospital setting constitute an important selective factor for their growth (Hakalehto, 2010). Similarly, the formation of different volatiles in the intestines (Hakalehto et al., 2008; Hakalehto et al., 2010) from blood samples (Hakalehto et al., 2009; Pesola and Hakalehto, 2011), and from the urological samples (Pesola et al., 2012) could form a sensitive means for the detection of harmful microbes. In addition to these detection principles, and the use of volatiles as basis for diagnostic operations, it could be well postulated that the presence and concentrations of different gases in the body fluids and organs could have a selective effect on the normal flora, commensal microbes, as well as on the pathogenic organisms.

Moreover, the gases emitted by microbes influence the pH, redox potential and enzymatic functions of the host. This could explain some observations associating the gastrointestinal strains with skin symptoms, such as rash and other dermatological damage.

Also the effect of oxygen treatments could be explained by the partial pressures of oxidative gaseous compounds inside the body. However, these effects can also be disastrous, but usually only when too high flow rates are applied for the treatments (Benditt, 2000). The generation of specific niches with distinctive gas conditions could explain the survival and effect of some lactic acid bacteria on the gastric epithelia (Hakalehto et al., 2011; Hakalehto et al., 2012), or in the mouth cavity (Hakalehto, 2011; Pesola et al., 2012).

In both of these instances it was possible to indicate the presence of probiotic micro-organisms regardless of the acidic pH or the antibiotic conditions, respectively.

In a similar fashion, the etiology of some microbial disease, such as tropical sprue (Ghoshal et al., 2014), or the irritable bowel disease (IBD) (Hakalehto et al., 2012; Jaakkola and Hakalehto, 2012), could relate with "unsuitable" or unhealthy gas condition created by the micro-organisms inside the body. In fact, it has been observed that some beneficial impacts of the LAB (Lactic Acid Bacteria) on the BIB (Bacterial Intestinal Balance) could be associated with the generation of CO_2 by these bacteria (Hakalehto and Hänninen, 2012). This effect could also play a role in the recovery of the gut microflora from the disturbances caused by the antibiotic treatments (Pesola and Hakalehto, 2011).

As a consequence of all the above-mentioned considerations, it is possible to further measure the volatiles liberated *in vivo* by the microflora in order to assess the health status of an individual. Then the monitored gases could be selected according to the diagnostic purpose.

1 total body gas emission (TBGE)
2 oral gas emission (OGE), and
3 respiratory gas emission (RGE)
4 intestinal gas emission (IGE)
5 fecal gas emission (FGE)

In this case the OGE, for example, should be taken during a breathless period of time, when the experimental patient is possibly subjected to a flushing of a carrier gas and is out of breath. This gas could potentially inflict a partial pressure of some gaseous components, which is standardizing the measurement.

It is of crucial importance to understand that in our body the microbes are facing variable oxidative or reductive conditions. Therefore, studying the pulmonary microbial diseases require careful consideration of the circumstances prevailing in any particular area of the respiratory tract. Obstruction caused by inflammation, for example, can change the gas conditions. If enrichment is needed for simulation, the cultivation conditions have to be critically evaluated. In the PMEU units it is possible to study the effect of some microbial emissions on other strains (Hakalehto and Hänninen, 2012), as well as in the complete anaerobiosis (Hell et al., 2010). Some strains are growing equally fast in anaerobiosis and in aerobic conditions (Hakalehto et al., 2007; Pesola et al., 2012). The effects of various gas concentrations on particular microbes can also be studied in the PMEU (Hakalehto, 2011).

10. Future Miniatyrized Microbiological MS Applications As Featured by Sensing with PMEU and Metal Oxide Probes

One of the most rapid and reliable means for monitoring micro-organisms and their metabolism is the screening of their volatiles. Whenever bacteria, moulds, yeasts, or other microbes onset their growth, they produce emissions detectable with the most sensitive sensors. As a model system for integrating enrichment cultivation with high-speed gas detection is demonstrated by PMEU Scentrion® equipment (Hakalehto et al., 2009) (for a Figure, see Chapter 1). This technology has been applied for:

1. detecting blood contamination
2. monitoring urinary tract infection
3. fecal microbiological analysis
4. screening hygiene indicators and pathogens in waters
5. air quality sampling (e.g., building damages caused by microbes)
6. simulating intestinal ecosystems
7. food microbiology

11. Metabolic Considerations

Although *Klebsiella aerogenes* has the biochemical potential to ferment glucose to acetate, 2,3-butanediol, ethanol, succinate, D-lactate and formate (or CO_2 and H_2), only acetate and ethanol are formed (together with the formate) in glucose limited chemostat cultures (Gottschalk, 1979). In all glucose sufficient conditions additional production of 2,3-butanediol, D-lactate and succinate occurred via a branched fermentation (Teixera de Mattos and Tempest, 1983). In anaerobic conditions under glycerol excess conditions *K. aerogenes* excreted high amounts of 1,3-propanediol (Streekstra et al., 1987). This production, even though partially considered as overflow metabolism in the glycerol excess condition, was a sign of potential faster metabolic route for glucose assimilation in the klebsiellas.

This metabolic activity is provoked by environmental stress, such as elevated osmotic pressure (Hakalehto et al., 2014). See also section 7 of this chapter.

12. From Cell Growth to Biofilm Structures

The bacterial and other microbial growth often has a tendency to root onto beneficial surfaces (Ellwood et al., 1982). It is fascinating to conceive the structural formation leading from the propagation of cell lines into sophisticated systems of microbial communities, and to biofilms (Costerton et al., 1999; Bernstein et al., 2014). The formation of a biofilm structure was photographed under our microscopic lenses (Figure 2 a-d). It has also been reported that some small molecules could, in turn, trigger the disassembly of the biofilms (Oppenheimer-Shaanan et al., 2013).

Bacterial attachment on mucosal membranes is often mediated by surface lectins specifically recognizing oligosaccharide receptors on glucolipids and glycoproteins (Svanborg et al., 1996). Quarum sensing phenomena which are related to the bacterial cell density, regulate the biofilm formation (Amara et al., 2009)

These lectins are often located in the protruding fimbrial or other adhesive structures. During the early development of neural or other tissues, novel receptors are exposed which can open up novel sites for bacterial attachment in the host body (Kouki et al., 2011).

The adhesion of human buccal cells to immobilized bacteria has been assayed (Sokuranko and Hasty, 1955). Then the *S. aureus* strain Cowan 1 and the *E. coli* strain CSH-50 were cultivated in the brain-heart-infusion (BHI) broth, and the *Streptococcus pyogenes* strain M5 on Todd-Hewitt broth (THB), and they were immobilized onto microplate walls. Then they were subjected to buccal cell suspension (50.000 cells/ml). The attached host cells were enumerated microscopically. Binding of the buccal cells onto layers of the *S. aureus* and *E. coli* were documented, whereas *S. pyogenes* had no such effect. In case of *E. coli*, mannose totally blocked the attachment. This reflects the mannose-sensitive binding of type-1-fimbriae onto host epithelia which has been described some 35 years ago (Korhonen et al., 1982).

13. Example of Potential Influences of Molecular Structures on the Human Host Etiology

The impact of beta-amyloid peptide on the onset of age-related senile dementia of Alzheimer's type (SDAT) has been for a long time under intensive investigations (Harman, 1996). Although these fibrils clearly correlate with the disease, their presence is not always leading to complications. We studied a striking similarity between the beta-amyloid peptides and some bacterial surface peptides in experimental animals (see below).

It was first found that some flagellin peptides of several eubacteria resembled the beta-A peptides in electron micrographs (Hakalehto et al., 1997). These peptides originated from the N-terminal end of the flagellar structure protein.

This part of the protein has been shown to be responsible for the coiling of the protein near the tip of the flagellin *in vivo* (Hakalehto, 2000).

Moreover, these organs are responsible for bacterial cell movement, chemotaxis, some aggregation and attachment reactions, and are strongly immunogenic. Their presence is relatively high, comprising some 5-10% of cellular proteins. Interestingly, the use of N-termini of rat encephalitogenic peptides as experimental inhaled vaccine a week before predisposing, the animals totally inhibited the disease by a single dose.

When a hybride peptide of Salmonella A8 and Pectinatus P13 was linked together, it caused first epileptic episodes for two rabbits used for immunizations studies (Hakalehto, 2000). The A8 peptide molecule derived from the immunogenic region of some Salmonella fimbrin structures, and P13 originated from *Pectinatus* flagellar N-termini, which had exhibited a tendency to form strong fibrous precipitates (Hakalehto et al., 1997). We then injected this hybrid peptide into 4 rats.

Both individual peptides were injected into 4 rats each, and 4 animals were kept as control. With about one year 3 out of 4 rats in the group injected with the hybrid peptide developed large skin lesions without hair formation, and eventually developed tumors into these areas and died (Table 1).

This strong reactivity in the animal body system of the relatively small peptides indicated the high risks and elevated pathogenic potential of miscellaneous peptides and other small proteins. This phenomenon could also relate to the occurrence of infective proteins, such as prions (Immel et al., 2007). Some skin peptides of frogs (and other reptiles) have a strong antimicrobial function, but they can also be toxic to the host cells (Samgina et al., 2012).

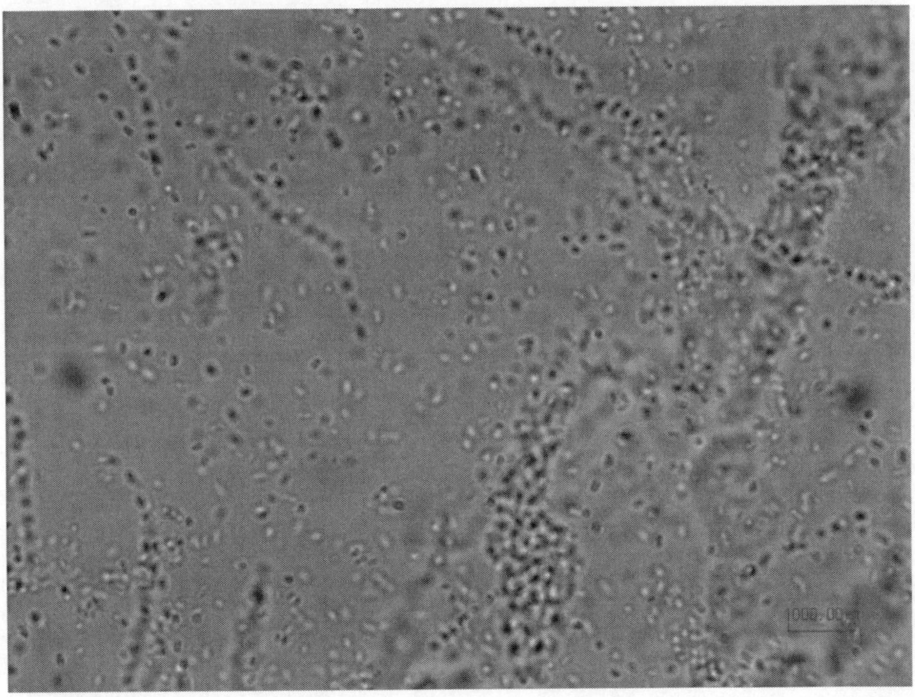

a

Figure 2. (Continued).

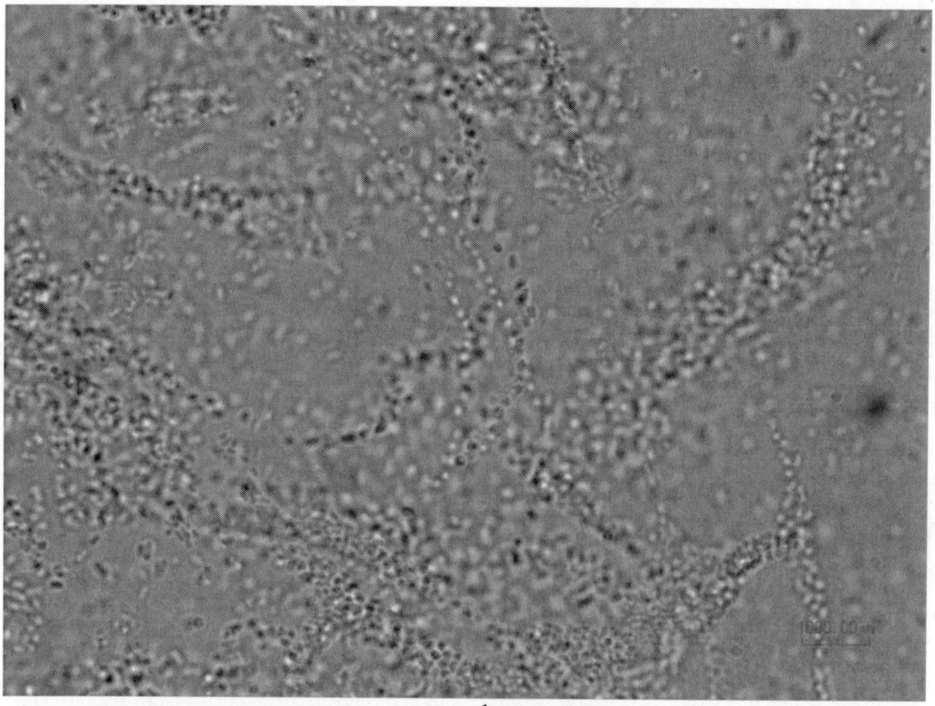

b

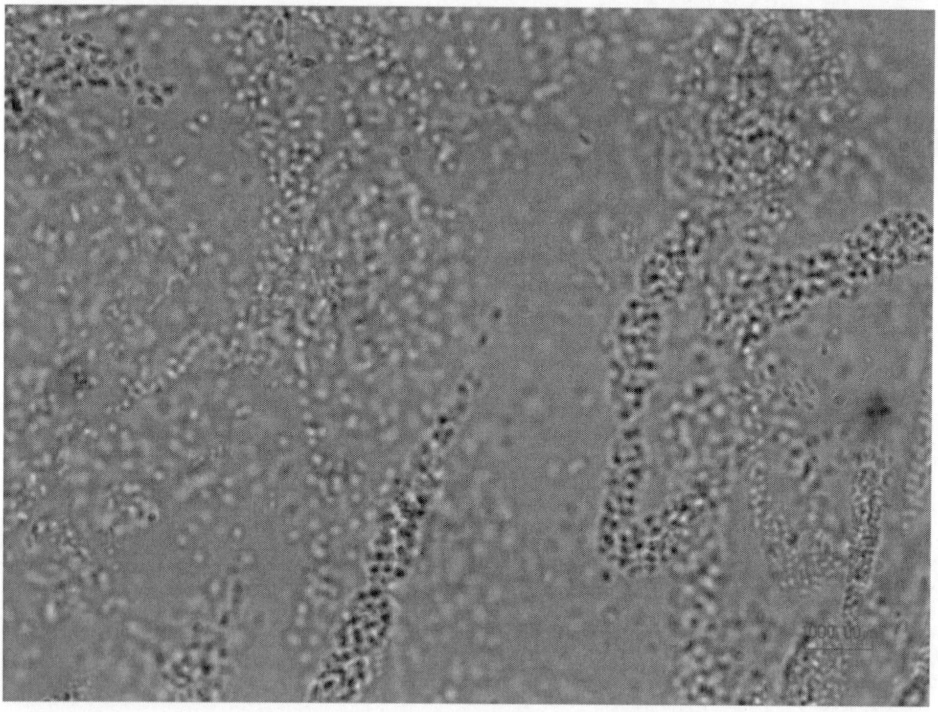

c

Figure 2. (Continued).

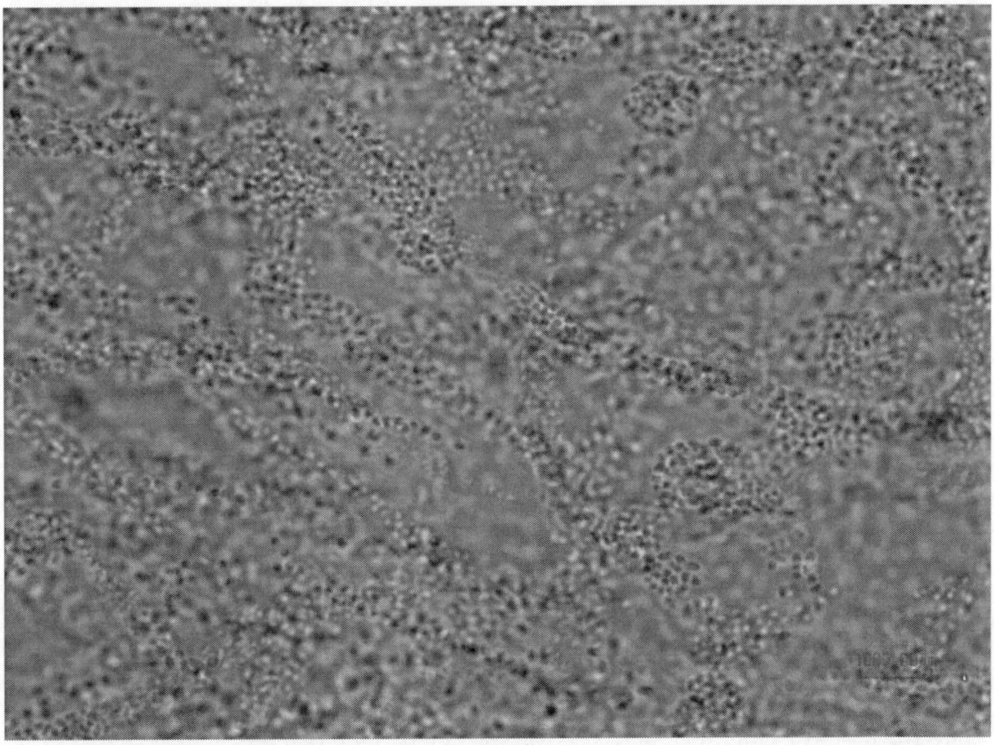

d

Micrographs are taken by Nikon CIL microscope in the laboratory of Finnoflag Oy by the author.

[a]In the early phases of nutrient exhaustion and/or attachment to the surfaces, bacterial cells form chains, or fibrious structures where cells aggregate to each other. Photo: Elias Hakalehto.

[b]Bacterial cell chains tend to spiral into thicker structures. Photo: Elias Hakalehto.

[c]The thicker strands formed by the bacterial cells. Photo: Elias Hakalehto.

[d]The stranded bacterial chains get organized into "textile-like" layers onto surfaces, thus forming the biofilms. This series of micrographs illustrates the gradual formation of biofilms which contain the necessary hollow spaces and holes for transporting nutrients into various parts of the microbial community, as well as the "molecular wastes" out of it.

Figure 2. A-D. The serial illustration of the sequence in formation of biofilm-like structures from a bacterial monoculture of an unspecified coccal strain. The rows of individual cells are twisted into chains and twines of several almost fibrous structures. This gives an idea on potential ways of biofilm formation on the intestinal surfaces. These often microscopic layers can thus have internal hollow-like structures. The physiological functions of these layers are well distinct from the populations traversing in the chyme. The latter ones are in fact going through a cultural growth cycles of some 6-7 hours during their passage through the small bowel (Hakalehto et al., 2008). On the way these microbes attach to the food particles and to each other but remain movable. The physiological distinction between the swarming and submerging cells and the cells in the layers is an essential characteristic for the digestive tract ecosystem. The formation of layered growth is restricted by the host in order to proportion their participation in the utilization of the nutrients in the chyme. On the other hand, the "attenuation" of the general growth of the intestinal community by its lactic acid (LAB) members has been shown to relate to the fibrous particle of e.g., crushed flax seeds (Hakalehto and Jaakkola, 2013). In the digestive tract some of the LAB could possibly derive from the gastric areas (Hakalehto et al., 2011). The transformation of the drifting cells e.g., of the salmonellas anchor on the new untouched sites for epithelial infection alongside the small intestines (Hakalehto et al., 2000).

Table 1. The effects of various cell surface peptides on the four series of four rats in each

Peptide	Symptomatic rats
1. Zero control (buffer)	0/4
2. *Salmonella* A8 fimbrial peptide	0/4
3. *Pectinatus* P13 flagellar N-terminal peptide	0/4
4. Conjugated hybride peptide of A8 and P13.	3/4

For explanations, see text.

Also the enzymatically dissociated derivatives of human, nutritive or microbial proteins could initiate pathological sequences of events in the tissues, even though no actual microbial presence could be demonstrated. They could also provoke immunological reactions, which might have a relative importance in case of many common diseases, such as arthritis and autoimmune symptoms.

It has been postulated, that autism could be caused by some food peptides that could be leaked into the body from the gut but more studies on this issue are needed.

In any case, gastrointestinal symptoms have been related to autism (Melmed et al., 2000).

Conclusion

Since the bacterial and other cells are in close contact with the human host epithelia, and many times also with deeper tissues, it is of essential importance to study their surfaces with respect to interactions. The structures and functions of the surface protrudements and compartments of microbial cells give us hints on their ways to influence our body organs. These structures are under continuous metabolically-related control by the microbes, and by our metabolism and defence functions. It is the borderline, and events thereoff, between the microbial kingdom and our body system which have the highest hygienic relevance. Biofilm formation plays a key role on these surfaces.

References

Amara, N., Mashiak, R., Amar, D., Krief, P., Spieser, S. A., Bottomley, M. J., Aharoni, A., Meijjler, M. M. Covalent inhibition of bacterial quorum sensing. *J. Am. Chem. Soc.*, 2009; 131, 10610-10619.

Back, W., Weiss, N., Seidel, H. Isolierung und systematische Zuordnung bierschadlicher gramnegativer Bakterien. II: Gramnegative anaerobe Stabchen/Anhang: aus Bier isolierte gramnegative fakultativ Stabchen. *Brauwissenschaft*, 1979; 32, 233-238.

Benditt, J. O. Adverse effects of low-flow oxygen therapy. *Respir. Care*, 2000; 45, 54-61.

Bernstein, R., Freger, J., Lee, J. H., King, Y. G., Lee, J., Herzberg, M. 'Should I stay or should I go?' Bacterial attachment vs biofilm formation on surface-modified membranes. *Biofouling*, 2014; 30, 367-376.

Buurman, E.T., Boiardi, J.L., Teixeira de Mattos, M.J., Neijssel, O.M. The role of magnesium and calcium ions in the glucose dehydrogenase activity of *Klebsiella pneumonia* NCTC 418. *Arch. Microbiol.*, 1990; 153, 502-505.

Buurman, E. T., ten Voorde, G. J., Teixeira de Mattos, M. J. The physiological function of periplasmic glucose ocidation in phosphate limited chemostat cultures of *Klebsiella pneumoniae* NCTC 418. *Microbiology*, 1994; 140, 2451-2458.

Costerton, J. W., Stewart, P. S., Greenberg, E. P. Bacterial biofilms, a common cause of persistent infections. *Science*, 1999; 248, 1318-1322.

Ellwood, D. C., Keevil, C. W., Marsh, P. D., Brown, C. M., Wardell, J. N. Surface-associated growth. In: Quayle, J. R., Bull, A. T., editors. New dimensions in microbiology: mixed substrates, mixed cultures and microbial communities. *Phil. Trans. R. Soc. Lond.*, 1982; B 297, 445-639.

Florence, A. T., Attwood, D., Editors. *Physicochemical principles of pharmacy.* 5th edition. Cornwall, UK: Pharmaceutical Press; 2006.

Ghoshal, U. C., Srivastava, D., Verma, A., Ghoshal, U. Tropical spruce in 2014: the new face of an old disease. Curr. Gastroenterol. Rep., 2014; 16, 391-393.

Gottschalk, G. Bacterial metabolism. In: Starr, M. P., editor. Springer series in microbiology. New York, US, Springer; 1979.

Haikara, A. The genera Pectinatus and Megasphaera, *In:* Balows, A., Trüper, G. H., Dworkin, M., Harder, W., Schleifer, K.-H., editors. The Prokaryotes. New York, US: Springer-Verlag; 1991; 1993-2004.

Hakalehto, E. Characterization of *Pectinatus cerevisiiphilus* and *P. frisingiensis* surface components. Use of synthetic peptides in the detection of some gram-negative bacteria. PhD Thesis. *Kuopio University Publications C, Natural and Environmental Sciences* 112; 2000.

Hakalehto, E. Hygiene monitoring with the Portable Microbe Enrichment Unit (PMEU). *41st R3 -Nordic Symposium. Cleanroom technology, contamination control and cleaning. VTT Publications 266.* Espoo, Finland: VTT (State Research Centre of Finland); 2010; 164-176.

Hakalehto, E. Simulation of enhanced growth and metabolism of intestinal *Escherichia coli* in the Portable Microbe Enrichment Unit (PMEU). In: Rogers, M. C., Peterson, N. D. editors. *E. coli infections: causes, treatment and prevention.* New York, US: Nova Science Publishers; 2011; 159-175.

Hakalehto, E, editor. *Alimentary microbiome - a PMEU approach.* New York, US: Nova Science Publishers, Inc.; 2012.

Hakalehto, E. Interactions of *Klebsiella* sp. with other intestinal flora. In: Pereira, L. A., Santos, A. editors. *Klebsiella infections: Epidemiology, pathogenesis and clinical outcomes.* New York, US: Nova Science Publishers, Inc.; 2013.

Hakalehto, E., Finne, J. Identification by immunoblot analysis of major antigenic determinants of the anaerobic beer spoilage bacterium genus *Pectinatus. FEMS Microbiol. Lett.,* 1990; 67, 307-312.

Hakalehto, E., Finne, J., inventors. Protein fragmets of *Pectinatus* bacteria (in Finnish). *Patent application* 924835; 1992.

Hakalehto, E., Hänninen, O. Gaseous CO_2 signal initiate growth of butyric acid producing *Clostridium butyricum* both in pure culture and in mixed cultures with *Lactobacillus brevis. Can. J. Microbiol.,* 2012; 58, 928-931.Hakalehto, E., Jaakkola, K. Synergistic effect of probiotics and prebiotic flax product on intestinal bacterial balance. *Clinical Nutrition,* 2013; 32, Suppl. 1, S200.

Hakalehto, E., Kuronen, I., inventors. A method for producing jelly sweets which contain antibodies. October, 1998. *Patent application nro WO/1998/043610.*

Hakalehto, E., Haikara, A., Lounatmaa, K., Enari, T.-M. Hydrochloric acid extractable protein patterns of *Pectinatus cerevisiophilus* strain. *Food Microbiol.*, 1984; 1, 209-216.

Hakalehto, E., Santa, H., Vepsäläinen, J., Laatikainen, R., Finne, J. Identification of a common structural motif in the disordered N-terminal region of bacterial flagellins. Evidence for a new class of fibril-forming peptides. *Eur. J. Biochem.,* 1997; 250, 19-29.

Hakalehto, E., Hujakka, H., Airaksinen, S., Ratilainen, J., Närvänen, A. Growth-phase limited expression and rapid detection of *Salmonella* type 1 fimbriae. In: Hakalehto, E. Characterization of *Pectinatus cerevisiiphilus* and *P. frisingiensis* surface components. Use of synthetic peptides in the detection of some gram-negative bacteria. PhD Thesis. *Kuopio University Publications C, Natural and Environmental Sciences* 112; 2000.

Hakalehto, E., Pesola, J., Heitto, L., Närvänen, A., Heitto, A. Aerobic and anaerobic growth modes and expression of type 1 fimbriae in *Salmonella*. *Pathophysiology*, 2007; 14, 61-69.

Hakalehto, E., Humppi, T., Paakkanen, H. Dualistic acidic and neutral glucose fermentation balance in small intestine: Simulation *in vitro*. *Pathophysiology*, 2008; 15, 211-220.

Hakalehto, E., Pesola, J., Heitto, A., Deo, B. B., Rissanen, K., Sankilampi, U., Humppi, T., Paakkanen, H. Fast detection of bacterial growth by using Portable Microbe Enrichment Unit (PMEU) and ChemPro100i® gas sensor. *Pathophysiology*, 2009; 16, 57-62.

Hakalehto, E., Hell, M., Bernhofer, C., Heitto, A., Pesola, J., Humppi, T., Paakkanen, H. Growth and gaseous emissions of pure and mixed small intestinal bacterial cultures: Effects of bile and vancomycin. *Pathophysiology*, 2010; 17, 45-53.

Hakalehto, E., Vilpponen-Salmela, T., Kinnunen, K., von Wright, A. Lactic acid bacteria enriched from human gastric biopsies. *ISRN Gastroenterol.,* 2011; 2011, 109183. doi: 10. 5402/2011/109183.

Hakalehto, E., Jääskeläinen, A., Humppi, T., Heitto, L. Production of energy and chemicals from biomasses by micro-organisms. In: Dalhquist, E. editor. *Biomass as energy source: resources, systems and applications*. CRC Press, Taylor and Francis Group, London, UK; 2012.

Hakalehto, E., Tiainen, M., Laatikainen, R., Paakkanen, H., Humppi, T., Hänninen, O. *Klebsiella* sp. Ferments hydrolyzed cellulose by overflow metabolism to 2,3-butanediol and ethanol by overflow metabolism to 2,3-butanediol and ethanol balancing pH and osmotic stress without bacterial growth. 2014. Manuscript in preparation.

Harman, D. A Hypothesis on the Pathogenesis of Alzheimer's Disease. *Proceedings of the sixth congress of the intervational association of biomedical gerontology*. New York: Annals of the New York Academy of Sciences, 1996 786, 152-168.

Helander, I., Hakalehto, E., Ahvenainen, J., Haikara, A. Characterization of lipopolysaccharides of Pectinatus cerevisiophilus, *FEMS Microbiol. Lett.*, 1983; 18, 223-226.

Helander, I., Saukkonen, K., Hakalehto, E., Vaara, M. Characterization of lipopolysaccharides of *Pectinatus cerevisiophilus*. *FEMS Microbiol. Lett.*, 1984; 24, 39-42.

Hell, M., Bernhofer, C., Huhulescu, S., Indra, A., Allerberger, F., Maass, M., Hakalehto, E. How safe is colonoscope-reprocessing regarding *Clostridium difficile* spores*? The Journal of Hospital Infection* Vol. 76, Supplement 1: Abstracts, 8th International Congress of the Hospital Infection Society, Liverpool, UK, 10-13 October 2010, 21-22.

Henriksson, E., Haikara, A. Airborne microorganisms in the brewery filling area and their effect on microbiological stability of beer. *Monatsschrift für Brauwissenschaft,* 1991; 44, 4-8.

Hewett, M. J., Knox, K. W., Bishop, D. G. Biochemical studies on lipopolysaccharides of *Veillonella. Eur. J. Biochem.*, 1971; 19, 169-175.

Immel, F., Jiang, Y., Wang, Y., Marchal, C., Maillet, L., Perrett, S., Cullin, C. *In vitro* analysis of SpUre2p, a prion-related protein, exemplifies the relationship between amyloid and prion. *J. Biol. Chem.*, 2007; 282, 7912-20.

Jaakkola, K., Hakalehto, E. Intestinal imbalances and diseases of the digestive tract. In: Hakalehto, E. editor. *Alimentary microbiome – A PMEU approach.* New York: Nova Science Puhlishers. 2012, 127-160.

Javersky, P., Lee, S. F., Gibbins, A. M., Forsberg, C. W. Extracellular β-galactosidase activity of a *Fibrobacter succinogenes* 885 mutant able to catabolize lactose. *Appl. Env. Microbiol.*, 1990; 56, 3657-3663.

Kim, P. S., Baldwin, R. L. Intermediates in the folding reactions of small proteins. *Annu. Rev. Biochem.,* 1990; 59, 631-660.

Korhonen, T. K., Väisänen, V., Kallio, P., Nurmiaho-Lassila, E. L., Ranta, H., Elo, J., Svensson, J. B., Svanborg-Eden, C. The role of pili in the in the adhesion of *Escherichia coli* to human urinary tract epithelial cells. *Scan. J. Infect. Dis.*, 1982; 33, 26-31.

Kouki, A., Haataja, S., Loimaranta, U., Pulliainen, A.T., Nilsson, U.J., Finne, J. Identification of a novel streptococcal adhesin P (SadP) protein recognizing galactosyl-α1-4-galactose-containing glycoconjugates: convergent evolution of bacterial pathogens to binding of the same host receptor. *J. Biol. Chem., 2011; 286, 38854-64.*

Knight, J., Reeves, J., Wakeman, M. ABEL-Sport Test for assessing overtraining syndrome and detecting infection. *Poster in: International Sports Science + Sports Medicine Conference, 2013.*

Le Bouguénec, C. Adhesins and invasins of pathogenic *Escherichia coli. International Journal of Medical Microbiology*, 2005; 295, 471-478.

Lee, C. A., Falkow, S. The ability of *Salmonella* to enter mammalian cells is affected by bacterial growth state. *PNAS*, 1990; 87, 4304-4308.

Melmed, R. D., Schneider, C. K., Fabes, R. A. Matabolic markers and gastrointestinal symptoms in children with autism and related disorders. *J. Pediatr. Gastroenterol. Nutr.,* 2000; 31, 31-32.

Midgley, M., Dawes, E. A. The regulation of transport of glucose and methyl α-glucoside in *Pseudomonas aeruginosa. Biochem. J.,* 1973; 132, 141-154.

Neijssel, O. M., Tempest, D. W., Postma, P. W., Duine, J. A., Frank Jzn, J. Glucose metabolism by K^+-limited *Klebsiella aerogenes*: evidence for the involvement of a quinoprotein glucose dehydrogenase. *FEMS Microbiol. Lett.*, 1983; 20, 35-39.Ofek, I, Hasty, D. L., Sharon, N. Anti-adhesion therapy of bacterial diseases: prospects and problems. *FEMS Immunol. Med. Microbiol.*, 2003; 38, 181-191.

Oppenheime-Shaanan, Y., Steinberg, N., Kolodkin-Gal, I. Small molecules are natural triggers for the disassembly of biofilms. *Trends Microbiol.,* 2013; 21, 594-601.

Pesola, I., Pesola, J., Kokki, H. Oral microbiology and human health. In: Hakalehto, E, editor. *Alimentary microbiome - a PMEU approach*. New York, US: Nova Science Publishers, Inc.; 2012.

Pesola, J., Hakalehto, E. Enterobacterial microflora in infancy - a case study with enhanced enrichment. *Indian J. Pediatr.,* 2011; 78, 562-568.

Pesola, J., Paakkanen, H., Hakalehto, E. Enhanced diagnostics of pyelonephritis – a case study. *Int. J. Med. Med. Sci.*, 2012; 2, 273-277.

Samgina, T., Vorontsov, E., Gorshkov, V., Hakalehto, E., Hänninen, O., Zubarev, R., Lebedev, A. Composition and antimicrobial activity of the skin peptidome of Russian brown frog *Rana temporaria. J Proteome Res*, 2012; 11, 6213-22.

Sokuranko, E. V., Hasty, D. L. Assay for adhesion of host cells to immobilized bacteria. In: Doyle, R. J., Ofek, I., editors. *Adhesion of microbial pathogens. Methods in enzymology*, San Diego, CA, US: Academic Press.; 1955; 253, 220-226.

Streekstra, H., Teixeira de Mattos, M. J., Neijssel, O. M., Tempest, D. W. Overflow metabolism during anaerobic growth of *Klebsiella aerogenes* NCTC 418 on glycerol and dihydroxyacetone in chemostat culture. *Arch. Microbiol.*, 1987; 147, 268-275.

Svanborg, C., Hedlund, M., Connell, H., Agace, W., Duan, R.-D., Nilsson, Å., Wullt, B. Bacterial adherence and mucosal cytokine responses – receptors and transmembrane signaling. In: Ades, E. W., Morse, S. A., Rest, R. F., Editors. *Microbial Pathogenesis and immune response II. Annals of the New York Academy of Sciences*, New York, US: The New York Academy of Sciences, 1996; 797, 177-190.

Teixera de Mattos, M. J., Tempest, D. W. Metabolic and energetic aspects of the growth of *Klebsiella aerogenes* NCTC 418 on glucose in anaerobic chemostat culture. *Arch. Microbiol.*, 1983; 134, 80-85.

Van Belkum, A., Durand, G., Peyret, M., Chatelier, S., Zambardi, G., Schrenzel, J., Shortridge, D., Engelhardt, A., Dunne Jr. W. M. Rapid clinical bacteriology and its future impact. *Ann. Lab. Med.,* 2013; 33, 14-27.

Van Gylswyk, N. O., Hippe, H., Rainey, F. A. *Schwartzia succinivorans* gen. nov., sp. nov., another ruminal bacterium utilizing succinate as the sole energy source. *IJSEM*, 1997; 47, 155-159.

Weiss, N., Seidel, H., Back, W. Isolierung und system-atische Zuordnung bierschadlicher Bakterien. I. Gram-negative, strikt anaerobe Kokken. *Brauwissenschaft*, 1979; 32,189-194.

Wells, W. F. *Airborne contagion and air hygiene: an ecological study of droplet infection.* Cambridge, MA: Harvard University Press; 1955.Wu, GD; Chen, J; Hoffmann, C; Bittinger, K; Chen, YY; Keilbaugh, SA; Bewtra, M; Knights, D; Walters, WA; Knight, R; Sinha, R; Gilroy, E; Gupta, K; Baldassano, R; Nessel, L; Li, H; Bushman, FD; Lewis, JD. Linking long-term dietary patterns with gut microbial enterotypes. *Science,* 2011; 334, 105-108.

In: Microbiological Clinical Hygiene
Editor: Eino Elias Hakalehto

ISBN: 978-1-63463-428-1

Chapter 3

Nosocomial Viruses

Robert Armon
Faculty of Civil & Environmental Eng., Technion, Haifa, Israel

Abstract

Viruses are perhaps the easiest microorganisms to be transmitted in hospital environments via aerosols, water, food and direct contact. Infected patients with those viruses are able to excrete large quantities of virions in their body fluids, urine and feces according to the viral species that they contracted. Hospitals being a closed and oftenly congested environment favor fast transmission of virion particles from one person to another. Another condition that favor viruses transmission in hospital milleu is the medical staff that come in a continuous contact with patients. Therefore severe prevention steps should be carried out to prevent the spread of any viral disease in hospitals as it has been only recently emphasized by the last Ebola outbreak.

1. Introduction

Perhaps the best definition for a virus is a "host dependent nano-organism" unable to multiply autonomously. Viruses are on the nano scale by size infecting all organisms' kingdoms such as: Archaebacteria - Eubacteria - Protista - Fungi - Plantae - Animalia (Figure 1). The smallest virus (Poliovirus) has a size of ~ 28 nm and once it was one of the dread hazards leaving many paralyzed children behind!; at present it is almost eradicated due to global vaccination, however it is still reported in various countries with poor hygiene. Among viruses some had a crucial role in population decimations across continents, e.g., the Spanish Flu of 1918 (Table 1).

The structural simplicity of viruses is amazing as they don't carry organelles but only a capsid, envelope, a nucleic acid (DNA or RNA) and sometimes an enzyme (e.g., a reverse transcriptase enzyme). They are able to survive but not to multiply in the environment (water, air or soil). Along their structural simplicity, they also carry genetic information to be used as a transfer reservoir for their hosts.

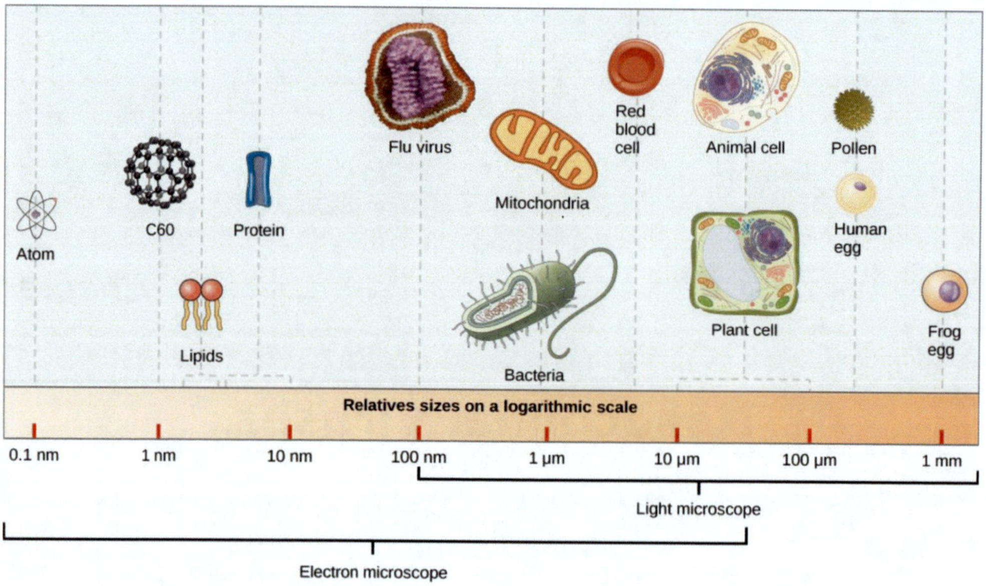

Figure 1. From atoms to multi cellular organisms: the relative size of viruses. (From http://cnx.org/content/m45541/latest/#fig-ch17_01_06).

Table 1. Major global pandemics since the last century

Pathogen	Year	Source	Disease	Data	Comments
Spanish Flu (mutated influenza viruses	1918	Unknown	Severe flu	20 million death in this pandemic ; 675,000 Americans	Taubenberger and Morens (2006)
Poliovirus	1952	Local	Poliomyelitis or child paralysis	In USA alone: 58,000 reported cases with3,145 fatalities	Source: Salk Institute; Melnick (1996)
Asian flu a subtype of type influenza virus A	1957	China	Severe Flu	In USA ~ 70,000 fatalities in this pandemic	Webby and Webster (2003); Ghendon (1994)
AIDS (acquired immune deficiency syndrome)	1980	Africa	Lung infection characterized by a weakened immune system	In USA > 650,000 fatalities (estimated)	Anonymous(b) (2013)

Environmentally, viruses are carried by infected individuals that excrete them into their environment (water, sewage, effluents, aerosols) through fecal material, puss, blood, sneeze or infected tissues. In hospitals patients infected with viruses are the main source of infection while doctors, nurses or other personnel use as carriers.

2. Virus Structure

A virus is assembled from a proteinaceous capsid in which a DNA/RNA strand single/double is coiled.

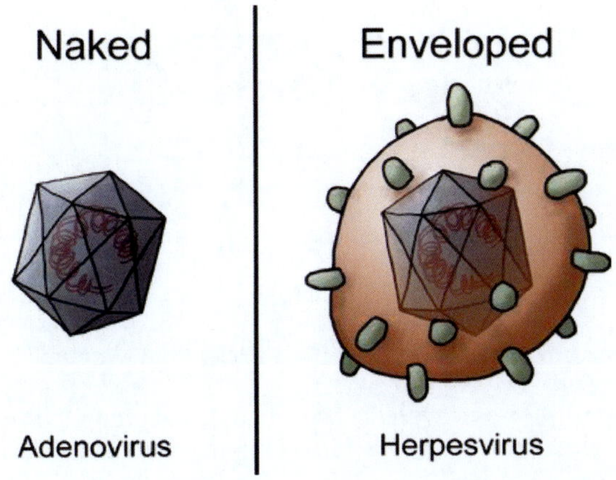

Figure 2. Two viral types according to their external structure (the genetic material is packed inside the capsid).

Some viral groups also contain an envelope (usually a part of its host membrane) that engulfs the capsid. The external structure defines two main groups of viruses: naked and enveloped (Figure 2). Some viruses (those that their genetic material is RNA) contain inside the capsid an enzyme called: reverse transcriptase (RT) used by virus to reverse-transcribe their RNA genomes into DNA, which is then integrated into the host genome and replicated along with it. Naked viruses are more resistant to environmental stresses in comparison with enveloped ones, consequently being spread by water and other environmental means.

3. Viruses Taxonomy

Currently, viruses are divided (according to Baltimore, 1971) in six groups based on their nucleic acid. A seventh group was added later, after its discovery (dsDNA-RT viruses, e.g., Hepadnaviruses-Hepatitis B virus). The groups are: I- ds-DNA; II-ss-DNA; III-ds-RNA; IV-ssRNA with positive strands (positive polarity); V-ss-RNA with negative strands (negative polarity); VI- ss-RNA associated with RT enzyme and VII-ds-DNA associated with RT enzyme (Figure 3).

An older taxonomic division by Lwoff et al (Lwoff et al., 1962) was based on the following criteria: the nature of the nucleic acid: RNA or DNA; capsid symmetry; presence/absence of envelope and virion and capsid's dimensions (Figure 4a-b) (Lwoff et al., 1962).

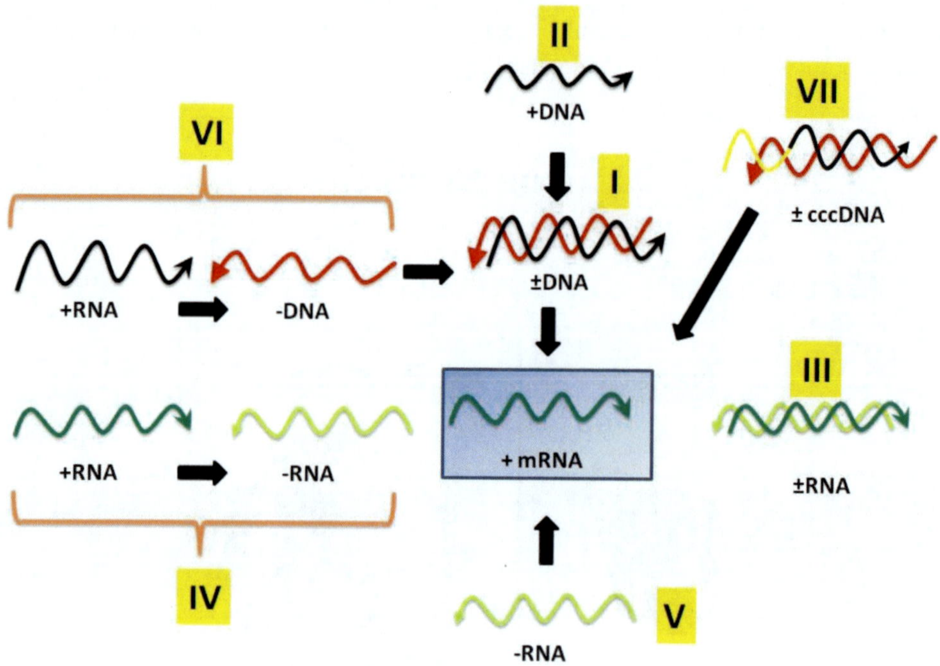

Figure 3. Baltimore taxonomy of viruses with the latest introduced group VII (Hepadnaviruses). (Adapted from http://www.virology.ws/2009/08/12/simplifying-virus-classification-the-baltimore-system/).

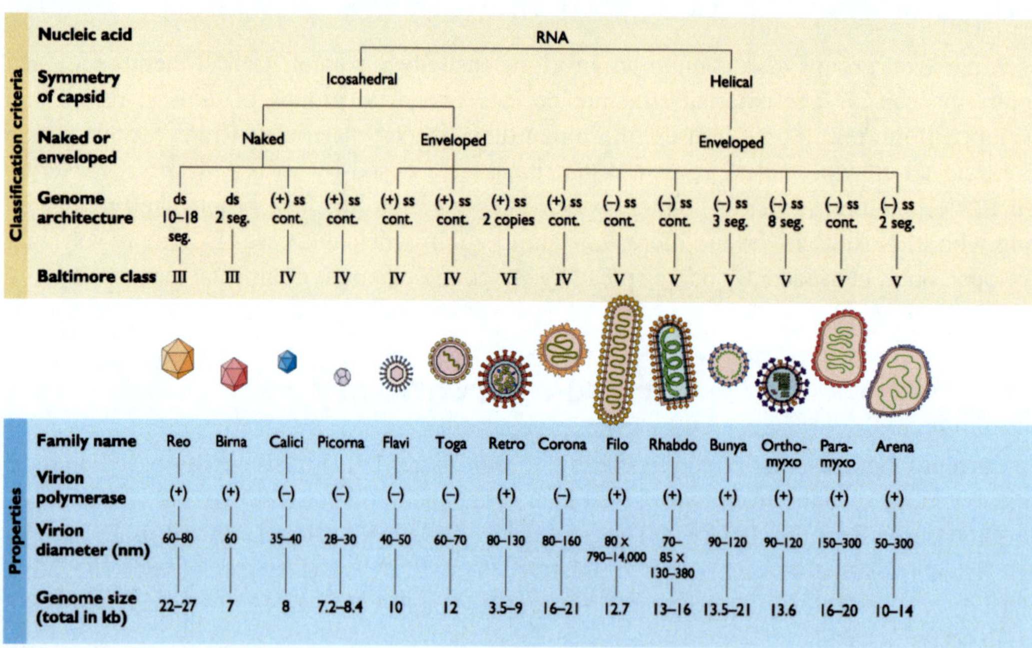

(a)

Figure 4a-b. (Continued).

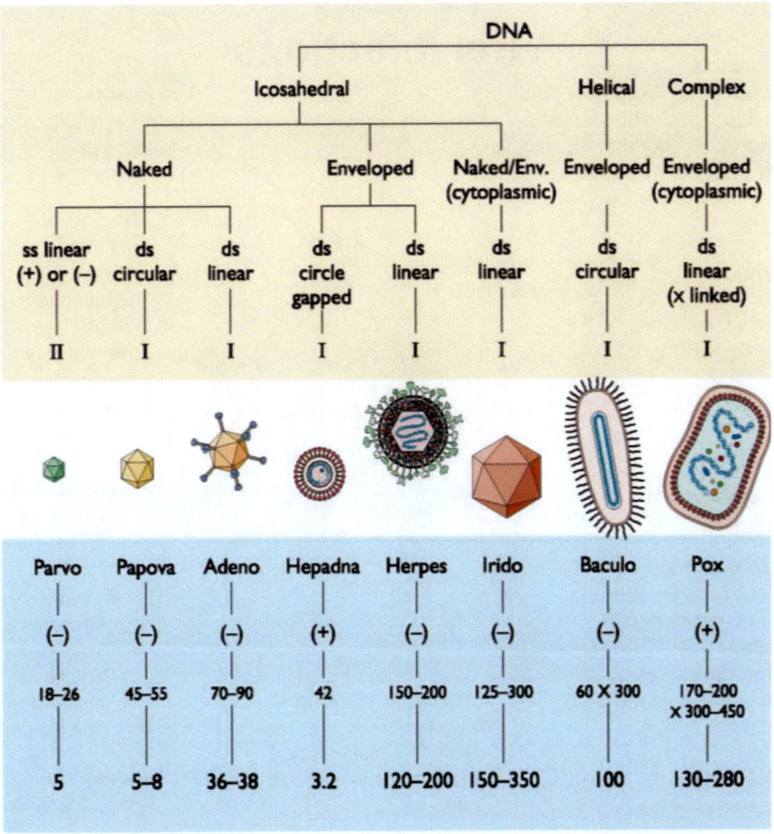

(b)

Figure 4a-b. The Lwoff et al (Lwoff et al., 1962) taxonomy of viruses. (From: http://www.nlv.ch /Virologytutorials/Classification.ht.

4. Human Viruses

Human viruses are diverse in their infection and entrance site (Figure 5). This chapter will not deal in particular with each human virus and its severity but will describe the hospital risk to contract those commonly found in health care institutions and ways to prevent nosocomial viral infections.

5. Viral Contagion

Human viruses are carried by infected persons that present or don't present symptoms. These people may excrete large numbers of viral particles into their feces, urine, saliva, blood, body fluids and aerosols produced via sneezing/coughing. Human viruses can be transmitted vertically or horizontally. The vertical transmission means from person to person (e.g., Hepatitis B virus or HIV) a good example are babies born already infected with the mentioned viruses (Fowler et al, 2007).

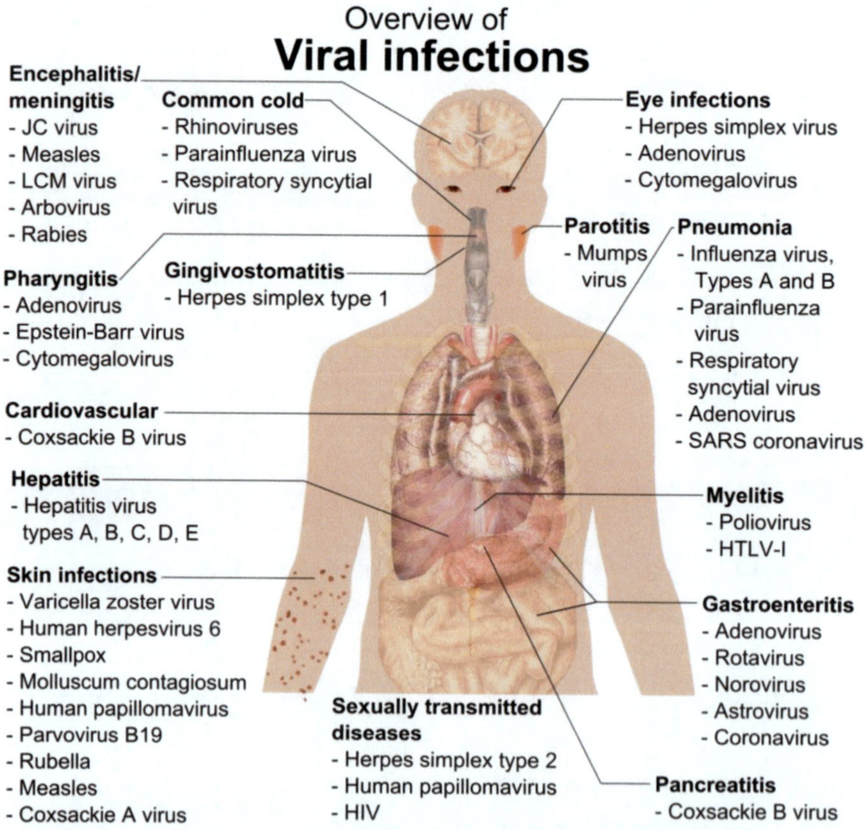

Figure 5. Human viral infections (From the medical gallery of Mikael Häggström).

In rare cases, varicella zoster virus (*Human herpesvirus 3* -HHV-3) that causes a moderately infection is fatal to foetus or new born babies (Sauerbrei and Wutzler, 2000).

Horizontal transmission is most frequent mechanism of virus transmission via person to person. As already mentioned, human excretions reach another person and viruses are ingested, inhaled or in contact with the body and cause infection. Examples of such "horizontal" viruses are: HIV (sexual contact), Hepatitis C (mouth contact), Epstein-Barr virus (human herpesvirus 4-HHV-4) (oral transfer of saliva and genital secretions, Noroviruses (water and food), Influenza virus (Orthomyxoviruses) (aerosols) and dengue (DENV) (mosquitoes).

Human infection with a virus has a so called incubation period with or without signs or symptoms. The incubation period can vary from days to weeks, an interval time which seems to be critical in health care institutions where patients are gathered for prolonged periods (Table 2) (Gelber and Ratner, 2002; Knipe et al., 2007). Following the incubation period but sometimes overlapping there is a period of communicability when the infected person is contagious.

At this point the infected person can transmit the virus to a large numbers of healthy people to develop into an outbreak (called by professionals an epidemic). The rate or speed of transmission of viral infections depends on factors such as population density, susceptible individuals in the population (i.e., immunocompromised persons or unvaccinated ones), the quality of healthcare and sometimes the weather.

Table 2. Incubation period and viral shedding (protracted in neonates) for nosocomial viral pathogens in the NICU. (adapted from Gelber and Ratner, 2002)

Virus	Incubation period	Viral Shedding (protracted in neonates)
Rotavirus	1-3 days	Up to 5 d after cessation of symptoms
Hepatitis A	2-5 weeks	2 wk prior to 1 wk after symptoms (infants likely asymptomatic)
Enteroviruses	3-6 days	3-4 d prior to 2 wk after symptoms (respiratory shedding < 1 wk)
RSV	2-8 days	3 d prior to until cessation of respiratory symptoms Infants 3d-4 wk
Influenza	1-3 days	1 d before symptoms appear through duration of svimptomatic period
Adenovirus	2-14 days (respiratory) 3-10 days (GI)	Several weeks possible
Parainfluenza	2-6 days	3-6 d prior to onset of Viral isolation symptoms until 10 d after rooolution
Varicella	10-21 days (up to 28)	4 d before to 5 d after rash appears
HSV	2 days to 2 weeks	Skin: lesion onset until crusting Disseminated or mucosal may be prolonged.
CMV	28-60 days, with an average of 40 days	Prolonged, intermittent

Hepatitis C virus is an excellent example of a virus carried by a large reservoir of asymptomatic chronically infected individuals from less developed countries (endemic areas) and immigration to less prevalent regions and needle sharing for intravenous drug use (IDU). Worldwide HCV data shows a prevalence of 2.27% or 160 million persons infected with this virus (Quer and Esteban Mur, 2014).

In hospitals, infection with any pathogenic microorganisms (virus, bacteria, protozoa or fungi) is called "hospital acquired infection" (HAI). In healthcare settings, viruses are commonly transmitted via: a) iatrogenic pathways e.g., transfusion of blood and blood products, an inanimate object (fomite) such as sharp instruments which penetrate the skin may carry infection (e.g., surgical instruments, syringes, razor blades, needles) for viruses like HCV, HIV, HBV Creutzfeldt-Jakob Disease (via injection of contaminated human growth hormone) and transplantation of infected organs (Quer and Esteban Mur, 2014; Anonymous(b), 2013); b) direct contact and airborne (e.g., agents present in nasopharynx or respiratory tract are disseminated in salivary droplets during coughing, sneezing or breathing) for example viruses like mumps, measles, chicken pox, colds, and influenza (viral) (La Rosa et al., 2013).

6. Viral Droplet Nuclei Transmission

People infected with common cold, influenza A & B, mumps, measles, rubella, SARS, etc. may transmit these viruses through coughing, sneezing, talking and breathing into the air. Mucus coated viruses are spread at a relative long distance (>6 m) during which mucus water evaporates pending temperature and humidity (the remaining virion is called droplet nucleus or quanta). In winter time, when the indoor temperature is high and humidity low, the droplet nuclei will remain floating in air due to their small volume and consequently infecting other people in close contact. Breath of these droplets by another person reaches their nose and mouse and further penetrate deeper in their lungs.

7. Fecal-Oral Transmission

In humans and especially in hospitals the direct route of fecal-oral transmission is rare (taking into account the medical hygiene procedures), however a more common route is the indirect one: through water and food. Contamination of hospital foodstuffs and water is merely produced by luck of hand washing by people involved in preparation procedures of the two. Examples of viruses transmitted this way are: Hepatitis A, Poliovirus and Rotavirus.

8. Cases of Acute Viral Outbreaks in Hospitals Respiratory Route

Among the most common respiratory viruses which spread easily and have a relatively short incubation time (typically between 1 and 8 days), one can find: RSV, influenza viruses A and B, parainfluenza viruses 1 to 3, rhinoviruses, and adenoviruses. The transmission may occur between patients through the hands of health care workers that fail to wash hands between patients. In contrast to most of nosocomial infections that occur throughout the year, respiratory viruses occur seasonal with a pick incidence in winter months reflecting community health status.

Prevention

Early prevention depends on the early diagnosis of the infection (Madge et al., 1992). In general, for respiratory syncytial virus (RSV) rapid laboratory diagnosis (direct antigen detection in nasopharyngeal cells), the wearing of aprons or gowns and gloves (for close contact with infected infants), and source isolation (or cohorting of infected patients) are essential (Aitken and Jeffries, 2001). In cases of suspected influenza viruses A and B similar precautions are required, but emphasis on droplet precautions, (including masks wearing) and isolation in a single room are much recommended (La Rosa et al, 2013). In parainfluenza infections, the above recommendations stand as well (interruption of droplet transmission and hand washing) including environmental cleaning with cleaners and disinfectants (available in each hospital) that should eliminate surface contamination. When Rhinoviruses and

Coronaviruses are involved, isolation and droplet precautions are the standard. Infected persons should be isolated in a single room, while care personnel should wear gloves and gowns when in contact or taking samples. Adenoviruses are highly stable therefore equipment decontamination is essential, particularly with ophthalmological equipment, by steam sterilization.

In case of "old common" viruses such as measles, mumps, and rubella the above measures apply for hospital patients as well beforehand vaccination of medical stuff as a must. When in contact with measles a person should be discharged home, and "should not have patient contact between days 5 and 21 after exposure" (Aitken and Jeffries, 2001). In cases of congenital rubella (rare cases) an infected infant excretes large amounts of rubella virus therefore isolation of both is recommended. The last important respiratory route transmitted virus, Parvovirus B19 which is associated with erythema infectiosum or fifth disease (slapped cheek syndrome) in children (Pattison, 1990), the U.S. Centers for Disease Control and Prevention (CDC) do not recommend any restrictions, not for regulars and not for pregnant, as the virus symptoms (rush appearance) occur after infectious period.

Fecal-Oral Route

Gastrointestinal viral infections are caused by: rotavirus, Small Round-Structured Viruses-SRSV (astroviruses, caliciviruses:e.g., Norwalk agent), enteric adenoviruses and parvovirus, Enteroviruses (e.g., coxsackieviruses A and B, echoviruses, polioviruses, and enteroviruses 68 to 71), Hepatitis A Virus-HAV, Hepatitis E virus-HEV, herpesvirus family: (e.g., herpes simplex virus-HSV types 1 and 2, Varicella-Zoster virus-VZV, Cytomegalovirus-CMV, Epstein Barr virus-EBV and human herpesviruses-HHVs 6, 7, and 8) (Kapikian et al., 1996, Cubitt, 1994). Transmission is predominantly by the fecal-oral route which include water, food, and personal contact (possible via contact with aerosols and/or contaminated fomites with vomit or aerosols) and infection through gastrointestinal track. For most of the above viruses the spread control is the set up of solitary room or cohort isolation with enteric precautions. To prevent patient-to-patient transmission, sodium hypochlorite is used for general disinfection and handwashing with 70 or 95% alcohol are recommended. Vaccination is recommended in case of efficient available vaccines on market. In case of HAV, HEV care should be taken in handling excreta, and single-room isolation is recommended due to maximum fecal shedding of virions occurring in the late incubation period.

Human Herpesviruses require good standard of hygiene such as frequent handwashing, gloves when handling infectious body fluids, patients with active lesions should be isolated and prevented to come in contact with high-risk groups (i.e., immunocompromised, neonates, patients with eczema or burns). Mothers with active lesions (mainly around the nipples) should be breast-feeding prevented. Acyclovir is a good therapy to reduce virus shedding period and for immunocompromised patients to prevent dissemination. Basic precautions used for contact with body fluids of all patients should be taken, i.e., gloves and apron or gown and personal contact with the other herpesvirus types (CMV, VZV, etc.).

Blood Route

Among the most known blood-borne viruses are: the Picornaviridae family genus Hepatovirus of Hepatitis B virus (HBV), Hepatitis C virus (HCV), and Retroviridae family, genus Lentivirus the Human Immunodeficiency Virus Type 1 (HIV-1) but some exotic viruses such as Viral hemorrhagic fevers (VHFs)(the filoviruses Ebola and Marburg virus, the arenaviruses particularly Lassa virus, the bunyavirus Congo Crimean hemorrhagic fever virus, and the flaviviridae Dengue virus 1–4) were reported in hospitals. Prevention of HBV, HCV and HIV is linked to transmission paths such as blood, tissue and body fluids transfer, from an infected to an uninfected individual, and patient-to-patient transmission in health care, therefore prevention of these activities is highly recommended. In case of the so called "exotic viruses" which are fatal if contracted, the prevention is very strict and requires the following logical steps (recommended by The U.S. Centers for Disease Control and Prevention-CDC and the UK Advisory Committee on Dangerous Pathogens-ACDP) (Berger et al., 2003; Anonymous(a), 2009; ACDP, 1996): "(1) environmental decontamination with household bleach (10,000 ppm available chlorine); (2) use of disposable linen (decontamination in an autoclave and washing in a washing machine with bleach are alternatives); (3) autoclaving, incineration, or treatment with household bleach for 5 min of all waste materials from the patients; (4) if a patient dies, the body should be handled minimally and placed in a sealable plastic body bag; it should be placed in a robust coffin and stored separately before burial or cremation; (5) persons with accidental percutaneous or mucous membrane exposure should wash the area immediately with copious amounts of soap and water" (Aitken and Jeffries, 2001). Possible prophylactic use of antiviral drugs should be sought urgently for those in contact with.

9. Viral Diagnosis

Isolation and Identification Methods

As mentioned above the sources of infectious viruses originate from their infection site (nasopharynx, oropharynx, laryngopharynx, gastrointestinal and genitals) or infected body parts such as: tissue, blood, urine, feces and other exudates. At laboratory level there a variety of methods to detect viruses.

Cell Culture

Cell culture has a major advantage over all other methods; it is the only method that indicates viral particles' viability. Other methods are based on molecular detection of various components of the virus, e.g., envelope, capsid or the genetic material (DNA/RNA). The sensitivity is relatively high, but pending on the virus type and its particle/plaque forming unit ratio_(Table 3). Another form of cell culture use is the cytopathic effect unit or endpoint dilution assay in which the viral last dilution that does not cause cytophatic effects is observed.

Table 3. Particle/plaque forming units for selected animal viruses (adapted from Flint et al., 2003; Benyesh-Melnick et al., 1966)

Virus	Particle/PFU ratio
Poliovirus	30-1000
Adenovirus	20-100
Herpes simplex virus	50-200
Papilloma virus	10,000
Semliki forest virus	1-2
Cytomegalovirus strain AD-169 strain C-87	 160-490 176-1,050
Influenza virus	20-50
Reovirus	10
Polyomavirus	38-50
Poxviridae	1-100

Antibody-Antigen Detection

Presently, highly specific antibodies such as monoclonal antibodies (MAb) that can detect a specific protein or glycoprotein on the outer viral coat are commercially available (immunofluorescence-IF). Infected cells containing viral particles can be labeled and microscopically visualized by epifluorescent microscopy. Another use of antibodies can be applied interlaced with tissue culture such as in neutralization tests. By applying antibodies to a viral particle, it can be neutralized therefore losing its infectivity as detected by plaque formation. Other methods are: immunoperoxidase (IP), enzyme-linked immunosorbent assay (ELISA), neutralization (NEUT), hemagglutination inhibition (HAI), passive agglutination (PA), radioimmunoassay, and immune adherence hemagglutination. Methods such as IF, IP, ELISA, and PA provide rapid and accurate virus identification, whereas NEUT and HAI, although accurate, are more costly and time consuming.

Non-Immunological Methods

Hemagglutination (HA) is an older method mostly used in the past for Myxoviruses (families Orthomyxoviridae-agents of influenza) and Paramyxoviridae. These viruses are studded with spike-like protein projections able to attach to molecules present on the surface of RBCs. As consequence at certain concentrations, a viral suspension may bind together (agglutinate) the RBCs, preventing them from settling out of suspension in a regular concentric button. Other non-immunological techniques are: histologic staining, electron microscopy, hemadsorption (HAD), challenged interference (CI), polymerase chain reaction (PCR) and DNA probes (Goldmann, 1987). HAD, HA, and CI are used primarily to detect non-cytopathogenic effect-producing viruses within cell cultures. PCR and DNA probes provide the most specific viral identification and will probably replace many traditional techniques (Mahony, 2008).

10. Case Studies and Confinement Measures

Dzelalija et al (Dzelalija et al., 2007) reported on an acute Norwalk like virus gastroenteritis outbreak in a Zadar hospital. The number of affected persons was 39 from which 22 inpatients and 17 healthcare workers. On the first day of the event recording, anti-epidemic measures were implemented (according to the source of infection detected and to the mechanisms of transmission). Epidemiological inspection continued for two more weeks following clinical symptoms in the last patient. The authors concluded "the necessity to rapidly inform the Hospital Infection Control Committee on the epidemic outbreak" in order to be effective in stopping the spread of acute gastroenteritis caused by Norwalk like viruses".

In case of hospital acute gastroenteritis caused by small round structured viruses (SRSVs) like in the previous case, Chadwick et al (Chadwick et al., 2000) based on outbreaks data suggested in details the following measures related to prevention, spread and confinement as related to two categories of recommendation: **Category I**- strongly recommended and strongly supported by well-designed experimental epidemiological studies; **Category II**-strongly recommended and viewed as effective by experts in the field and by the working group, based on strong rationale and suggestive evidence, even though definitive studies may not have been done and **No Category**: an unresolved issue as there is insufficient evidence or consensus regarding efficacy.

11. Spread Prevention

1) Staff working in affected areas must not then work in unaffected areas of 48h (includes agency and bank staff) (Category II).
2) Avoid patient movements to unaffected areas (unless medically urgent and after consultation with infection control staff) and other institutions (Category II).

12. Control Measures for SRSVs Within Affected Clinical Areas (confinement) at Ward Level

1) Cohort nurse or isolate symptomatic individuals (Category II)
2) Wear gloves and apron for contact with an affected patient or environment (Category II)
3) Wash hands with soap and water after contact with an affected patient or environment, after removing gloves and apron (Category I)
4) Remove exposed food such as fruit (No Category)
5) Consider use of antiemetics for patients with vomiting (No Category)
6) Exclude affected staff from the ward immediately and until 48 h symptom-free (Category II)
7) Close the ward to prevent the introduction of new susceptibles. Avoid transfer to unaffected wards or departments (unless medically urgent and after consultation with infection control staff). The priority is to stop spread of the virus to other areas (Category II).

8) Exclude non-essential personnel from the ward (Category II)
9) Caution visitors and emphasize hand hygiene (Category II)
10) Clean and disinfect vomit and faeces spillages promptly: Appendix B* (Category II)
11) Increase the frequency of routine ward, bathroom and toilet cleaning (Category II)
12) Use freshly prepared 0.1% (1000 ppm) hypochlorite to disinfect hard surfaces after cleaning (Category II)
13) The ward should not be re-opened until 72 h after the last new case and 72 h after uncontained vomiting and diarrhoea (Category II)
14) Thoroughly clean the ward and change the bed curtains before re-opening (Category II)
15) Clean carpets and soft furnishings with hot water and detergent, or steam clean. Vacuum cleaning is not recommended (No Category)

*Appendix B: Guidance on Cleaning Up Vomit and Faeces (Detailed Procedure)

The following precautions should be used by individuals who clean up vomit or faeces in order to minimize the risk of infection to them.

1. Wear disposable gloves and apron.
2. Use paper towels to soak up excess liquid. Transfer these and any solid matter directly into a clinical waste bag.
3. Clean the soiled area with detergent and hot water, using a disposable cloth.
4. Disinfect the contaminated area with freshly made 1000 ppm (0.1%) hypochlorite solution. Note that hypochlorite is corrosive and may bleach furnishings and fabrics.
5. Dispose of gloves, apron and cloths into the clinical waste bag.
6. Wash hands thoroughly using soap and water and dry them.

13. Laboratory Diagnosis

In spite of advanced molecular technology advancement the electron microscopy remains the first line diagnostic method for SRSVs. In parallel, the reverse transcription polymerase chain reaction (RT-PCR) methodology is presently developed for a variety of SRSVs. On the other hand, RT-PCR is not yet a routine diagnostic method because not all strains can be amplified in the currently described assays.

The added sensitivity of RT-PCR over EM is likely to extend the diagnostic window beyond 48 h for these viruses and they will be the next routine lab testing in every hospital. According to electron microscopy the following policy has been recommended (Curry et al., 1999):

1. Only unformed faecal specimens from symptomatic individuals within three days of onset should be referred for examination
2. An initial batch of up to six specimens will be examined

3. A further batch of four specimens will be examined if less than two are positive
4. Not all specimens from an outbreak will necessarily be examined
5. New cases on a different ward will be regarded as a potentially distinct outbreak

14. Hospital Function during Fatal Virus Outbreak

An interesting issue related to nosocomial infection and hospital function during fatal epidemics like in the case of Ebola virus (Hall et al., 2008). The Kikwit Ebola outbreak of 1995 was one of the most well studied infectious epidemics and one of the first times that the Ebola virus was treated in a hospital setting (CDC, 1995). Due to lack of knowledge, many difficulties were revealed during this outbreak. It should be reminded that the mortality rate of Ebola virus is 50-70%.

The lessons learned from this outbreak are important especially for developing countries as well for developed ones (in emergency cases such as hurricanes or terrorists attack). The main problems raised throughout this outbreak were typical to countries with poor health expressed as: severely hampered treatment due to issues of contagion; initial poor records keeping; disinfection problems and limited medical equipment (intravenous medications and hydration not available due to both the lack of supplies and the risk/fear of staff being exposed to blood); the majority of the patients' daily needs (feeding and bathing) were performed by family members and worst those family members slept in the bed with the infected patient, putting them at risk. Finally, patients discharged from the convalescent ward would often return to the hospital after they were physically attacked or shunned by their neighbors! (Thacker, 2003). Hall et al (Hall et al., 2008) concluded the Kikwit outbreak in these words: "General lessons from the outbreak include the importance of having simple, well-defined triage procedures; staff who are flexible and able to adapt to situations with unknowns; and the need to protect staff physically and emotionally to ensure a sustained effort to provide care".

Conclusion

The present chapter described nosocomial viral infections in hospitals, their spread and the damage to patients beside the life loss, high cost of treatment and undesired effects. In order to summarize the measures to control nosocomial viral infections in hospitals the following recommendations seem to be valid for all cases no matter of transmission route (minor changes should be regarded to time intervals, as each virus has its own incubation time):

- Cohort nurse or isolate symptomatic individuals
- Emphasize the importance of handwashing
- Wash and dry hands before and after patient/environmental contacts
- Wear gloves and aprons for contact with infected patients/environment

- Avoid transfer to unaffected wards or departments (unless medically urgent and after consultation with infection control staff). The priority is to stop spread of the virus to other areas
- Minimize movements of staff between affected and unaffected wards
- Exclude affected staff until symptom-free for 48 h
- Caution visitors that they may be exposed to infection
- Wherever possible, exclude children from visiting affected wards
- Advise relatives not to visit if they are feeling unwell or have D&V.
- Use 1000 ppm hypochlorite to disinfect contaminated environmental surfaces.
- Thoroughly clean the ward and change curtains before re-opening to admissions (usually 72 h after symptoms have subsided). This will be arranged by the infection control team.
- Refer to enteric precautions and the outbreak policy in the infection control folder.
- Remember always to inform the infection control team of any unexpected vomiting or diarrhoea among patients or staff in your area (Chadwick et al., 2000).

References

ACDP. Management and control of viral hemorrhagic fevers. London Stationery Office, London, United Kingdom. 1996.

Aitken, C; Jeffries, DJ. Nosocomial Spread of Viral Disease. *Clin. Microbiol. Rev.*, 2001; 14(3), 528-546.

Anonymous(a). Exotic Animal Disease Risk Pathways & Countermeasures Final Report. Published by Department for Environment, Food and Rural Affairs (DEFRA), UK. 2009; 129.

Anonymous(b). "The HIV/AIDS Epidemic in the United States". Kaiser Family Foundation. March 22, 2013. Retrieved June 14, 2014.

Baltimore, D. Expression of animal virus genomes. *Bacteriological reviews,* 1971; 35 (3), 235-241.

Benyesh-Melnick, M; Probstmeyer, F: Mccombs, R; Brunschwig, JP; Vonka, V. Correlation between infectivity and physical virus particles in human cytomegalovirus. *J. Bacteriol.,* 1966; 92(5), 1555-1561.

Berger, SA; Calisher, CH; Keystone, JS. Exotic Viral Diseases: A Global Guide. Hamilton, Ontario: BC Decker, Inc.; 2003; 252.

CDC. Update: outbreak of Ebola viral hemorrhagic fever-Zaire. Morb. Mortal. Wkly. Rep. 1995; 44:468–469, 475.

Chadwick, PR; Beards, G; Brown, D; Caul, EO; Cheesebough, J; Clarke, I; Curry, A; O'Brien, S; Quigley, K; Sellwood, J; Westmoreland, D. Management of hospital outbreaks of gastro-enteritis due to small round structured viruses. *J. Hosp. Infect.,* 2000; 45, 1–10.

Cubitt, WD. Caliciviruses. In: Kapikian AZ, editor. Viral infections of the gastrointestinal tract. New York, N.Y.: Marcel Dekker; 1994; 549-568.

Curry, A; Bryden, A; Morgan-Capner, P; Fox, A; Guiver, M; Martin, L; Mutton, K; Wright, P; Mannion, P; Wastwell, A; Cheesebrough, J; Ashton, I; Blackley, A. A rationalized virological electron microscope specimen testing policy. PHLS North West Viral Gastroenteritis and Electron Microscopy Subcommitee. *J. Clin. Pathol.*, 1999 52, 471–474.

Dzelalija, B; Medic, A; Leto, I; Seric, J; Juric, M. The outbreak of acute gastroenteritis caused by Norwalk like viruses in Zadar general hospital (2007) *Acta. Med. Croat.,* 2008; 62(3), 305-308.

Flint, SJ; Enquist, LW; Racaniello, VR; Skalka, AM. Principles of Virology: Molecular Biology, Pathogenesis, and Control of Animal Viruses. 2nd Edition. Washington DC: ASM Press; 2003.

Fowler, MG; Lampe, MA; Jamieson, DJ; Kourtis, AP; Rogers, MF. Reducing the risk of mother-to-child human immunodeficiency virus transmission: past successes, current progress and challenges, and future directions. *Am. J. Obstet. Gynecol.*, 2007; 197(3 Suppl), S3–S9.

Gelber, SE; Ratner, AJ.Hospital-acquired Viral Pathogens in the Neonatal Intensive Care Unit. *Semin Perinatol,* 2002; 6(5), 346-356.

Ghendon, Y. Introduction to Pandemic Influenza through History. *Europ. J. Epidemiol.,* 1994; 10 (4), 451-453.

Goldmann, DA. New Microbiological Techniques for Hospital Epidemiology. *Eur. J. Clin. Microbiol.,* 1987; 6(3), 344-347.

Hall, RC; Hall, RC; Chapman, MJ. The 1995 Kikwit Ebola outbreak: lessons hospitals and physicians can apply to future viral epidemics. *Gen. Hosp. Psychiat.,* 2008; 30, 446–452.

Kapikian, AZ; Estes, MK; Chanock, RM. Norwalk group of viruses. In: Fields BN, Knipe DM, Howley PM editors. Fields virology, 3rd ed. Philadelphia, PA: Lippincott-Raven; 1996; 783-810.

Knipe, DM; Howley, PM; Griffin, DE; Lamb, RA; Martin, MA; Roizman, B; Straus, SE. *Fields Virology*. Philadelphia, PA: Lippincott Williams & Wilkins; 2007.

La Rosa, G; Fratini, M; Della Libera, S; Iaconelli, M; Muscillo, M. Viral infections acquired indoors through airborne, droplet or contact transmission. *Ann. Ist. Super Sanità,* 2013; 49(2), 124-132.

Lwoff, A; Horne, R; Tournier, P. "A system of viruses". Cold Spring Harb. *Symp. Quant Biol.,* 1962; 27, 51–55.

Madge, P; Paton, J; McColl, H; Mackie, PLK. Prospective controlled study of four infection-control procedures to prevent nosocomial infection with respiratory syncytial virus. *Lancet,* 1992; 340, 1079–1083.

Mahony, JB. Detection of Respiratory Viruses by Molecular Methods. *Clin. Microbiol. Rev.,* 2008; 21(4): 716–747.

Melnick, J. Current status of poliovirus infections. *Clin. Microbiol. Rev.,* 1996; 9 (3), 293–300.

Pattison, JR. Parvovirus: medical and biological aspects. In: Fields BN, Knipe DM editors. *Virology.* New York, NY: Raven Press; 1990; 1765-1786.

Quer, J; Esteban Mur, JI. Chapter 17: Epidemiology and prevention. In: Thomas HC, Lok ASF, Locarinini SA, Zuckerman AJ editors. Viral Hepatitis, 4th Edition. John Wiley & Sons, Ltd.; 2014; 246-265.

Sauerbrei, A; Wutzler, P. The congenital varicella syndrome. *J. Perinatol.,* 2000; 20(8 Pt 1), 548–554.

Taubenberger, JK; Morens, DM. 1918 Influenza: the Mother of All Pandemics. Centers for Disease Control and Prevention. 2006. Retrieved, 2014-06-19.

Thacker, PD. An Ebola epidemic simmers in Africa: in remote region, outbreak shows staying power. *JAMA*, 2003; 290, 317–319.

Webby, RJ; Webster, RG. (2003) Are We Ready for Pandemic Influenza? *Science,* 2003; 302(5650), 1519-1522.

In: Microbiological Clinical Hygiene
Editor: Eino Elias Hakalehto

ISBN: 978-1-63463-428-1

Chapter 4

Some Common Mild and More Serious Respiratory Infections

***Kaarlo Jaakkola*[1] *and Elias Hakalehto*[2]**
[1] Kruunuhaka Medical Center, Helsinki, Finland
[2] Department of Environmental Sciences,
University of Eastern Finland, Kuopio, Finland

Abstract

Human respiratory tract is a complex organ system. One of its main functions is to regulate essential gas balances for our entire body system. The pulmonary and other parts of this region are relatively sensitive and vulnerable tissues. Together with skin, as well as intestinal and other epithelia they represent the major barriers into our body system. These borderlines have to carry out sieve functions at the same time as the gas exchange is continuously performed by the lungs. This gas flow also supports microbial growth inside the system, since it is maintaining relatively stable conditions which promote the microbial metabolism. On the other hand, the partial pressures of different gases and other circumstances that favor some microbes more than others, and are thus very selective ones. Moreover, any partial obstruction in the respiratory airways can cause altered pressure conditions, and may increase the risks of infections in the affected areas..

In this chapter several pulmonary and other respiratory problems are reviewed from the microbiological point of view, together with some potential cures for them. Some ideas regarding hygiene management are also introduced. In practical clinical care even minor respiratory illnesses cause a physiological stress and could initiate inflammations, which lower the general status of patients. These initially minor health problems also involve risks of inducing more serious diseases. In hospital environment, it is also of crucial importance to distinct the cases of mild respiratory infections from other more severe sicknesses, whose symptoms can often initially resemble them.

1. Introduction

In the community and inside the healthcare units many common viral respiratory illnesses cause huge financial losses in the form of lost working days only. On individual level, they can also damage the respiratory airways, which potentially leads to more severe consequences. Bacterial infection is often initiated by a viral one, or courses of bacterial and viral illnesses are overlapping. In order to avoid unnecessary spreading of *e.g.,* the flu epidemics, standard hygienic practices have to be maintained in hand hygiene (Appendix II) and in the hospital premises including the air phase.

Preventive and curing measures for the mild viral diseases, or for these diseases combined with some bacteriological components, have been traditionally developed in all cultures. These treatments include various nutritive, herbal and natural antioxidant medications. More profound virological considerations are presented in Chapter 3. Antibiotic treatments are important remedies for more severe bacterial infections, but they can have side-effects and provoke resistance. Therefore, it is important to properly evaluate the need for antibiotic treatments, and to use them in case of a verified need only. For this purpose, new methods and devices are warranted, as presented in Chapters 1, 6, 18 and 19, for instance.

Pneumonia, along with influenza, was the eight leading cause of mortality in the USA in 2005 (National Center for Health Statistics, USA, 2008). These infections are, unfortunately, also subjected to the generation of antibiotic resistant strains (Jones et al., 2010). In any case, proper treatment for pneumonia, or pneumonia as a sequela for influenza, requires antibiotics.

2. Respiratory Diseases Outline

Respiratory infections are the world's most common infections. They are divided into upper and lower respiratory infections. Bronchitis and pneumonia belong to the latter. Numerous respiratory infections also occur in small children. The current understanding is that the majority of lower respiratory infections are mixed infections caused by several various microbes. Basic useful lines of treatment regarding the treatment of upper respiratory infections are postulated in Table 1.

Common diseases or symptoms of the respiratory tract include:

- influenza
- common cold
- nasopharyngeal mucus
- sinusitis
- throat infections
- tonsillitis
- cough
- bronchitis
- pneumonia
- allergic cold
- asthma

Table 1. Lines of treatment for upper respiratory tract infections

The common scientific basic view is: "one airway and one illness".
Upper and lower respiratory infections occur uniformly.
The respiratory tract is attempted to be treated as a whole

3. Nasopharyngeal Mucus and Cilia

Upper respiratory diseases such as prolonged cold and sinusitis, as well as reflux disease in the digestive tract can be the cause for extensive mucus occurring in the nasopharyngeal tract. Reflux disease means the rising of gastric fluid into the esophagus, pharynx and occasionally the respiratory tract. Nasopharyngeal mucus is a fairly little-known syndrome by Finnish doctors. In English it is known as postnasal drip. Instead of this, nowadays the concept of upper airway cough syndrome has been introduced for wider use.

In the respiratory area cilia are acting as means for protection. The task of the cilia is to transport the mucus on cell surfaces and particles stuck to it upwards into the pharynx (Sleigh et al., 1988). Cilia move 12 to 14 times per second in which case mucus moves 100 micrometers per second (6 mm/minute). The liquid envelope capsuling the epithelial cells is indispensable to the efficient activity of cilia.

Infections in the nose and sinus and during nasopharyngeal diseases cause mucus to trickle into the pharynx. This is also stacking the movements of the cilia. The rise of gastric fluid into the esophagus and pharynx may cause nasopharyngeal mucus either alone or together with upper respiratory diseases.

Prolonged cold occurs often simultaneously together with prolonged sinusitis. In this case the term rhinosinusitis, the infection of the nose and sinuses, is used. Maxillary sinusitis is the most common sinusitis. The trickle of mucus into the pharynx occurs in 80 % of patients with prolonged cough. It causes coughing with mechanisms disseminated either directly, by blood flow or by the nervous system. Mechanical stress caused by coughing also damages the cilia.

4. Heartburn Increases Symptoms

It is estimated that every tenth Finn has daily heartburn and/or the rise of bitters into the mouth. With every third asthmatic patient, gastric fluid with hydrochloric acid flows abnormally abundantly backwards, occasionally without reflux symptoms. So-called proton pump inhibitor drugs decrease the symptoms of patients and also nightly asthma symptoms as a sign that there is a reflux disease in the background. Reflux is common in children with occurrence between 34-89% (Sinitchi and Stanchi, 1990). Children's reflux has the tendency of ameliorating by itself when the confluence of the esophagus and stomach begins to develop.

5. Chronic Infections of Upper Airways

A chronic infection in the nasal passage and sinusitis may lead to nasal polyposis.

Approximately half of those who suffer from prolonged cold are allergic persons. Prolonged cold may be roughly categorized into three groups:

- allergic
- infectious, i.e., caused by microbe infections
- the group where there is no evidence of neither allergy nor microbial infection

In the treatment of chronic allergic cold, common allergens are avoided and additionally symptoms are relieved with antihistamine products and nose sprays. If medication does not have an effect the doctor must find out if the main cause for the trickle of mucus symptoms is reflux disease. If the symptoms of cough and mucus trickle into the nasopharyngeal is prolonged, it is recommended to perform an endoscopic examination of the esophagus and if necessary pH measurement of the esophagus.

In the treatment of prolonged cough, prolonged sinusitis and mucus of the nasopharyngeal, all background disease processes should be clarified. Often it is important that an ear, nose and throat specialist adequately examines whether there are nasal polyposis that can be operated or chronic sinusitis that can be remedied with an operation, in the background.

6. Common Cold Is Known to All of Us

Common cold is an acute infection of the upper respiratory tract caused by a virus and it lasts for 5 to 10 days. Good immunity helps in recovering from a common cold caused by a virus normally in about 2 weeks. A common cold is normally not dangerous, one can recover from it by staying out of work for a couple of days and even easier with effective supportive treatment. These infections occur around the year and there is no vaccine against them. The common cold is easily confused with influenza which is a serious epidemic caused by viruses.

Common cold symptoms are a sore throat, cough and feeling cold. The incubation time for a cold is normally 1 to 3 days. A typical initial symptom is a sore throat. The cold and nasal congestion gradually get worse and are at worst within 2 to 4 days. The cough appears normally within 4 to 5 days. It can, however, last for several weeks. Symptoms vary according to the pathogen in question. The common cold normally heals fairly well by itself after lasting an average of 10 days. Every third patient's symptoms may continue up to 3 weeks.

When a doctor examines the oral cavity and pharynx of a patient with common cold, the mucous membranes appear more erythematous and swollen than normally. The cold is a fairly common illness that account for over 20% of acute illnesses and 40% of respiratory infections. Adults have a common cold in average 1 to 6 times and small children 5 to 10 times a year. Infections are pivotal illnesses that burden healthcare services and cause sickness absences.

In Table 2 different mechanisms of the body's defenses against viruses is presented.

Table 2.

The body's defense against viruses
- In large epidemics and pandemics most people survive with mild symptoms.
- The condition of mucous membranes is the decisive factor.
- The function of the immune system is crucial.
- The formation of antibodies in lymph nodes may prevent the virus from spreading.
- Immune response forms in 7 to 14 days.
- The strength of the gained immunity varies.

7. How Does the Common Cold Transmit?

There are more than 200 known cold causing viruses. Rhinoviruses cause about a half of all viral illnesses. During the autumn over 90% of all cases are caused by rhinoviruses. Also enteroviruses often cause common cold. Respiratory infection causing viruses appear mostly during the autumn and winter months. In Table 3 the prevalence of different viruses is described.

Most viruses transmit mainly in close contact. Rhinoviruses transmit mostly through infected secretions via hands. When common cold patients blow or touch their nose, the secretion comes in contact with the hand. From there the viruses may transmit to the next person's hands and further to the nose and even eyes. In the beginning of a common cold, during the first days, rhinoviruses move to the nasopharyngeal. A rhinovirus can also stick to the eye's conjunctival epithelial cells and transmit from there to the nasopharyngeal.

The reproduction of viruses frees infection transmitters which are often the cause of the symptoms of contagion in the common cold.

Table 3.

Common cold viruses
- The most important cause of the flu is rhinovirus (30-50%)
- coronavirus causes 5-30%
- RS-virus about 10%
- adenovirus about 8%

8. Viruses and Bacteria on the Move

A couple of hundred different viruses, including their subtypes, are known. Many viruses are able to genetically transform with time.

Rhinovirus

The rhinovirus, i.e., common cold virus that belongs to the picornaviruses causes nearly half of all illnesses of this type. The disease transmits via the upper respiratory tract to mucous membranes as droplet infection. Sequelae that can follow a prolonged common cold are sinusitis, ear infections and bronchitis. Annually, the rhinovirus causes 30 to 50% of those infections that are called common colds.

RSV Virus

RSV, respiratory syncytial virus causes respiratory infections especially among small children. In care facilities for the elderly extensive RSV epidemics may appear. RSV may cause respiratory infections to people of all ages. Based on only a disease description, an illness caused by RSV cannot be distinguished from other respiratory infections. RSV may also cause bronchitis, and it is a major cause of lower respiratory tract infections, *e.g.,* bronchiolitis. Hospital treatment for this disease includes supplemental oxygen, nasal suctioning, fluids to prevent dehydration, and other supportive therapies (Steiner, 2004).

Adenoviruses

57 types of adenoviruses are known. Some of them cause respiratory infections, some intestinal, eye or other infections. Adenoviruses often cause diseases to children that are nursing and other small children, but are less common among adults.

In 2012 almost 700 confirmed adenovirus infections were noted in Finland. Most of the incidences were in those patients under 5 years of age, but many also with 15 to 24 year olds. It is noteworthy, that most cases of relatively mild viral infections remain undiagnosed.

Mycoplasma Bacteria

Mycoplasma belongs to the significant microbes that cause respiratory infections. This bacteria causes respiratory infections especially to school aged children and young adults but also to people of all ages. Infections caused by mycoplasma may lead to a severe chronic fatigue syndrome (CFS) (Endresen, 2003). At its worse, the fatigue may be so difficult that the patient is not able to walk even a short distance. A severe infection may destroy the quality of life and even shorten life span significantly.

Mycoplasma transmits in respiratory secretions. The incubation time from contagion to the beginning of symptoms is 1 to 14 days. The disease causes respiratory infection symptoms: fever, coughing, nausea and headache. Prolonged irritant coughing may occur for a long time during the healing time. At worst, mycoplasma may cause serious bronchitis or pneumonia. During the mycoplasma epidemic in Finland in 2011, over 7800 cases were verified and in 2012 4600 more. The earlier mycoplasma epidemics is included in a survey (Polkowska et al., 2012).

Based on treatment outcomes of patients we have experienced, that in the recovery from a mycoplasma caused respiratory infection the patient may get significant help with extensive and individual measurement based drug dose level nutrition therapy (Dr. Kaarlo Jaakkola, personal communication).

Viruses are highly contagious pathogens (La Rosa et al., 2013). When a family member falls ill with a respiratory infection, approximately 13-54% of other family members get the infection, too. In most cases, the symptoms begin within a few days from the time the first family member's symptoms began. The more severe the symptoms of common cold are, the more likely it is that other people in close contact fall also ill. Rhinoviruses transmit especially via hands but also as droplet transmission. The contagion is possible also when an object that is "contaminated" with nose secretion is touched soon. The contagion is unlikely if the secretion has already dried. RS virus is believed to transmit above all through direct contact with a secretion, while influenza and adenoviruses transmit efficiently also as droplet transmission. One cough or blow of the nose spreads up to a million aerosol droplets that will remain in the vicinity for quite a long time. Managing hand hygiene is regarded as an important prevention of spreading the common cold.

Rhinoviruses are amply found in secretions during the first days of the illness but the excretion may continue up to two weeks. In adults RS virus can normally be detected during a few days but with nursing children the virus may excrete for several weeks. A patient with the common cold can apparently transmit for a longer time than was previously thought. Some viruses excrete for a child's respiratory tract up to a month from the beginning of symptoms. The beginning phase of an illness is more contagious than later phases but generally speaking the saying that "an old cold doesn't transmit" is not correct when it comes to many viruses.

9. Ciliary Activity Weakens

During a common cold infectious cells gather to the mucous membranes of the respiratory tract and the submucosal space. The body's defense mechanisms, cause severe damage to the mucous membrane and weakens the ciliary activity (Gudis et al., 2012).

In respiratory tract illnesses, natural cleansing mechanisms, i.e., the excretion of mucus and ciliary activity are disturbed. The infection changes the composition and amount of the respiratory tract mucus. Less mucus may form as a consequence of high fever or general dehydration. Inadequate hydration, severe infection, smoking and dry breathing air may increase the stringiness of the mucus. Thus the moving out of the mucus from the respiratory tract becomes more difficult. Impaired mucus activity works as a growth base for microbes thus increasing the infection problems. In the lower respiratory tract the exiting of air and weakened ciliary activity shows as coughing and shortness of breath. In the upper respiratory tract it causes nose stuffiness, cold, coughing and irritation of the larynx and nasopharyngeal. In addition to catarrhs, i.e., coughs and increased mucus caused by respiratory tract inflammation, there is inflammation reaction in the area. Related to common cold is often the sensitization of cough receptors, contraction of the bronchi and heavy mucus excretion which causes coughing.

10. Prolonged Inflammation

Inflammation caused by respiratory infection may be prolonged as a sequel to common cold. It affects especially in long-term chronic diseases such as asthma, chronic bronchitis, chronic obstructive pulmonary disease and bronchiectasis. A long-term inflammation factor causes often local and general pain feelings. The background to this is the weakened cleansing of the airways through air and cilia.

In prolonged upper respiratory inflammations and severe lung inflammation, a so-called biofilm, i.e., polysaccharide structured protective film, may have been developed to protect bacteria. Its forming slows down healing because the biofilm protects bacteria from the effect of antibiotics and the patient's own defense mechanisms. In acute, for example virus based respiratory tract infections and chronic inflammations, a mucus loosening drug, decreases the stringiness of mucus and makes the activity of cilia more effective. Some agents with surfactant activity have also been studied for this purpose (Rosen et al., 2013).

11. Virus Infection Treatments

When to take a child to a doctor?
Example of situations where a child with common cold should be taken to a doctor:

- When the child has pain or starts to wake during the night
- The common cold lasts over two weeks
- Fever lasts over 5 days
- Fever subsides but then rises again.
- The child has high fever and is weary.
- Eyes begin to discharge

An adult should go to a doctor if the illness that started with common cold symptoms includes high fever and a severe exhaustion. If breathing is clearly difficult, it is useful to visit a doctor to ensure that it is not an onset of bacterial pneumonia. If the disease has clearly already been healing and the symptoms reappear within a week or two, it should be ensured that it is not a secondary bacterial disease. If the coughing lasts over three weeks and is disturbing, it is good to visit a doctor.

12. Are Common Cold Treatments Effective?

In the treatment of common cold, physical means such as cooling the environment, a change of clothes or cooling drinks and anti-inflammatory drugs have been used. Coughing has been tried to restrain with water vapor and drugs. Drugs and product combinations for the secretion of mucus have a questionable effect.

Common cold has been tried to medicate by orally administered antihistamine products, drug products that contract local blood vessels and saline drops or sprays. The effect of these is questionable and drug products for contracting local blood vessels weaken ciliary activity.

Vitamin C has been administered as medium strength pharmacological doses (1 to 3 g per day). This is estimated to relieve and shorten symptoms but there is controversy on the effects. Kedar N. Prasad has noted that nutrition therapy with a single micro-nutritional factor, even the famous vitamin C, is not adequate treatment, instead nutrition therapy should be implemented as combination medication of key micro-nutritional factors (Prasad et al., 1999a). In case of standard cancer therapies, high doses of antioxidants including vitamin C do not decrease the efficiency of chemotherapy (Prasad et al., 1999b).

On the surface of the epithelial cells of the respiratory tract, there is a liquid envelope on whose surface is covered with a thin mucus layer. Numerous antioxidants such as vitamins C and E, and enzymes have been found in it. Impurities in breathing air stick to the mucus layers and the antioxidants of the liquid envelope "neutralize" impurities, free radicals and other air pollution.

The task of the cilia is to transport the mucus on cell surfaces and particles stuck to it upwards into the pharynx (Sleigh et al., 1988). Cilia move 12 to 14 times per second in which case mucus moves 100 micrometers per second (6mm/minute). The liquid envelope capsuling the epithelial cells is indispensable to the efficient activity of cilia.

13. Problems of New Treatments

Medicine has tried to develop new treatments for common cold. Locally administered interferon alpha has been tested in the treatment and prevention of rhinovirus infections (Winther et al., 1998). Results demonstrate that large doses may relieve symptoms and shorten the excretion time of viruses. The problem, however, is that interferon easily causes mucous membrane ulcers. The local efficacy of corticosteroid products is not convincing either.

Several antiviral drugs have been developed. Up to now, the results have not been convincing. Drugs suitable for rhinovirus infections are not in clinical use. The purpose of antiviral drugs is to prevent the reproduction of viruses. At the stage when symptoms appear, the reproduction of viruses on mucous membranes is already almost over. As the common cold is a virus disease, antibiotics or other microbe drugs do not expedite healing from it. Only when, and in the case of a few per cent of patients with common cold, a clear bacterial sequel develops (such as sinusitis, otitis media or pneumonia) is antibiotic medication necessary. Passive immunization with therapeutic antibodies could help the body system to eradicate pathogens (Hakalehto and Kuronen, 1998).

14. Supportive Medication Interrupts Recurring Common Cold

A healthy lifestyle enhances the immunity of the body. Fresh air and exercise improve it. Smoking should be avoided. Individuals that exercise regularly have less infections than others. Immunity weakens in dwellings that are too warm and dry. A wide spectrum supportive medication prescribed by a doctor, comprising micronutritional factors and medicament products, has shown to be an effective treatment that relieves the course of the common cold disease. Supportive medication may also prevent the outbreak of ancillary diseases. The medication is prescribed individually based on what measurement data from blood tests tell about the nutrient status of the patient's body. The treatment is prescribed by a doctor specialized in this area.

The most important antioxidants include the necessary micronutrients, i.e., vitamins, trace elements, amino acids and fatty acids. Supportive medication, with which the patient is treated with individually selected micro nutrients, may boost the body's antioxidant and immunity systems so that viruses cannot reproduce without control in the body. If the defense of the cell state is in order, one can cope with an infection with minor symptoms, a short bed rest and sick leave. Self-care with nutritional and medicament products is different than supportive medication prescribed by a doctor. Self-care with various products is common and popular. Certain products can be trialled as self-care for the treatment of common cold. They may relieve symptoms and sooth the feeling.

15. Lactic Acid Bacteria Maintain Immunity

Stomach microbes are the foundation of the defense mechanism. The microbes of an adult's digestive tract regulate the development and action of the immunological defense mechanism. This way they also influence the development of respiratory diseases.

In supportive medication, probiotic products are used to increase the production of lactic acid bacteria that strengthen the body's immunity. Probiotics are living micro-organisms that in adequate quantities and taken orally cause effects that are beneficial for the health (FAO/WHO 2001). Probiotics are important for example in the prevention of infections. They can be combined with so called prebiotics for an anhanced effect (Hakalehto and Jaakkola, 2013).

16. Risks of Antibiotics

Most dramatic changes in the bowel bacteria take place during antibiotic treatments. When the bacteria sensitive to the antibiotic diminish, the bacteria that are resistant to antibiotics gain more space to live. After antibiotic treatment it takes several weeks, even months for the normal bacteria to recover (Reid et al., 2011). The weakening of bacteria compromises health. When antibiotics reduce the normal bacteria of the bowel, a new infection forms easier as much less disease-causing bacteria are needed than in a healthy bowel.

Unusual microbe flora composition has been connected for instance with constipation, diarrhea, formation of gases, infections, liver damage and exposure to cancer and allergies.

In chronic infections bacteria excrete for their safety a biofilm, i.e., a protective cover of mucus, under which the bacteria are many times more resistant than those living freely. For example the dental plaque on the surface of a tooth is a biofilm excreted by differently sized bacteria. Also pneumococcal bacteria (*Streptococcus pneumonia*) forms biofilm to the extent that pneumococcal strains may cause ear infections, pneumonia, blood poisonings and meningitis (Moscoso et al., 2009). Also the background for chronic sinus infections may be the biofilm formation. Repeated ear infections may be caused by this protective film around bacteria. Samples of bacterial strains taken from patients with chronic respiratory diseases may be exceptionally slimy. It is believed that normal microflora prevents the growth of harmful bacteria on intestine surfaces and the penetration of these bacteria through the intestine surface. Without microbial growth, the immune system of a small child will not develop normally. In adulthood the useful intestinal microbial flora is important in maintaining general immunity and in the exploitation of nutrients.

Unusual microflora composition has been associated for instance with constipation, diarrhea, formation of gases, infections, liver damage and exposure to cancer and allergies.

Lactic acid bacteria as cure assisting remedies:

- Prebiotics: enhance the growth of bacteria that produce lactic acid for example in case when breast milk is given to a small baby
- food products into which probiotics have been added
- flax groats as prebiotics
- oat as fiber forming substance

Probiotics: living micro-organisms, often belong to lactic acid bacteria. For example

- lactobacilli
- bifidobacteria

Combination Product That Contains Both Pre- and Probiotics

Grocery stores sell numerous dairy products, berry soups and juices and sour vegetable products (*e.g.,* sauerkraut and sour cucumber) that have been leavened or to which both probiotics and prebiotics have been added. A properly produced commercial foodstuff may improve the viability of useful microbes and their adhesion to the intestines. Food or foodstuff that contain enough prebiotics enhance especially the growth of bacteria that produce lactic acid such as bifidobacteria and lactobacilli. Healthy intestinal or digestive microflora will help the body system to defend itself against respiratory pathogens, too.

The metabolism of intestinal bacteria can fairly efficiently be balanced with food. Leavened products such as sour vegetables contain lactic acid bacteria. It is important that the composition of the diet is such that the body is able to produce enough short-chain fatty acids. For example the good-quality fibers of flax groats and oat enhance the growth of lactic acid bacteria (Hakalehto and Jaakkola, 2013). It is important that food is rich in fiber and contains whole grain products, vegetables, root vegetables, fruit and berries. These guarantee a good growth environment for probiotic bacteria. For a more profound survey about the aspects related to probiotic treatments, see Chapter 17.

17. Undisputed Health Impacts

The health impacts of probiotic lactic acid bacteria are undisputed provided that they are

- of human origin
- harmless
- can spread into the intestines in adequate quantities
- can attach to the epithelial cells of the intestines

Probiotics are living micro-organisms that in adequate amounts orally taken cause effects that are beneficial for the health (FAO/WHO 2001). Probiotics are of great significance for example in the prevention of infections. See also Chapter 17.

Probiotics have been used as medication already for several decades. The probiotic bacteria that are used for medication are mainly lactobacilli and bifidobacteria; these are called probiotic lactic acid bacteria. Probiotic products are classified as foodstuff.

The useful effects of probiotic lactic acid bacteria may be based on the functions created by living bacteria. They can remove harmful microbes from the mucous membranes of the intestines and protect the mucous membranes from harmful microbes. From the viewpoint of this ability to occupy, the ability of the probiotic to attach to the mucous membrane of the intestine is important. It can weaken the disease causing ability of many harmful intestinal bacteria.

Certain probiotics progress through the human digestive tract alive. They attach to the digestive tract temporarily when the bacteria is taken orally for several days and the doses are large enough, i.e., at least 100 million bacteria per day. After ending the use of the product, the appearance of many probiotics in the stool ends in about a week. Adequate medicinal probiotic doses may repair the long-term side effects of antibiotic treatments. The use of probiotics pursues to strengthen the immune response by affecting the immune system functioning on the intestinal mucous membrane. Antibiotic medication decreases the amount of normal bacteria in the intestines thus weakening immunity. Repeated antibiotic treatments can clearly increase the infection sensitivity of the patient.

Nowadays the subject of research is the affects of probiotics to allergies and chronic inflammatory intestinal diseases as well as respiratory tract infections (Popova et al., 2012).

18. Experiences in the Use of Strong Probiotics

The strongest dose of medically used products is a probiotic sachet that contains 30 billion probiotic bacteria. The bacteria of this probiotic sachet are separately microcapsuled, i.e., the bacteria are covered with a protective casing. The purpose of large quantities of probiotics is to quickly occupy the top layers of the intestinal mucous membranes as habitat. Most likely they ae able to remove harmful bacteria and yeasts from mucous membrane surfaces and they also promote the removal of harmful bacteria from the intestines together with the stool. This "counterrevolution" succeeds the better, the larger the probiotic dose is in the beginning of the medication. The ability to attach efficiently onto the surface of the mucous membranes of the colon refers to an extra protective layer that probiotic bacteria form which can prevent the harmful substances of the bowel contents from penetrating through the bowel wall into blood circulation and that way to different parts of the body. This "cobblestone-like" protective layer formed by probiotic bacteria is thought to prevent the onset of leaky gut syndrome.

19. Which Type of Product?

- high enough original concentration
- safe (neutral strains)
- remains active for a long time before use(in the bowels (pH, gall bladder)
- high enough bowel concentrations are achieved
- probiotic's own protection (microcapsulation)
- better therapeutic effect
- results are more regular
- results are achieved faster

The probiotic dose can normally be decreased within a couple of days and continue the medication with a probiotic capsule that contains 20 000 million *Lactobacillus acidophilus* and 4000 million *Bifidobacterium bifidum* bacteria, for example. Together a capsule contains approximately 30 000 million microcapsuled bacteria.

Later the dose can be further decreased to a probiotic product (10 000 million cells) every other or every third day, if the disease is chronic or easily renewable. Based on experience in patient care, there is a common understanding, that in order to achieve good treatment results the probiotic product must contain adequately large amounts of microcapsuled lactic acid bacteria. Without side effects, lactic acid bacteria have been prescribed to the elderly, small children and pregnant women. Even so, undesirable effects may occur also when using probiotic products. Some lactobacilli may cause infection if the patient has a disease or medication that greatly weakens immunity. Instead, bifidobacteria are safe. Some outlines for probiotic therapies are presented in Chapter 17.

20. Sinusitis

Sinusitis means the infection of the sinuses, specifically an infection of the mucous membrane that covers the walls of them. Usually there is a bacterial inflammation of the sinuses, but also allergic mucous membrane damage on the epithelia predisposed to microbe infections. Infections lasting less than 2 weeks are acute while infections lasting at least for 2-3 weeks are considered as either subacute or chronic. Chronic infections may worsen other respiratory tract illnesses such as asthma. Mucous membrane infections are often associated with virus infections. Sinusitis is a typical consequential disease of common cold. Approximately 0.5-5% of common cold patients also get sinusitis. Approximately 5-10% of sinusitis cases are developed as a consequence of an infection with dental origin. Other predisposing factors are allergic rhinitis, a large amount of amalgam fillings, the inclination of the nasal septum and nasopharyngeal aperture stenosis.

Of bacteria, pneumococci, *Haemophilus influenzae* and *Branhamella* sp. are the most important sinusitis causing bacteria (Anon, 2010). Other causative bacteria are *e.g.,* group A beta-haemolytic streptococci and *Staphylococcus aureus.*

The mucous membranes of sinuses have an efficient ciliary action that cleans them normally. An acute virus infection causes edema and damage to the mucous membranes. In this case the ciliary action weakens. The opening between the nasal cavity and paranasal sinuses may be blocked. As a consequence the partial oxygen pressure of the sinuses is often reduced which further weakens the ciliary action.

Pus forms into sinuses when bacteria remain in the sinuses and start an infective reaction. Large amounts of white blood cells that participate in the formation of pus gather into the cavity secretion from which infection mediators and enzymes that break down proteins are released. They damage the deeper layers of the mucous membrane. Sinus secretion normally contains large amounts of bacteria.

Symptoms and Diagnosis of the Sinusitis

Sinusitis symptoms are nose stuffiness, cold in the head and cough. These are found in 80-90% of sinusitis patients. Coughing occurs at all times of the day but becomes more severe during the night time. Fever may be periodic or continuous and is found in about half of the patients. Almost half of child patients have headache. Local pain and ache occurs in the facial area and half of the patients have sensation of heaviness in the cheekbones, periorbital edema and bad breath. A sure diagnostic indication of sinusitis is the suppurative secretion obtained in a puncture. However, punctures are less frequent so one must often rely on medical history, clinical examination, echo examination and x-rays. When the patient has a sudden fever, runny nose and sensation of heaviness and ache in the cheekbones, the diagnosis is rather clear and other examinations are not necessary.

To the doctor the distinction between sinusitis and virus infection may be a diagnostic problem. Cold in the head and a cough that occurs especially during the night and morning, periodical fever that lasts over 2 weeks and cankerous secretion in the nose and pharynx indicate sinusitis. A sign of frontal sinusitis is mostly pain in the forehead and head.

Prolonged Cold and Sinusitis

Prolonged cold and sinusitis infection cause typical mucus to trickle into the nasopharyngeal tract. Prolonged cold can be roughly divided into three groups:

1. allergic
2. infectious, caused by an infection
3. non-allergic and non-infectious

Some aspects of sinusitis:

- Chronic infection in the nasal passage and sinus cause nasal polyposis
- Approximately half of those suffering from prolonged cold are allergics

- Prolonged cold occurs simultaneously with prolonged sinusitis
- In this case a better name is rhinosinusitis. About half of rhinosinusitis patients have asthma.

Traditional Treatments of Sinusitis

Many infections heal spontaneously and antibiotic medication should not easily be started. The general medical opinion is that antimicrobial medication of acute sinusitis speeds up healing and decreases complications (Mandal et al., 2012). Therefore a 7 to 10 day antibiotic medication is recommended.

When a patient has recurring sinusitises it is important to examine the predisposing factors. Normally the nasal passage and tonsil of children are x-rayed. An ear specialist examines the nasal passage and sinuses to clarify if the patient has polypes or inclination of the nasal septum.

A sinusitis that continues for 2 to 3 months is considered chronic. The mucous membrane of the sinus cilia has been replaced by squamous which is the consequence of a long term bacterial infection. In some patients constant pus is noted but often the case is mainly a chronic mucous membrane infection and edema. Especially allergy patients can have their condition developed into chronic sinusitis. Symptoms of chronic sinusitis are continued cold and stuffiness, hoarseness, headache and local sensations. In the treatment of a chronic infection, operations by ear specialists are often needed.

21. Influenza

An influenza that spreads as an epidemic is totally different than a regular common cold, even though both of them are viral diseases.

Protection against influenza has been tried to bolster with vaccines but the best safeguard is a good basic immunity. The thousands of viruses that cause influenza change quickly. Influenza spreads during coughing, sneezing and talking as a droplet infection. In the target cell the virus attaches to certain surface proteins that are called receptors. The receptors contain cyanic acid to which the virus attaches. Normally the influenza virus attaches to the cells on the surface of the respiratory tract.

Michael Osterholm, a public health expert at the University of Minnesota expressed his worries regarding the global influenza threat according to “Foreign Affairs” (Nov./Dec. 2013 number) by saying: “ Many other agents worked on within BSL-4 (“Biosafety level”) labs do not have that transmissibility what we see with influenza. I cannot think of any that have the potential to be transmitted around the world as with influenza.” (Garrett, 2013). It is also worth mentioning here that in case of vital pandemics, often the accompanying bacterial diseases, such as pneumococcal infections during the “Spanish disease” almost 100 years ago, cause the biggest death tolls. Therefore, the alertness for respiratory infections have to take into account both viral and bacterial components of the epidemics.

Is Vaccination Necessary?

Influenza vaccination is not necessary but it is recommended to those belonging to certain risk groups to prevent influenza. The Finnish vaccination program covers *e.g.,* those over 65 years of age, children between 6 and 35 months of age, who are starting their military service, who are pregnant, who because of chronic heart or lung disease or diabetes are in regular medical care, who have hepatic impairment, who have weak immunity or a disease or medication that weakens immunity or immune deficiency or corticosteroid therapy. Also those who are close to those exposed to influenza, such as under 6 month old babies, those who are pregnant, elderly and chronically ill, belong to the risk group. Risk groups receive free vaccination at health centers. Healthy working people may acquire influenza vaccination from a pharmacy by mid-September. Because of the transformation of viruses, the composition of the vaccination is checked every year. The vaccine contains two different A viruses and one B virus. The protective efficacy ranges from 70 to 90 per cent in those of working age and normally the vaccine at least relieves the disease symptoms.

Influenza Viruses Change Continuously

Influenza viruses travel the world like migrating birds. Every winter the infections caused by them knock down people to the sick bed.

Occasionally in the winter the epidemics are so bad that they can cause death to those in poor conditions. The danger of epidemic influenzas vary. The Spanish fever in 1918 caused the death of over 20 million people, including about 10,000 Finns. Nowadays the epidemics are usually more tame ones but they last longer than before. Annually, about 1,000 Finns loose their lives because of influenza and its sequela.

Influenza viruses are divided into three types: A, B and C. They are distantly related to each other.

Influenza viruses have the ability to transform their surface structures. If the change is minimal, the virus infection seldom kills. If the change is big, an epidemic that kills tens of millions of people with the efficacy of a world war, may be born. Influenza viruses transmit very easily from person to person as a droplet infection. They travel from one side of the earth to another by human contacts.

An influenza virus in itself is easy to destroy as it dies already in a temperature under 100 °C. Because viruses change all the time, immunity from an earlier influenza illness does not always protect from a new infection. Therefore vaccines need to be changed.

Influenza A and B

In 2012 5,960 influenza A findings were reported to the infectious disease register in Finland. By August of 2013 there were 5,653 influenza A findings before the autumn epidemic season. In August 2013 1,609 influenza B findings were reported which is more than during 2012 with 462 cases. During the peak year, there were 3,444 influenza B virus infections. Influenza epidemics cause death especially among the elderly and those in the risk groups.

Typical influenza symptoms are sudden, often high fever, muscle aches and severe upper respiratory tract symptoms. Influenza viruses typically secrete 5 to 7 days. The illness lasts normally 6 to 8 days.

A death caused by influenza virus may be a result of a bacterial sequel such as pneumonia. Also, numerous cases of myocarditis and neural symptoms also occur as sequel. Special risk factors are serious basic illnesses such as heart and kidney malfunctions, chronic lung diseases, severe diabetes.

22. Parainfluenza

The parainfluenza virus transmits typically as a droplet and contact infection. Parainfluenza is found in all age groups. The largest number of infections occur normally in April and May.

The disease causes sensation of heaviness in the chest, high fever and other flu symptoms. In 2012 401 parainfluenza infections were confirmed in Finland. The majority of these were in the 0 to 4 years age group. Parainfluenza viruses normally secrete 3 to 10 days.

23. Lower Respiratory Tract Infections

Acute Bronchitis

Lower respiratory tract infections include bronchitis and pneumonia. In small children also infection of the small bronchi, i.e., bronchiolitis occur. According to current understanding the majority of lower respiratory tract infections are mixed infections caused by many microbes.

In acute bronchitis the infection is normally caused by a virus such as influenza A and B, RSV, parainfluenza, adenovirus or rhinovirus. The key infection causing bacteria are *Mycoplasma pneumoniae*, *Chlamydia pneumoniae*, *Streptococcus pneumoniae* and *Haemophilus influenzae*.

Acute bronchitis is a fairly common disease. An average of 10 cases per 100 persons are noted per year. The occurrence is even greater in children than among adults.

Severe Coughing Spells

Smoking, pollution, immune deficiencies, allergies and other lung diseases expose to bronchitis. The disease typically begins with upper respiratory tract symptoms such as sore throat and a cold. When the disease moves to the lower respiratory tract, symptoms are coughing and mucus secretion from the bronchus. Occasionally there is blood in the sputum. Symptoms are fever, muscle pains and other general symptoms. In the case of whooping cough, the disease begins slowly. In this case the patient has respiratory tract symptoms such as a sore throat and a cold, hacking cough and mild fever. The whooping means the wheezing sound when inhaling. Coughing spells may be severe. The cough may last for months.

The diagnosis of an acute bronchitis is clinical examination. Lung x-ray findings are generally normal. In laboratory testing the value of C-reactive protein (CRP) may rise over 100 mg/l. If the value is well over 100 mg/l a heart and lung x-ray is taken to exclude a bacterial infection.

Treatment According to Symptoms

Treatment is according to symptoms. The significance of general cough medicines is controversial. If the coughing disturbs the patients sleep medication that relieve irritant coughing should be used. If the disease is prolonged then antibiotics are needed.

One example of a herbal medicine for respiratory tract problems is Carolus Mixtura™ by Biomed Oy, Helsinki, Finland. It contains 8 different herbs: sundew, salvia, thyme, anis, peppermint, lavendel, clove and carmellose. This mixture is kept in mouth for about two minutes, which spreads the calming effects onto the epithelia by diffusion. This is not a traditional kind of cough medicine, but extends the treatment into the entire upper respiratory tract.

If an efficient medicament combination product is used when the symptoms start it is possible that the course of the disease is interrupted and a severe bronchitis does not develop. This can possibly prevent longer than normal sick leaves and antibiotic medication. If antibiotic medication is needed macrolides, tetracycline derivatives and penicillin or its derivatives can often be recommended.

A Liquid Jacket Protects the Respiratory Tract

The deficiencies of the individual micronutritional factors of cell nutrition have a significant effect to the severity and recovery of diseases. The ability of the body to protect the epithelium and ability to repair damage that has already occurred is directly dependent on whether a person gets enough micronutrients that are necessary for the body (Roscioli et al., 2013).

The epithelial cells on the surface of the respiratory tract have a biochemical protective system and also the ability to repair damage formed to the epithelium. One central defense mechanism is the liquid jacket that covers the epithelial cells and which is about 10 micrometers thick. Any substitutions, such as the passive immunization with IgY antibodies can rapidly move on this jacket to all parts of the respiratory system (Hakalehto and Kuronen, 1998).

Numerous antioxidants and proteins that have an antioxidative effect as well as vitamins E and C have been found in the liquid layer covering the epithelium. The epithelial cells and the antioxidants in the liquid layer that cover the cells have a central task in defending body against oxidative stress. The majority of foreign matter that increase oxidative stress spread into the body through the respiratory tract.

Many irritants increase the secretion of mucus. External irritants include cigarette smoke and sulfur oxide. Moreover, individual internal causes can increase mucus secretion. Inflammation reactions are associated with many respiratory tract diseases.

The most significant threats to the cells of the respiratory tract are the toxic byproducts of oxygen metabolism, the so-called free radicals: the oxidizing components of cigarette smoke, pollution and the free radicals production of inflammatory cells that increase with inflammation. Free radicals are born intracellularly *e.g.,* as a byproduct of cell respiration and as the function of intracellular enzymes.

Respiratory Cilia Need Antioxidants

Especially in the large areas of the respiratory tract such as trachea there are cells with cilia. The movement of the cilia requires energy. Particles that have attached to the liquid and mucus on the surface of epithelial cells move upward in the respiratory tract.

The liquid jacket that covers the epithelial cells is necessary for the efficient function of the cilia. The function of the cilia is the transport the liquid and mucus on the cell surface and particles that have attached to it. The cilia move 12 to 14 times per second which makes the mucus to move about 100 micrometers per second.

The cilia movement happens in the liquid layer beneath the mucus layer. At the same time the mucus that covers the liquid helps the movement of foreign particles that have stuck to it. The ciliary action will be paralyzed with too little liquid or too much mucus secretion and accumulate a lot of mucus can consequently accumulate into the respiratory tract. This happens *e.g.,* in chronic bronchitis.

An adequate intake of antioxidants is the prerequisite to efficient ciliary action. Of hereditary structural and functional defects *e.g.,* the rare immotile cilia disease is known. A child patient who had been diagnosed with this disease was healed with antioxidants. When personalized antioxidant medication was prescribed for the child the respiratory tract symptoms ended. In traditional medicine it has long been thought that hereditary diseases cannot effectively be influenced with any treatment. Antioxidants thus have a potential to repair weakened ciliary action whether it is caused by hereditary or acquired reasons or both.

During any acute mucosal inflammation more than normal amounts of acidic mucopolysaccharides and different harmful compounds produced by the inflammation reaction, i.e., protein-carbohydrate compounds are being freed. The secretions of the irritant mucous membrane cells, i.e., epithelium, are often very stringy which in turn prevents the ciliary action in the bronchus. In this case the cilia cannot transport the secretions upwards towards the throat efficiently enough.

The stringiness of secretions can be reduced with plant medicaments. Some medicaments form a protective additional layer on the mucous membranes so that they do not prevent the mucus from exiting. Evaporating oils in phytotherapeutic cough medicines often increase salivation. Increase swallowing relieves coughing and the dryness of the mucous membrane of the mouth. Evaporating oils in small doses accelerate the function of epithelial cells and alveoles while large doses may prevent it.

24. Lung Tissue and Its Microflora

Lung tissue consists mainly of alveoli (Fig. 1) that are filled with breathed air. There are 300 million of them. Their combined surface area compares to a large apartment. An alveoli is a small bag. It is in connection with the bronchus through which outside air can reach the alveolar bag whose diameter is about a tenth of a millimeter. During inhalation the size of the lungs doubles.

The wall of the alveolar is very thin. Surrounding it there is a dense network of capillaries. Breathing air gets to less than a thousandth of a millimeter from the capillary blood which is poor in oxygen and has carbon dioxide and which the heart's right ventricle pumps from the veins. The blood and air meet at the wall of the alveolar for the exchange of gases.

The walls of both the alveoli and the capillaries consist of specialized flat surface cells, i.e., epithelial cells. Between them is only a thin membrane. The anatomical structures enable fast exchange of gases. The partial pressure of the oxygen in the blood that comes into the alveolar is more than twice that of the blood in the vein. Thus oxygen transfers efficiently to the blood.

In the opposite direction the difference in pressure of the carbon dioxide is registered in the alveoli and in the junction of external and internal carotid artery. These react sensitively to the increase of carbon dioxide in the blood in the veins and send information of it via nerves to the medulla oblongata. From the adjustment center there, information via other nerves are sent to the breathing muscles. The chest expands and we inhale air into our lungs. These actions are delicately adjusted so that a special reflex in the breathing center stops the inhaling.

Carbon dioxide is a central and important regulator of breathing, more important than oxygen. The lungs have approximately an area of 100 m^2 for the exchange of gases. The water that the alveoli contain, approximately 1 deciliter, when spread to such a large area, forms a water film that is barely the thickness of a red blood cell. This film changes every second.

During normal breathing the lungs pump air about 12 to 14 times per minute. The air that is poor in oxygen but contains a lot of carbon dioxide exits and new air replaces it. During physical exercise this ventilation multiplies. The lungs are an airtight bag that expands and collapses. Expanding lungs suck air inside and collapsing lungs push it out. The chest is the structure for the pleura. A very important organ in breathing is the diaphragm, a "muscle plate" between the abdominal cavity and chest.

The capacity of adult healthy lungs is about 4 liters of air at one time (during inhalation). This amount is only needed during heavy exercise. During rest, the suction of about half a liter of air into the lungs is enough. During the course of a day about 10,000 liters, i.e., 10 m^3 of air passes through the lungs of an adult. The sensitive cell layer that covers the inside of the bronchus does not tolerate impurities. For example when food is swallowed, it passes over the opening of the respiratory tubing to the esophagus behind it. During this it is possible that the food or drink moving in the pharynx gets into the respiratory tract. To prevent this epiglottis closes tightly when swallowing. At the same time the vestibular valves nestle tightly against each other. Thus extra substances only occasionally get into the trachea.

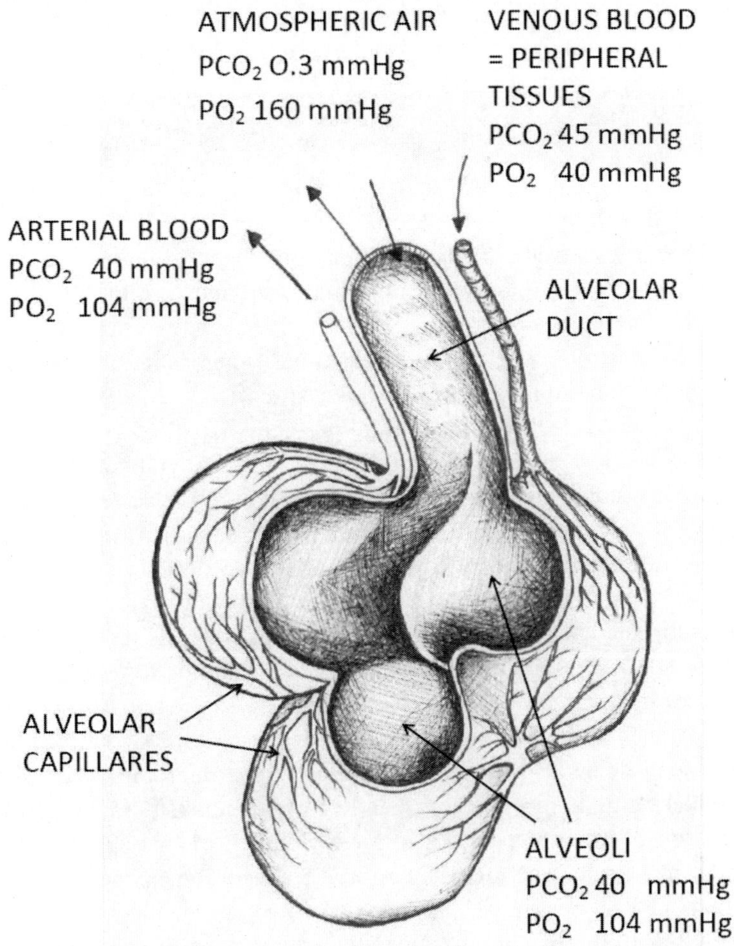

Figure 1. Partial pressures of O_2 and CO_2 during the human respiratory function and gas exchange. Especially, the CO_2 concentration is regulating many body functions, such as blood acidity. In the hemic molecular structure, some traces of CO_3^{2-} are demanded for maintaining correct protein conformation for oxygen binding. This is a sensitive mechanism behind the essential respiratory functions, and any microbial disturbance of it could cause systematic effects on well-being.

If, however, food does get to slip into the trachea, in a blink a reflex that mobilizes the entire body in order to remove the trash, starts. The immediate reflex closes the vestibular valves and epiglottis and strain the respiratory muscles used in out-breathing to the extreme. Thus the reflex suddenly opens a way for air to get out as a coughing spell that blows at the speed of stormy wind, with the help of the coughing reflex removes the extra objects from the respiratory tract.

The partial pressures of various gases inside the lungs are differing from the atmospheric pressures (Silverthorn, 2014). The partial pressure of oxygen is about 30-40 percent less and the partial pressure of carbon dioxide is around one hundred sixty times more in the alveoles than in the atmosphere (Fig. 1). In the human body only seven percent of the carbon dioxide remains dissolved in plasma, whereas the rest is inside the cells. There it mostly exists as bicarbonates (70 %). These bicarbonates neutralize the metabolic acids inside the cells. It can well be asked if the same function is fulfilled in the bacterial and other microbial cells. In human body system hemoglobin is buffering the hydrogen ions which prevent large changes in the pH inside the body system. If carbon dioxide levels rice up high enough it will cause a phenomenon called respiratory acidosis where excess hydrogen ions accumulate in the plasma.

In microbial world, many bacterial cells secrete acids as the final products of their metabolic actions. This serves as a method for maintaining balance inside their cells. Moreover, many bacterial species are able to liberate hydrogen in the molecular form. In the intestinal milieu, the gaseous substances, mainly hydrogen and carbon dioxide, produced by the intestinal bacteria will affect the redox potential of the body system. Carbon dioxide is coming out from the digestion along the intestinal canal, whereas hydrogen can be supposed to penetrate into the body and to be partially liberated trough the human tissues.

All bacterial strains have their optimal partial pressures for the essential gases. These are subjected to some variation according to the other conditions around the cells. In all circumstances, it is of crucial importance for the bacterial cell to maintain the intracellular conditions suitable for the metabolic actions. Therefore, the bacteria often carry out metabolic functions which are designated as overflow metabolism. (Neijssel and Tempest, 1973). In practice this means, that the bacterial cells are not multiplying, but the stored metabolic energies from the substrate are converted into such a form which is more beneficial for their survival. This is a somewhat neglected subject in microbiological studies, but it is the mechanism which guarantees various bacterial strains the option to survive in drastically changing conditions, such as in the respiratory or the digestive tract. We must keep in mind that all reactions take place swiftly in these conditions. These microbiological phenomena are more deeply introduced e.g., in the Chapters 2 and 14 of this book.

It's beneficial for all microbial strains to have as much metabolic capacity as possible available for quick metabolic reactions. Therefore, co-operation between various strains is most abundant. It is also a prerequisite for survival for different members of the microbial communities. In these conditions various substrates are overwhelmingly arriving into the gut where they have to be digested and used quickly in order to maintain the activity of digestive system and its microflora. This is important both for man and his microbiota. If these molecular mechanisms are disturbed, this could cause several consequences and pathological developments. For example, in the case of carbon dioxide production from the lactic acid bacteria it has been documented that gas information is activating other components of the microflora (Hakalehto and Hänninen, 2012). The continuous gas flow is also keeping enough surface area between liquid and gas phases inside the chyme suspension.

In the respiratory tract, less nutrients are available than in the gut. However, similar laws of gas exchange are prevailing. It is descriptive of the microbial world that a common bacterial species, *Klebsiella pneumonia*, is often considered as a pathogen in the lungs, but a harmless, or beneficial member of the normal flora in the intestines (Hakalehto, 2013). In the lungs any obstructions can cause adverse effects on the gas flows and on their exchange. This, in turn, is provoking inflammation and gives more several infections room for conquering the space in the lungs. Mycobacterial infections, such as tuberculosis, are a good example on this kind of pathogenic development inside the lungs, where the airways are getting narrowed till the alveoles in the "tip" of the gas leading tubular system (Fig. 2.). More information on slowly developing pulmonary infections by *Legionella* sp. (Chapter 7) and *Mycobacterium tuberculosis* (Chapter 9) are presented elsewhere in this book. The slow growth of these pathogens could be related to the low amounts of quickly utilizable nutrients in the respiratory tract, in comparison with the alimentary system.

Similar phenomena that are occurring in the digestive tract can also take place in the lungs. However, the amount of microbes is not as high as it is in the intestines. The conditions are rapidly fluctuating (gas volumes and the partial pressures of the gases) which has to be coped with by the micro-organisms that are functioning in the pulmonary tract. They have to possess means for maintaining their intracellular pH. , If the airwaves are obstructed the pressure is growing which is easily causing disformation inside the lungs. This could be the one of the root causes for the development of respiratory infections.

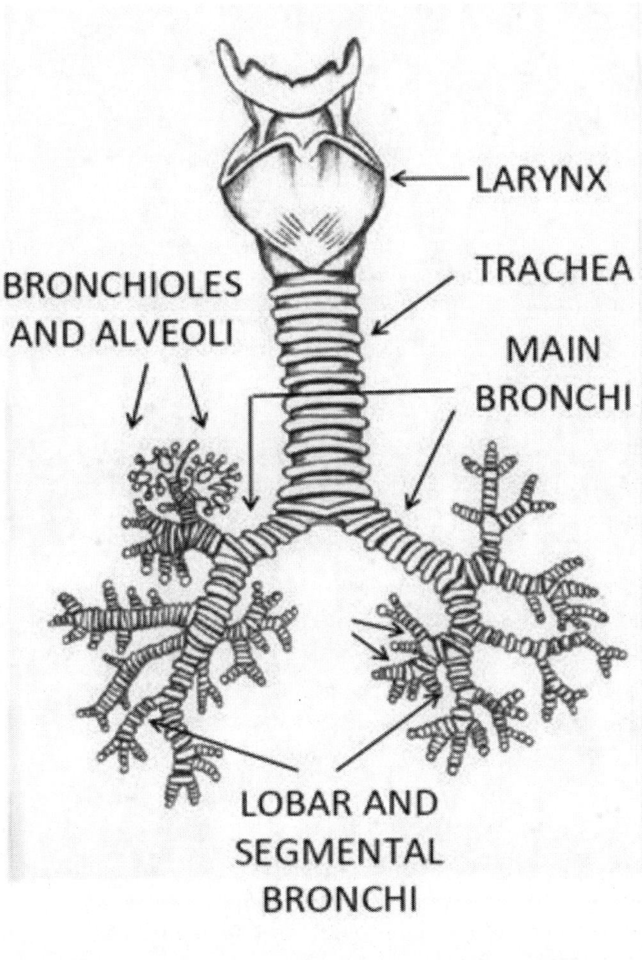

Figure 2. All pulmonary airways get thinner towards the alveoli. It is of crucial importance to prevent obstruction caused by infections and inflammations. Such mechanisms include mucin formation, antibiotics and defensins, ciliary movements as well as biosurfactant layer on the alveolar surfaces. The last one is forming in fetal lungs at the age of about 8 months for supporting the thin alveolar walls against the pressures and for reducing the surface tension right after the birth when the amniotic fluid should be removed from the airways. Any infection or inflammation causes additional pressure against the lung confinements. The bacterial volatile organic compounds and gas emissions strain the pulmonary tubings.

Conclusion

Any inflammation in the respiratory tract, and especially in the lungs, could lead to narrowing of the air space. This, in turn, can provoke inflammation and infections. Many natural and antioxidant therapies could be healing this root cause of many lung problems. Microbes can cause worsening of the situation if they increase the pressure, and cause inflammation. Viruses destroy the ciliary structure, which makes room for more serious bacterial infections. As usual, the remedies consist of many factors influencing toward the positive direction. Good general health, with strong immunodefences, combined with adequate supply of trace elements and antioxidants, supports the host body against intruders coming in via the airways.

References

Anon, J. B. Upper respiratory infections. *Am. J. Med.*, 2010; 123 (4 Suppl), S16-25.

Endresen, G. K. Mycoplasma blood infection in chronic fatigue and fibromyalgia syndromes. *Rheumatol. Int.*, 2003; 23, 211-215.

Garrett, L. Biology's brave new world. *Foreign Affairs*, 2013; 92, 28-46.

Gudis, D., Zhao, K. Q., Cohen, N. A. Acquired cilia dysfunction in chronic rhinosinusitis. Am. J. Rhinol. Allergy, 2012; 26, 1-6.

Hakalehto, E. Interactions of *Klebsiella* sp. with other intestinal flora. In: Pereira, L. A., Santos, A., editors. *Klebsiella infections: epidemiology, pathogenesis and clinical outcomes*. New York, USA: Nova Science Publishers, Inc.; 2013; pp. 1-33.

Hakalehto, E., Hänninen, O. (2012). Gaseous CO_2 signal initiate growth of butyric acid producing *Clostridium butyricum* both in pure culture and in mixed cultures with *Lactobacillus brevis*. *Can. J. Microbiol.,* 2012; 58, 928-931.

Hakalehto, E., Jaakkola, K. Synergistic effect of probiotics and prebiotic flax product on intestinal bacterial balance. *Clinical Nutrition,* 2013; 32, Suppl. 1, S200.

Hakalehto, E., Kuronen, I. A method for producing jelly sweets, which contain antibodies. WIPO Patent Application WO/1998/043610; 1998.

Jones, R. N., Jacobs, M. R., Sader, H. S. Evolving trends in *Streptococcus pneumonia* resistance: implications for therapy of community-acquired bacterial pneumonia. *Int. J. Antimicrob. Agents*, 2010; 36, 197-204.

La Rosa, G., Fratini, M., Della Libera, S., Iaconelli, M., Muscillo, M. HYPERLINK "http://www.ncbi.nlm.nih.gov.ezproxy.uef.fi:2048/pubmed/23771256" Viral infections acquired indoors through airborne, droplet or contact transmission. *Ann. Ist. Super. Sanita,*. 2013; 49, 124-132.

Mandal, R., Patel, N., Ferguson, B. J. Role of antibiotics in sinusitis. *Curr. Opin. Infect. Dis.*, 2012; 25, 183-192.

Moscoso, M., García, E., López, R. Pneumococcal biofilms. *Int. Microbiol.*, 2009; 12, 77-85.

National Center for Health Statistics, USA, with special feature on health of young adults; 2008.

Neijssel, E. W., Tempest, D. W. The role of energy-spilling reactions in the growth of *Klebsiella aerogenes* NCTC 418 in aerobic chemostat culture. *Arch. Microbiol.*, 1973; 110, 305-311.

Polkowska, A., Harjunpää, A., Toikkanen, S., Lappalainen M., Vuento, R., Vuorinen, T., Kauppinen, J., Flinck, H., Lyytikäinen, O. Increased incidence of *Mycoplasma pneumoniae* infection in Finland, 2010-2011. *Euro Surveill.*, 2012; 17. pii: 20072..

Popova, M., Molimard, P., Courau, S., Crociani, J., Dufour, C., Le Vacon, F., Carton, T. Beneficial effects of probiotics in upper respiratory tract infections and their mechanical actions to antagonize pathogens. *J. Appl. Microbiol.*, 2012; 113, 1305-1318.

Prasad, K. N., Cole, W.C., Prasad, J. E. Multiple antioxidant vitamins as an adjunct to standard and experimental cancer therapies. *Z. Onkol. / J. Oncol.*, 1999a; 31.

Prasad, K. N., Kumar, A., Kochupillai, V., Cole, W. C. High doses of multiple antioxidant vitamins: Essential ingredients in improving the efficacy of standard cancer therapy. *J. Am. Coll. Nutr.*, 1999b; 18, 13-25.

Reid, G., Younes, J. A., Van der Mei, H. C., Gloor, G. B., Knight, R., Busscher, H. J. Microbiota restoration: natural and supplemented recovery of human microbial communities. *Nat. Rev. Microbiol.,* 2011; 9: 27-38.

Roscioli, E., Hamon, R., Lester, S., Murgia, C., Grant, J., Zalewski, P. Zinc-rich inhibitor of apoptosis proteins (IAPs) as regulatory factors in the epithelium of normal and inflamed airways. *Biometals*, 2013; 26, 205-227.

Rosen, P. L., Palmer, J. N., O'Malley, B. W. Jr., Cohen, N. A. Surfactants in the management of rhinopathologies. *Am. J. Rhinol. Allergy*, 2013; 27, 177-180.

Silverthorn; DU. *Human Physiology*. United Kingdom: Pearson and Harlow; 2014.

Sinitchi, G; Stanchi, C. The bronchial asthma-gastroesophaged reflux association. *Rev. Med. Chir. Soc. Med. Nat. Iasi*, 1990 94, 75-78.

Sleigh, MA; Blake, JR; Liron, N. The propulsion of mucus by cilia. *Am. Rev. Respir. Dis.*, 1988 137, 726-741.

Steiner, RWP. Treating acute bronchiolitis associated with RSV. *Am. Fam. Physician*, 2004 69, 325-330.

Winther, B., Gwaltney, J. M. Jr., Mygind, N., Hendley, J. O. Viral-induced rhinitis. *Am. J. Rhinol.,* 1998; 12, 17-20.

In: Microbiological Clinical Hygiene
Editor: Eino Elias Hakalehto
ISBN: 978-1-63463-428-1

Chapter 5

Planning and Construction of Healthcare Facilities – A Case Evaluation on Hygienic Aspects

***Elias Hakalehto*[1]*, Markus Hell*[2] *and Anneli Heitto*[3]**
[1]Department of Environmental Sciences,
University of Eastern Finland, Kuopio, Finland
[2]Zentrum für Krankenhaushygiene und Infektionskontrolle
der SALK, Universitätsklinikum Salzburg, Salzburg, Austria
[3]Anneli Heitto, Finnoflag Oy, Kuopio, Finland

Abstract

Microbiological conditions in the care facilities have a remarkable contribution to the recovery of the patients and the well-being of the personnel. During the years of intensive use the hospitals and clinics are subjected to remarkable microbial loads. Also the building materials can contain rooted contaminations in the worst case, or offer platform for microbial growth. The alterations in the hygienic situation should be continuously monitored and risks avoided by careful planning of both the construction or renovation work and the daily work in the departments. Moisture damages should be prevented, or if already happened, they should be contained and repaired. This is highly important, since many toxic or contagious microbes may hide in the structures. Many molds and bacteria also disseminate toxins, or are toxigenic themselves, which could compromise the hygienic quality of the air in the care unit. In this case report an investigation on a "diseased building" is introduced as a "warning example".

1. Introduction

Risk assessment regarding the microbiological parameters during the construction period is an essential phase for the proper functioning of a modern hospital.

Inside the ready-made premises several factors might influence transmission of infection, some of which are listed below (modified from Ransjö and Popp, 2011):

- Numbers of patient and staff
- Numbers and types of procedures and examinations
- Available space, also airspace
- Numbers and types of rooms
- Number of beds in a room
- Floors and surfaces, material choices
- Water, electricity, and sanitation
- Ventilation and air quality
- Handling of used and unused medical equipment
- Handling of food, laundry, and waste.

In all considerations, basic knowledge about microbial physiology and other microbiological parameters is of paramount importance. Some results from either prudent or negligent planning can be seen during everyday operations from the very beginning of the lifespan of a new hospital or other healthcare facility. However, many consequences of bad material choices, inadequate thinking etc. come across only after some years of pursuing the clinical activities. This can come out as a building mold problem, or other throughout contamination of the unit with e.g., antibiotic resistant strains.

In long-term healthcare facilities also the medical devices tend to get contaminated by the microbes (Mutters et al., 2014). One such bacterial contaminant spreading into patients from the equipment is *Enterobacter cloacae* (Hakalehto, 2011; Laitiomäki et al., 2014).

A typical identifiable risk and preventable type of contamination is the *Clostridium difficile* spreading with endoscopes and colonoscopes (Hell et al., 2010).

The influence of design and construction of care facilities on healthcare-associated infections (HAI) is difficult to evaluate. Published references on this topic are rare so far. To identify environmental contributions to a risk-adjusted rate, such as surgical site infection (SSI), is even more challenging. Microbial counts in air or water can be used for estimating microbial occupation of:

1 space
2 surfaces, and
3 structures

The topic of hospital design as an important factor behind future hygienic standards has been recently reviewed. One such piece of work is presented in the IFIC Basic Concepts of Infection Control (Friedman and Newsom, 2011), which is also recommended by the authors of this chapter.

In this chapter we focus on a case of mold and bacterial contamination of hospital premises as an example of long-term microbial rooting into the building subjected to moisture and microbial load. In this model study we used the PMEU method for monitoring the surfaces. The results indicate the risks of also the strains of human origin to prevail and even spread in the structures.

2. A Case Evaluation: Mold and Bacterial Sampling on Moist Surfaces

Specimens were collected from an underground waiting room, where modest to severe moisture was detected. Sampling with cotton swab (standard method) was compared with a procedure with PMEU (Portable Microbe Enrichment Unit) sampling, cultivation and detection syringes (Hakalehto, 1998; Hakalehto and Heitto, 2012).

The basic structure of the syringe surface sampler is introduced in Chapter 6.

In the standard protocol, samples were taken by cotton swabs wetted in saline. In the PMEU method, the surface was wiped swiftly with moist surfaces of the PMEU syringe pistons. After specimen collection, the piston was positioned into the syringe, and the microbes detached from the adsorbing surface into 5 ml of saline. In case of the standard method the collected micro-organisms were suspended into 5 ml of saline in a test tube.

Sampling sites:

1 Wall surface in the underground hallway. Sampling areas were A. an intact painted wall surface, and B. cement surface underneath the detached paint. Sampling areas 1.5 x 22 cm.
2 WC wall specimens, sampling areas as above, 1.5 x 45 cm.
3 Cellar room cement wall, unpainted with visible damages caused by the moisture, areas 1.5 x 36 cm.
4 Cellar cement floor in the same condition as the walls, area 1.5 cm x 20 cm. Only PMEU syringe samples were used for collecting the sample no. 4.

Thenafter, microbiological dilution series was produced from all samples in the Finnoflag Oy laboratory. Cultivation on TYG (Tryptone, Yeast extract, Glucose) and Malt extract plates (the latter for microfungi, the former a generalized medium for bacterial cultivation). The inoculated dilutions were in case of TYG plates: -1, -2 and -3, whereas the dilutions for malt extract plates were -1, -2, -3, -4 and -5.

All plates were cultivated in the laboratory of the National Institute of Health and Welfare in Kuopio, Finland at 25 °C for 7 days (malt extract plates), or at room temperature for 5 days (TYG plates). After the cultivations, the colonies were counted, and they were identified with microscopy.

The results from this survey are presented in Table 1.

Some samples of both standard and syringe sample type were enriched in the PMEU at Finnoflag Oy's laboratory using TYG broth as the liquid medium (2 ml of sample suspension in 10 ml of TYG in each syringe). The samples were cultivated until the microbial growth was visible. Samples 2 – 4 became turbid in 10 – 12,5 hours, and sample 1 in 21 hours in the PMEU cultivation at 25 °C with air bubble flow.

Culture fluid samples were spread onto TYG plates, and after 2 days of incubation at 25 °C, further samples were picked up from the colonies thereof onto the following medias:

1 CHROMagar Orientation™ plates (Becton Dickinson, US)
2 *Staphylococcus* medium 110 (Oxoid, England)

Table 1. Cfu (colony forming unit) numbers of mold spores and bacteria (cfu/cm^2)

	Mesofilic fungi (cfu/cm²)		Mesofilic bacteria (cfu/cm²)	
	2% malt exract		TYG medium	
Sample 1	TOTAL CONSENTRATION (TC)	49	TOTAL CONSENTRATION (TC)	21
	CLA	<1		
	ACR	49		
Sample 1E	TC	347	TC	298
	CLA	14	ACT	46
	ACR	41	OTH	252
	TUN	293		
Sample 2	TC	383	TC	406
	ACR	153		
	STA	230		
Sample 2E	TC	2 072	TC	691
	ACR	45		
	STA	2 027		
Sample 3	TC	5 815	TC	42 000
	PEN	5	ACT	28 200
	CLA	901	OTH	13 800
	ACR	4 910		
Sample 3E	TC	3 605	TC	42 800
	PEN	1	ACT	17 000
	CLA	450	OTH	25 800
	ACR	1 712		
	TUN	1 441		
Sample 4E	TC	349	TC	5 550
	PEN	7	ACT	232
	STE	167	OTH	5 318
	SCO	41		
	AVER	135		

E = enriched in PMEU, CLA = *Cladosporium,* ACR = *Acremonium,* TUN = unidentified, STA = *Stachybotrys,* PEN = *Penicillium,* STE = sterile, SCO = *Scopulariopsis,* AVER = *Aspergillus versicolor,* ACT = *Actinomycetes,* OTH = other bacteria.

After some days of cultivation on these most common bacterial group turned out to be *Actinomycetes*. In all samples lesser amounts of potentially ill health causing mold species, such as *Aspergillus versicolor*, *Cladosporium* sp. and *Penicillium* sp., were detected. Aspergillus fumigatus emissions from construction sites exhibit an increased risk for nearby departments of immunocompromised patients (Vonberg and Gastmeier, 2006). Most serious contaminants were the *Acremonium* and *Stachybotrus*. Symptoms of *Stachybotrys* exposure include the following:

- strong fatigue, tiredness
- chronic fatigue syndrome (CFS)

- nausea, vomiting, abdominal pain, diarrhea
- nose bleeds, bleeding gums, coughing up blood
- gynecological bleeding, and bleeding disorders
- headache, general ill feeling
- redness, irritation, rash
- neurological symptoms, memory impairment, inability to concentrate, lack of initiative
- sore throat, runny nose, cough, pain in the chest
- muscle and joint pain
- pneumonia, neonatal hemorrhagic pneumonitis

This list indicates the potential of ”diseased buildings” to cause various indications of compromised health.

These impacts can be caused by poor control of contaminations in hospital premises, as well as in the homes, offices, school, day care centers and other public buildings.

Conclusion

Since the hygienic condition of the hospital and other clinical premises can be estimated from the microbial contaminations on the surfaces of the permanent structures, we performed this case evaluation in a waiting room area which was under renovation.

Some microbiological signs of severe mold contaminations (e.g., *Stachybotrys* sp., *Acremonium* sp.) were detected. From most specimens PMEU syringe samples produced higher estimates on microbial numbers than the standard cotton swab. With the PMEU samples, more unidentifiable colonies were spotted.

In the enrichment with the PMEU, some staphylococcal growth was verified under the paint layer indicating the penetration of bacterial strains into the wall structures. By correct hygiene maintenance measures and careful planning of the construction phase and operation of the clinical units, most hygienic problems could be prevented.

Effective hygiene monitoring, in turn, makes it possible to eradicate the grown-in problems in due time. This is also protecting the patients from the threats form the “diseased” buildings.

References

Friedman, C., Newsom, W., editors. *IFIC Basic Concepts of Infection Control* (2nd Edition - Revised 2011). Portadown, North Ireland, UK: International Federation of Infection Control; 2011; pp. 349-359.

Hakalehto, E. Syringe for collecting microbiological sweep samples. *US Patent 5846209 A, 1998.*

Hakalehto, E. Antibiotic resistance traits of facultative *Enterobacter cloacae* strain studied with the PMEU (Portable Microbe Enrichment Unit). In: Méndez-Vilas, A., editor. *Science against microbial pathogens: communicating current research and technological advances*. Microbiology Series No: 3, vol. 2. Badajoz, Spain: Formatex Research Center; 2011; pp. 786-796.

Hakalehto, E., Heitto, L. Minute microbial levels detection in water samples by Portable Microbe Enrichment Unit Technology. *Environment and Natural Resources Research,* 2012; 2, 80-88.

Hell, M., Bernhofer, C., Huhulescu, S., Indra, A., Allerberger, F., Maass, M., Hakalehto, E. How safe is colonoscope-reprocessing regarding *Clostridium difficile* spores*? The Journal of Hospital Infection,* 2010, 76 (Suppl. 1): Abstracts, 8th International Congress of the Hospital Infection Society, 10-13 October 2010, Liverpool, UK, S21-22.

Laitiomäki, E., Pesola, J., Hakalehto, E. *Projected improvement in the fast microbiological analysis of neonatal blood samples; 2014*. Submitted for publication.

Mutters, N. T., Günther, F., Heininger, A., Frank, U. Device-related infections in long-term healthcare facilities: the challenge of prevention. *Future Microbiol.*, 2014; 9, 487-495.

Ransjö, U., Popp, W. Health Care Facility Design, Construction, and Renovation. In: Friedman, C., Newsom, W., editors. *IFIC Basic Concepts of Infection Control*, 2nd Edition - Revised 2011. Portadown, North Ireland, UK: International Federation of Infection Control; 2011; pp. 349-359.

Vonberg, R. P., Gastmeier, P. Nosocomial aspergillosis in outbreak settings. *J. Hosp. Infect.,* 2006; 63, 246-254.

In: Microbiological Clinical Hygiene
Editor: Eino Elias Hakalehto

ISBN: 978-1-63463-428-1

Chapter 6

Environmental Sampling and Sample Processing in Hospitals

***Elias Hakalehto*[1]*, Jouni Pesola*[2] *and Lauri Heitto*[3]**
[1]Department of Environmental Sciences, University of Eastern Finland, Kuopio, Finland
[2]Department of Pediatrics, Kuopio University Hospital, Kuopio, Finland
[3]Environmental Research of Savo-Karjala, Kuopio, Finland

Abstract

Different hospital areas, such as operation theatres, overpressured patient rooms, cohort units for isolation, and intensive care units (ICVs), should be continuously monitored on their air outlets with selective techniques. This arrangement could make it possible to get early warnings or alarms on

- distribution of hazardous pathogens
- emerging antibiotic resistant strains
- increasing hygienic problems

The results from continuously monitoring PMEU (Portable Microbe Enrichment Unit) units produce data for decision making on the hospital hygiene management. The purpose is to limit the potential problems, and also to prevent the spreading out of contagious microbial diseases. With any screening method, the sampling procedures are the foundation of acquiring relevant information. Both air and surface sampling are to be performed on an undisturbed basis every day.

Aerial maps of the hospital and its hygienic situation could be presented. In the case of epidemics, a rapid view on the situation is thus created. Similarly, any object of interest could be hygienically monitored. As a result, a broad view on the whole microbiological situation of a ward, a clinic or in the entire hospital could be effectively formed. Basic building blocks for this high level of hygienic control practices are outlined.

1. Introduction

Nowadays, broad clinical hygienie analysis is performed only on special situations, *e.g.*, when large-scale hospital infection is occurring, or during pre-determined follow up with regular intervals. Then the main purpose is often to obey the instructions for everyday surveillance work, if such ones are existing in the particular situation. However, when dealing with dangerous infections and health deteriorating contaminations, our level of awareness should be elevated. – In fact, this is the situation in every hospital on every day. – The future developments of rapid clinical bacteriology are prognosed to cause a "second revolution" in hospital diagnostics (van Belkum et al. 2013).

This revolution will be based on the earlier phases of the progress in the microbial detection technologies, and will combine culture techniques with molecular biology, and with the latest progress of such methods as mass spectroscopy (MS).

Sampling is the beginning of the process of the microbiological analysis. In every case of investigation it has to be a successful one for the analysis chain not to produce misinformation or misintepretations. Some recommendations on mindset related questions with respect to the sampling plan:

- from where?
- when?
- by whom?

Various samples include e.g., surface samples and air samples, both of which require specific attention regarding the ways of their collection. In these sampling situations it is of crucial importance to get as many strains of the relevant microbes to recover as possible. If the objects and specimens are screened with genetic techniques *only*, the relative importance of the findings may also become unclear.

In case of epidemics, hazardous or fast-spreading infections, and other alarming microbiological threats, it is increasingly important to make a fast plan for a strategy for the sampling and the subsequent analysis. Samples from outside the hospitals, or between the laboratories, could be sent using innovative techniques, such as secured mailing bag for biomaterials by Biosafe Ab (Halstahammar, Sweden).

2. Microbial Detection Is a Chain of Events

In pharmaceutical industries, the Process Analytical Technology (PAT) is a key tool for better characterization of the manufacturing process. It is crucial for the successful implementation of the PAT to arrange a timely acquisition of data by monitoring all critical parameters relevant to process quality and performance (Ball 2006). This is in line with the use of the PMEU in hospitals or industries (Hakalehto 2010). Further citation from Dr. Ball: "Microbiological test methods have changed little since the 1890's. They can only detect a restricted range of replicating organisms that are recovered on the limited range of culture media and incubation temperatures routinely used. The current compendial methods are operator-dependent and hence to a degree are subjective and they are far from real time methods, needing between 5 and 14 days (or more) to produce a result acceptable to the regulators. This reality is being increasingly exposed as the amount of manufacturing and regulatory focus on PAT has grown."

Nowadays, more attention is given to the development of process microbiology. Nevertheless, the actual microbiological detection itself is a process. Although all steps of this process are important, the final verification steps (detection-identification-characterization) are still often the most intensively developed part of the chain (Figure 1).

More focus should be directed into the balancing of the entire diagnostic process.

The logic of rapid microbiology (according to Ball 2006) is that it can:

- provide rapid results that permit an early response to any apparent process deviations.
- offer the potential for simpler methods that require less highly trained operators.
- can increase the number of samples that can be processed

However, while the regulations are improving the monitoring of the methods they sometimes end up making up obstacles for the development. In the PDA Technical Report 33 (Revised 2013) the key aspects for alternative or rapid microbiology are presented.

- accuracy
- sensitivity
- linearity (primarily relevant for methods that count bacteria)
- reproducibility

Already in year 1992 we compiled a questionnaire to be used as an inquiry among Finnish microbiological laboratories about their expectations with respect to future rapid microbiological methods. The four major attributes highlighted in this study were:

- speed
- reliability / accuracy
- sensitivity
- easiness for use

3. Equipment Development Could Serve the Patients

In a lecture on personalized medicine advancements given by Prof. Feng Lu ("Biotech Japan 2014" Conference, Tokyo, May 2014) he stated that new devices for diagnosis or treatments do not reach the patient application level quickly enough in many countries. This could also be a bottleneck in the healthcare development. In Japan, the trend is toward more rapid acquisition of the permission for novel instruments. The period of time required for the permission is intended to get shortened by new legislation.

SAMPLING ⇨ PRE-TREATMENT ⇨ TRANSPORT & STORAGE ⇨ PRE-ENRICHMENT ⇨ ENRICHMENT ⇨ DETECTION ⇨ IDENTIFICATION ⇨ CHARACTERIZATION

Figure 1. Stepwise presentation of unit tools in microbiological hygiene analysis.

In 2013, 104 new medical devices were introduced to the market in Japan, whereas this number was only 13 in 2009. In anyway, for the manufacturer it is important to understand what is in the regulators mind. The goal is to maintain a balance between protection of patients on one hand and promotion of new technologies on the other.

Microbial distribution inside the hospitals has been studied with the Portable Microbe Enrichment Unit (PMEU) (Hakalehto 2006, 2010). PMEU equipment as either versatile laboratory tool, or field instrument, was first suggested to be used widely in the control of hospital hygiene. The PMEU method could actualize the various needs for developing hospital hygiene monitoring, and microbiological screening in the entire healthcare system as presented earlier (Hakalehto 2011a). Different hospital areas, as well as separated spaces or confinements, such as operation theatres, overpressured patient rooms, cohort units for isolation as well as intensive case units, could be continuously monitored with selective PMEU units on the air outlets (Hakalehto et al., 2009). This arrangement makes it possible to get early warnings or alarms on

- the distribution of hazardous pathogens
- the emerging antibiotic resistant strains
- the worsening overall hygienic situation

Results from the continuously monitoring with PMEU units produce data for decision making in the hospital management in real-time. The purpose is to limit potential problems, and prevent the spreading of contagious microbial diseases, and antibiotic resistant strains. Aerial maps of the hospital and its hygienic situation could be presented. In the case of epidemics, a rapid view on the situation could be created. Similarly, any object of interest could be hygienically monitored. Also, any trend or tendency of the spreading of unwanted agents could be screened with the PMEU technology.

Any clinical entity, organization or situation requires determined microbiological follow up of the premises, equipment, personnel and patients (Hakalehto 2006). The PMEU technology provides solutions for combined laboratory and in field or point-of-care (POC) hygiene management. All critically ill infection patients could be screened and followed up using this method (Pesola et al., 2012; Laitiomäki et al., 2014). The results could be updated in real-time with equipment dedicated to *e.g.,* any particular patient, hospital room, emergency unit, or other clinical setting.

In developing areas, or during crisis or catastrophes, it would be extremely important to use modern microbiology effectively also when proper infrastructure is not existing. The PMEU has been operational also in safeguarding water, clinical and food hygiene in Mosambik, South China or in the southern Spain, respectively. Thus, it has been operable in various geographical areas. It has been used in field condition in many other locations, especially in Finland during all seasons with temperature varying from -25°C to +40°C. The PMEU platform offers excellent means for simulating the behavior of microbes and their communities *in vivo*. More recently, the PMEU technologies have been used for identifying the hygiene control of water and food-chain in Burkina Faso, East Africa (Hakalehto et al., 2014a). Food samples from the market, and patient samples from the pediatric hospital, were screened and identical genotypes were detected in them. For example, identical *Campylobacter* sp. genotypes were found both in the local market chicken products and in the nearby pediatric hospital.

Some functions of the PMEU are listed below:

1) microbial verification
    a. pre-enrichment
        i. speed
        ii. accuracy
        iii. reliability
    b. metabolic studies / markers
        i. evaporated compounds
        ii. changes in culture conditions
        iii. mixed cultures
    c. source tracing
        i. routes of contamination
        ii. contaminating strains
2) studying interactions
    a. host-microbe
        i. hormones
        ii. messengers, signals
        iii. symbiosis, normal flora
        iv. pathogenic "balances"
    b. microbe-microbe
        i. balances
        ii. intra- and interspecies signals
        iii. genetic recombination
        iv. formation of biofilms
3) microbial exploitation
        i. disease markers
        ii. probiotics
        iii. functional foods
        iv. biotechnology / biorefineries
        v. purification

4. Sampling Areas and Microbiological "Mapping"

Applications of the PMEU technologies in the hospital is offering means for centralized data handling of microbiological results. Patients, personel and visitors carry their microbes, which constitute a potential source for contaminations or infections. Moreover, microbes may spread into hospitals with air, water, food sources, equipment, consumables, chemicals, building materials etc. In general terms, it has been stated that if the versatility of microbiological isolates in the hospital remains high, this is a sign of somewhat positive hygienic situation, whereas any development into the direction of monotonous flora could indicate worsening of the hygienic condition.

Handling various hygienic samples; water, air, surface, device, patient samples etc. on continuous basis is a key to successful microbial monitoring in the hospital environment.

Their simultaneous surveillance could give useful views on the overall situation. For example, spreading contaminations, or routes for contaminations, can be mapped inside the units. This may cause additional costs, but could also cause savings in the total budget as the hygienic problems are getting limited or solved on early stages, which will eventually lead to improved cure results. By this kind of "mapping" approach on microbiological conditions in various parts of the hospital, it is possible to aquire early warnings on the emerging threats. Similarly, antibiotic resistances can be screened on-line.

On individual level, when researching patient samples from skin, respiratory, urinary or alimentary traits, genital areas, or elsewhere, several deductions can be made on.

1. balances of microflora
2. potentially harmful microbial strains

Particularly from samples of normally sterile body regions, such as bladder, blood cerebrospinal fluid, can give rapidly useful alarms on life threatening situations.

PMEU method has been used for surveing the sterility of research instruments, for example in case of colonoscopes (Hell et al., 2010). Equally well it is possibly to study the purity of blood specimens, or blood products (Hakalehto et al., 2009).

Potential hospital uses of the PMEU

1. Critically ill patients
    - POC (Point-Of-Care) analysis
    - guick estimation
    - treatment plan
    - follow up
    - "one PMEU per patient" -> human and economic gains
2. Emergency transportations
3. Remote control and access to the information on results
    - access to real-time results
    - antibiotic treatments screened; aerial follow up of resistance ("resistance maps")
    - epidemics
4. Cohorts
    - typing of the strains
    - risk assessment
5. Microbial ecosystems and natural protection

5. Indicator Bacteria Applied for Hygiene Monitoring

Human feces contain huge amount of microbes, of which some may be pathogenic, such as *Salmonella* and other intestinal bacterial pathogens, different viruses, protozoa or parasites. These pathogens may also be found in the feces of many warm-blooded animal. It is very important for general human health to know if there is any risk for fecal contamination in the environment (Hakalehto, 2014). Surveillance on the hygienic indicator could be combined also with screening of the antibiotic resistance (Hakalehto, 2011a).

Since each pathogen needs its own methods for identification, and is detected relatively scarcely, the concept of indicator bacteria has been widely accepted in environmental monitoring as an "early-warning approach." In the following paragraphs some early history of the concept has been outlined (Heitto et al. 2012).

The use of bacteria as indicators of the sanitary quality of water probably dates back to 1880 when Von Fritsch described *Klebsiella pneumoniae* and *K.rhinoscleromatis* as micro-organisms characteristically found in human feces. In 1885, Percy and Grace Frankland started the first routine bacteriological examination of water in London, using Robert Koch's solid gelatine media to count bacteria. Also in 1885, Escherich described *Bacillus coli* (renamed *Escherichia coli* by Castellani and Chalmers (1919)) from the feces of breast-fed infants. In 1891, the Franklands came up with the concept that organisms characteristic of sewage must be identified to provide evidence of potentially dangerous pollution. By 1893, the 'Wurtz method' of enumerating *B. coli* by direct plating of water samples on litmus lactose agar was being used by sanitary bacteriologists, using the concept of acid from lactose as a diagnostic feature. This was followed by gas production, with the introduction of the Durham tube. The concept of 'coliform' bacteria, those bacteria resembling *B. coli*, was in use in Britain in 1901. The colony count for bacteria in water, however, was not formally introduced until the first Report 71. Nowadays, the coliforms from water samples can be monitored with the PMEU applications (Hakalehto, 2011b; Hakalehto and Heitto, 2012; Hakalehto et al., 2013).

Therefore, the sanitary significance of finding various coliforms along with streptococci and *C. perfringens* was recognised by bacteriologists by the start of the twentieth century. It was not until 1905, however, that MacConkey described his now famous MacConkey's broth, which was a diagnostic tool for enumerating lactose-fermenting bacteria tolerant of bile salts. Nonetheless, *coli-forms* were still considered to be a heterogeneous group of organisms, many of which were not of fecal origin. The origins of the critical observation that *B. coli* was largely fecal in origin while other coliforms were not, could be claimed by Winslow and Walker (1907).

Parallel to the work on coliforms, a group of Gram-positive coccoid bacteria known as fecal streptococci (FS) were being investigated as important pollution indicator bacteria. Problems in differentiating fecal from non-fecal streptococci, however, initially impeded their use. It was not until 1957, however, with the availability of the selective medium of Slanetz and Bartley that enumeration of FS became popular.

According to Ashbolt et al. (2001) indicator bacteria can be divided into three groups, process indicators, fecal indicators, and index and model organisms. Process indicators demonstrate the efficiency of a process, e.g, total coliforms for chlorine disinfection. Fecal indicators indicate the presence of fecal contamination. Nowadays the most commonly used bacteria for fecal indicators are *E. coli* and fecal enterococci (earlier fecal streptococci). Interestingly, they are among the most resistant microbes against bile acids, and therefore most frequent members of the duodenal flora and in the biliary tract. Consequently, they are colonizing the entire length of the intestines (Hakalehto et al., 2008, 2010; Hakalehto, 2014). Index and model organisms are species that indicate pathogen presence and behavior, respectively, e.g., *E coli* is an index for *Salmonella* (Hakalehto et al., 2011).

6. The Airborne Contagion and Air Hygiene

The brilliant postulates and other paradigms presented by William Firth Wells (Wells, 1955) are incorporated into this book (Appendix I).

Some comments arise from these ideas. First of all, the laws of physics are determining the fate of aerosols, vapours or particles in the atmosphere. When these materials are of biological origin it is crucial for their viability to maintain the integrity and characteristics required for initiating new microbial growth or novel activities in the object or target surfaces, or tissues. It is generally known that if the diameter of a particle is less than ten microns it will move in the atmosphere according to the up or downward (lateral) air flows and without the interference of any gravitational forces. Consequently, microbes can move across borders and they are able to travel long distances in the air. However, it should be kept in mind that in the atmosphere there are many factors which are diminishing the chances of airborne microbes for staying viable. Ultraviolet radiation is rapidly disinfecting air masses especially at high altitudes and during daytime. This effect is also influencing the contagion levels of many viruses and as an example it has been given a thumb rule that staying away some one and half meter away from a diseased person could lower the risk of catching respiratory viral infection significantly. Movements of big air masses can transmit diseased of both human and zoonotic origin as well as plant diseases vast distances away from their origins (Hakalehto, 2014).

Besides the ultraviolet radiation in the atmosphere also air humidity (or dryness in the form of dehydration) has effects on the survival of micro-organisms. Often the microbes are aggregated or at least attached to some other particles and surrounded by some humidity. The formation of such integrated particles or droplets is depending on the humidity of the atmosphere (Wells, 1955). In collecting microbiological air samples we come across with the survival rate issue. Whether the microbes we have studied are able to continue their lives after the travel in the air and what would be the proportion of the so called colony forming units of the total populations if sample collection on microbiological plates is used. This question has a partially methodological answer. In fact, it is a known fact that the techniques chosen for the collection of the air samples are influencing significantly on the result from the hygienic study (Hakalehto, 2014). For example, if air filter systems are used the microbes attached on the filter are subjected to remarkable dehydration which is causing osmotic pressures that easily can break many cell types. For example, in the air sampling at the height of one kilometer on such filters under a jet plane was producing mostly growth of mold colonies when the filters were studied on plate cultures. This was obviously due to the fact in the air remarkable amounts of mold spores existed even at higher altitudes, and they were able to sustain the dehydrating air flow across the filter during the sampling procedure. They also were floating in the air as robust spores.

On the surfaces of "diseased buildings" the sampling has to be considered carefully. Important finding in many studies has been the outstanding performance of impinger techniques in the recovery of germs, and thus in getting reliable results on the airborne micro-organisms (Thomas et al., 1981; Dolan et al., 2011; Hakalehto, 2014).

One possibility is also to study the microbial content of the fallouts using surface plate method or an equivalent technique for investigating the cumulative fallout onto the surfaces. This is an easy-to-do method for hygienic studies regarding air quality and it can be carried out anywhere where it is possible to produce sterile culture plates with relevant growth medium. Hygienic quality of air is often related to water microbiological qualities, and *vice versa* (Dneker, 2012). As an example of our studies on microbiological aerosols, we investigated A. the air in an apartment and took samples also from B. the respiratory tract of the inhabitants as well as from C. the air humidifying system. The same strain of staphylococci was found in all of these three objects. This indicated once again, how man is connected with the environment via his or her microflora (Hakalehto, 2014).

In another unpublished study it was found out that many bacterial strains were staying viable inside the brick wall. Moreover, when these sampling efforts were directed to this wall and aseptic samples were taken from inside the tiles it was observed that even there viable bacteria were found, for example, some strains of *Microbacterium* sp. Consequently, it is possible to postulate that whatever goes into the air, it will eventually land up to surfaces where it is possible for the microbes in the particles to continue their lives under favorable conditions for an undetermined period of time. This means that in practice any building, such as a hospital department, will eventually get contaminated by the bacterial and other microbial emissions from the patients and other people in there. Therefore, the surface hygienic treatments are important factors in preventing contaminations of the building materials, equipment, and other surfaces and materials. One example of a diseased building case is presented in Chapter 5.

Several ways to produce antimicrobial surface materials have been developed (Varghese et al., 2013). Also medical devices can be protected with various coatings against contamination (Evliyaoğlu et al., 2011, Sileika et al., 2011). However, with respect to antimicrobial surfaces; they should not replace proper hygienic measures or cleaning. In Salzburg hospital in Austria (SALK) silver-impregnated central line catheters are used only at ICU (Intensive Care Unit) where the highest infection rates usually occur (2-3 infections/1000 central line days) (Dr. Markus Hell, personal information).

In modern days, when the contamination problem has each and every year become more serious inside the hospitals and other healthcare units, new methodology and equipment have been introduced for fighting back the risky situation. These methods include various devices for disinfecting entire wards, or buildings, but we do not go into details of these commercially available techniques in here. For an overview see Chapter 7.

By using the above-mentioned techniques it is possible to safeguard the patients and personnel inside the hospital buildings, *e.g.,* patient rooms, operation theatres, and in public spaces of the hospitals. In case of some epidemics, cohort approach has been chosen, which means that new premises are taken into use in order to replace the contaminated hospital or clinic. Costs of such approach in case of multi-drug resistant tuberculosis (MDR) have recently been estimated (Wingfield et al., 2014). These premises are then to be hygienized by an effective approach and then returned back to normal use after some inspections. It is recommendable, however, that during any common operations or any active period of health care unit the air quality is to be continnously monitored by effective techniques (Hakalehto, 2010).

7. Surface Sampling and Analysis

Artificially contaminated laboratory surfaces have been studied with the PMEU syringe sampler (Figure 2. a-f) (Hakalehto, 1998), and the growth of the attached microbes thereof was recorded with PMEU Spectrion®. Relatively late onset of the growth was detected (Hakalehto, 2010). This indicated low survival rate of the organisms and is probably due to the surface tension and dehydration on the metallic and other surfaces. Encountering positively charged surface may cause the microbial cell inactivation and even rupture as a result from electrostatic and other forces on the surfaces. Many metals are also toxic to the microbial cells whose iron pumps on the membranes may be interfered by the charges on the metallic surfaces. This could incapacitate the cells since their intracellular pH, redox and osmotic statuses get out of balance on these surfaces. Therefore, it can be difficult for individual bacterial cells, for example, to survive on even surfaces which do not provide protection of uneven microstructure or any protective debris or previously existing microcolonies on the surfaces. Consequently, in order to overcome these repulsive forces, microbes tend to form biofilms (Costerton and Lappin-Scott, 1987). This biofilm formation is a widely studied, but complex phenomenon. The biofilms can have sophisticated structures with holes and cavities or even inner "airways" for the gas emission. Photographs of the formation of biofilm can be seen in Chapter 2 of this book.

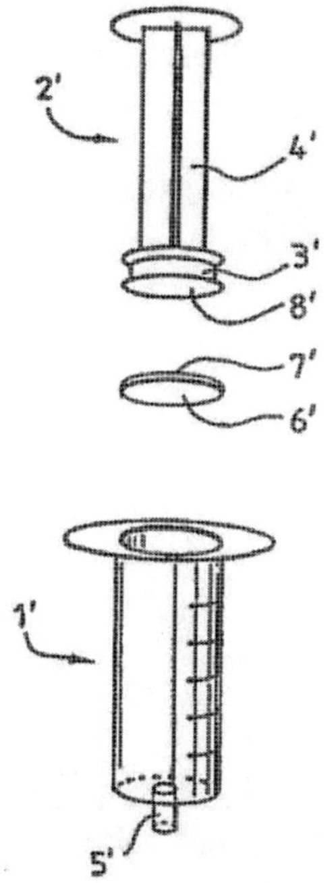

a.

Figure 2. (Continued).

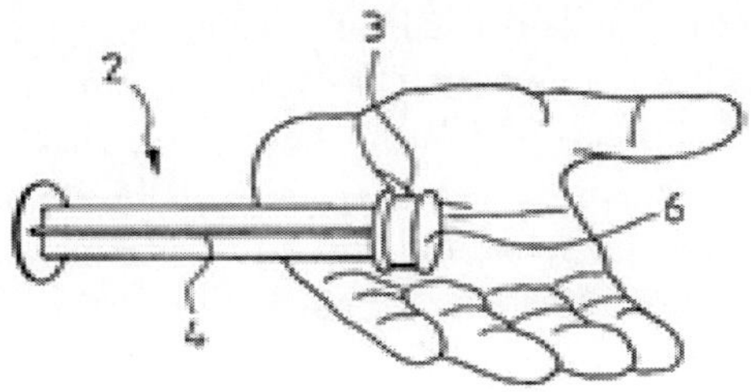

b.

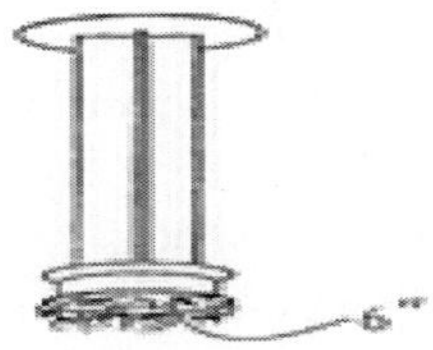

c.

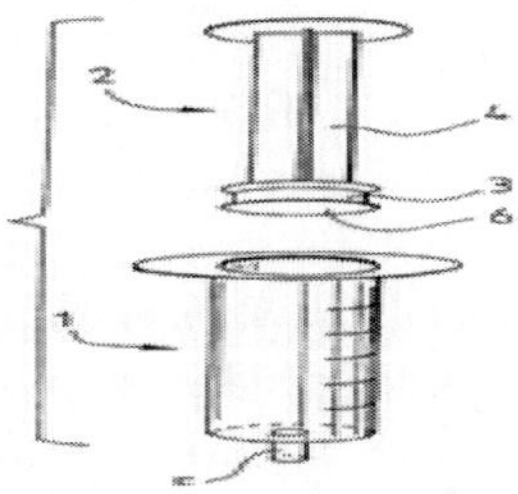

d.

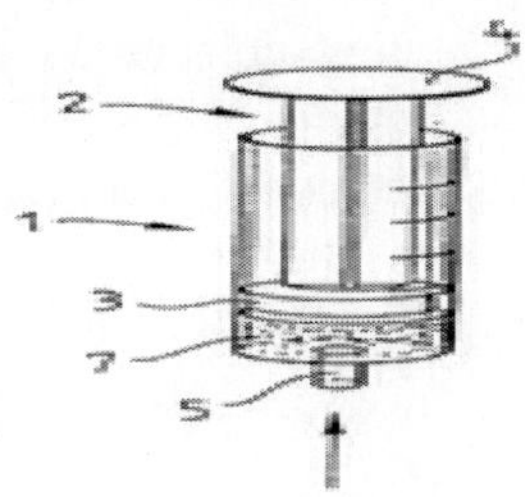

e.

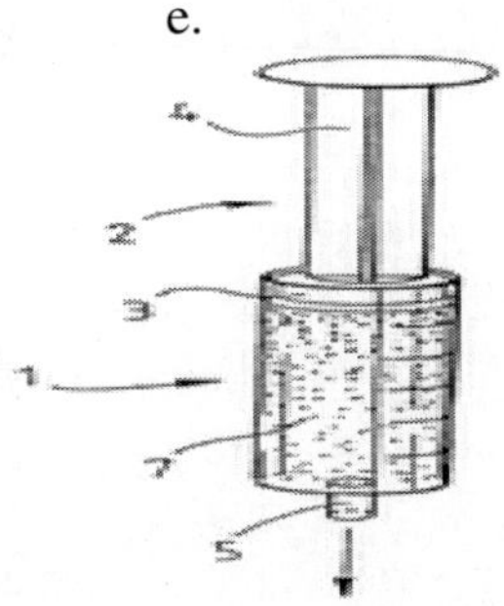

f.

Figure 2. Illustrations of the PMEU syringe sampler (Hakalehto, 1998). a-c. the tip of the piston is equipped with a special sampling surface; d-f. the syringe sampler can be used as a lab tube or container both for surface samples and for liquid samples. Further samples can be dispensed from it e.g., after cultivation in the PMEU.

The outflow of gaseous substances is needed for maintaining the integrity of the biofilms. The distribution of nutrients is possible only if the structures are prevailing in a shape which allows effective diffusion of nutrients and metabolic wastes. There is also a clear metabolic difference between swarming cells in solution and the cells inside the biofilm layers, even if they were representing only one genotype. In case of mucosal membranes in the body, it has been documented in many studies that the commensal microflora is competing with the pathogens for the nutrients (Smith, 1982). In case of gnotobiotic animals, the caecal microbial contents of normal mice (100 various strains pooled) restricted the growth of a specific *E. coli* strain and *Shigellae* 10-1000 –fold (Freter and Abrams, 1972). Equal 10-100 –fold "attenuation" of *E. coli* and klebsiellas was detected by lactic acid bacteria in specific conditions (Hakalehto and Jaakkola, 2013) (See also the Chapter 17 of this book). Correspondingly, a 5-fold simultaneous decrease was detected in the PMEU in case of mixed culture of *E. coli* and klebsiellas when newcoming other strains (*S. aureus* and *B. cereus*) were inoculated to the culture (Hakalehto et al., 2010). However, when *E. coli* and *Klebsiella mobilis* (or *K. pneumoniae*) grew together they did not restrict the growth of each other (Hakalehto et al., 2008). This indicates that the klebsiellas are exploiting acetic acid residues formed by the *E. coli* strain (Hakalehto et al., 2010). It is evident that *Klebsiella* sp. can utilize also the acetic acid produced by themselves, and convert it into ethanol or 2,3-butanediol in anaerobiosis, thus compensating the pH drop caused by the acidic compounds (Hakalehto et al., 2014). In natural ecosystems microbial activities are often associated with the presence of surface structures (Ellwood et al. 1982). Especially in low-nutrient environments that seems to be the case. On the other hand, in the intestinal epithelia such pathogenic bacteria as salmonellas seem to stay in suspension long as they find a suitable site for attachment with adequate nutrients present and growth factors available (Hakalehto et al., 2000). They express the type 1 fimbriae in less than 4 hours in a submerged culture where the nutrients are still present, but these appendices are detached when the nutritional prerequisities for growth are exhausted. The above-mentioned consideration is illustrating the influence of cellular metabolic status and surface structures on the attachment onto the different surfaces. This matter is discussed more deeply in Chapter 2 of this book.

8. Viable but Non-Culturable Bacteria

Viable but non-culturable (VNC) bacterial findings include strains of many common or severe pathogens, such as *E. coli* 0157:H7 (Makino et al. 2000), *Vibrio cholerae* (Xu et al. 1982, Sharan et al., 2011), *Salmonella typhi* (Sharan et al., 2011) and *Campylobacter jejuni* (Rollins and Colwell 1986). In hospital hygiene and during patient monitoring, the cultivation of these strains should be arranged. Related issues:

1. Improved recovery of bacterial strains from a particular sample
2. More effective and representative sampling
3. Less delay in starting the sample processing

The first aim could be achieved eg. with improved culture media or supplementation (Siegrist J, Product Manager, Sigma-Aldrich, www.sigma-aldrich.com/microbiology). In cultivating *Salmonella* sp., *Staphylococcus aureus* or *Yersinia enterocolitica*, Ferrioxamine E was used for reactivating damaged bacterial cells and for shortening the lag period. In case of *S. aureus* (MRSA), ferrioxamine could be combined with desferrioxamine B. These substances utilize specific features of the iron metabolism of various bacteria, and could also offer selection. The PMEU method was shown to increase the number of intestinal isolates belonging to the family *Enterobacteriaceae* 2.6-fold (Pesola and Hakalehto 2011). In case of *Bacillus* sp. the concentrations of the selective antibiotics in the PMEU culture media could be adjusted to even ¼ of the corresponding concentrations in the standard medium in order to achieve the optimal results (Mentu et al. 2009). This could form a remarkable advantage in controlling both disease-causing as well as antibiotic resistant bacterial strains (Luna et al. 2006). Smaller concentrations of antibiotics needed for actual selection could offer better resolution in the analysis. In case of campylobacteria, this observation was confirmed (Pitkänen et al. 2009). In this study conducted by the Finnish Institute of Health and Welfare the PMEU method was stated to be significantly more effective than the corresponding ISO method for the detection of water pathogens. This high effectiveness of the PMEU was also established in the case of mycobacterial isolates from water (Hakalehto 2013, Hakalehto et al., 2014b).

9. Microbiological Results from around the Patient Could Help in Diagnosing the Diseases

Some sentences from the New York Times bestseller "How Doctors Think" (Groopman, 2007). "After you determine your patient's primary complaint, you must then decide what blood tests and x-rays to order, if any." Then a specialist's viewed: "He told me that he emphasizes to his interns and residents in the emergency department there that they should not order a test unless they know how that test performs in a patient with the condition they assume he has. That way, they can properly weigh the result in their assessment. This is not as easy as it may sound." - In addition to careful planning of the tests it is of utmost importance to avoid mistakes caused by errors in the performance of the test, or in the interpretation of any results. "Other errors can be more subtle, like taking a chest x-ray when the patient has not held his breath. This can cause white streaking in the lower lungs, a sign of pneumonia."

Even more acute question would be, in case of real pneumonia, what is the causative organisms, and what are its basic characteristics. In microbiology minimalization of diagnostic performance is seldom fruitful. This is a consequence of the multi-factorial causes of infections and inflammations. The microbiological factors behind the condition are often considered to be the root cause of the disease. Therefore, an adequate coverage of microbiological analysis is warranted for the optimal treatment. Without more advanced personalized health care with individual analysis of normal flora it is difficult to give accurate diagnosis or statements about such complications as irritable bowel disease (IBD). If the surroundings of critically ill patients were monitored continuously (air, surfaces), it could

1. give leads for detecting the pathogens
2. add safety to everyone in the hospital surroundings

The modern methods could make it economically feasible enough to establish an ideal hospital also from microbiological point of view (van Belkum et al. 2013).

10. Bioagent Threat Monitoring

Biologically hazardous agents which could be used in the terrorism have been divided into three categories (according to Moran et al. 2008):

A – Easy to disseminate; cause high morbidity and mortality; and require specific enhancements of CDC's diagnostic capacity and enhanced disease surveillance.

Antrax
Plaque
Smallpox
Hemorrhagic Fevers
Botulism
Tularemia

B – Somewhat easy to disseminate; cause moderate morbidity and low mortality; and require specific enhancement of CDC's diagnostic capacity and enhanced disease surveillance.

Coxiella burnetii (Q fever)
Brucella species (brucellosis)
Burkholderia mallei (glanders)
Alphaviruses
Venezuelan encephalomyelitis
Eastern and Western equine encephalomyelitis
Ricin toxin from *Ricinus communis* (castor beans)
Epsilon toxin of *Clostridium perfringens*
Staphylococcus enterotoxin B
Food or waterborne agents
Salmonella species
Shigella dysenteria
Escherichia coli O157:H7
Vibrio cholera
Cryptosporidium parvum

C – Emerging pathogens that could be engineered for mass dissemination in the future because of availability; ease of production and dissemination; and potential for high morbidity and mortality and major health impact

Nipah virus
Hantaviruses
Tickborne hemorrhagic fever viruses

Tickborne encephalitis fever viruses
Yellow fever
Multidrug-resistant tuberculosis

The emerging antibiotic resistance could cause additional risks due to speed of distribution of these infections.

11. HACCP Practices and Microbiological Screening

The HACCP (Hazard Analysis and Critical Control Points) system is widely used in the food industries. There the main shortcomings of the approach include difficulties in estimating the extent and risk of the occurrence of any specific hazard. Therefore, a system for microbial diagnostics, such as the PMEU, could serve as basis for determining the actual risk levels (Hakalehto, Lecture in Labdagarna (Swedish Laboratory Days) in Stockholm, December 2012).

An assessment of risks of VTEC (Verocytotoxin producing *Escherichia coli*) in fermented sausages has been carried out in Sweden and elsewhere (Quinto et al., 2014). Depending on the VTEC strain contaminating the new material, there was a variation in the survival rate of VTEC in the sausages. The reduction of VTEC in the product was evaluated as a function of various parameters, such as temperature. The models show that the pH, as well as active water and lactic acid concentrations are additional parameters influencing the potential for bacterial growth, besides the temperature. Comparable to the food industry cases, the HACCP could be applied to the clinical mindset (Kramer et al. 2011). It can be implemented into hygiene control as a stepwise quality assurance protocol (Hübner et al. 2011). In the proposal for alternative system based on HACCP principles, the authors pay attention to also system wide audits (structure, process, outcome) of the entire healthcare "chain" consisting of sequential transfer of patients:

1. General practitioner
2. Specialist
3. Ward
4. Operation room
5. Intensive care unit
6. Rehabilitation

In practice, one PMEU device could be dedicated to a single patient in need for his or her entire care period (Hakalehto 2011). This is particularly desirable in cases where the outcome from infection treatments needs to be followed up. A schematic presentation on the ideas of the PMEU system in monitoring both hospital hygiene and patient samples is presented in Chapter 18.

12. Maintaining the Hygienic Levels on the Basis of Analysis

Strategies for the maintenance of favorable hospital environment for patient recovery are described in several guidelines proposed by different committees (e.g., Rutala and Weber 2008). In modern days, when the contamination problem has every year grown worse inside the hospitals and other health care units, new methodology and equipment have been introduced for fighting back the problematic situations. For surfaces with blood contamination, a disinfectant with activity against tuberculosis and hepatitis B virus or HIV a 5.25% bleach solution, at a final dilution of 1:10, can be used (Rutala and Weber, 2001). The methods for preventing the contaminations are reviewed by Abreu et al. (2013). They include:

- antimicrobial chemicals
    - quaternary ammonium compounds
    - aldehydes
    - alcohols
    - halogens
- radiation
- heat
- antimicrobial surfaces, some examples
    - Surfacine - incorporates an antimicrobial compound (silver iodide) in a surface-immobilized coating (a modified polyhexamethylenebiguanide) (Rutala and Weber 2001)
    - Microban® - contains triclosan [5-chloro-2-(2,4-dichlorophenoxy)-phenol] as the antimicrobial agent, making the surface resistant to the growth of microorganisms (Additives for Polymers, vol. 2009)
- vapour systems
    - steam vapour disinfection
    - hydrogen peroxide vapour
- UV-C light
- gas plasma
    - consists of a mixture of photons, electrons, ions, atoms and radicals (*e.g.,* atomic oxygen, ozone, nitrogen oxides, hydroxyl and superoxide) (Cotter et al. 2011; Moreau et al. 2008).

Conclusion

In modern hospital units, careful planning of sampling and sample processing is required. The strategies evolve from the previous experience, directives and local conditions. Such systems as HACCP (Hazard Analysis and Critical Control Points) or PAT (Process Analytical Technology) have been developed in order to deal with big pictures of health care hygiene control. Novel methods, such as the PMEU (Portable Microbe Enrichment Unit) technology could provide tools for enhancing the microbe detection processes in various clinical environments, and with respect to the patient-environment interface.

References

Ashbolt, N. J.; Grabow, W. O. K.; Snozzi, M. Indicators of microbial water quality. In: Fewtrell L., Bartram J., editors. World Health Organization (WHO). Water Quality: Guidelines, Standards and Health. London, UK.: IWA Publishing; 2001; 289-315.

Ball, P. How does rapid microbiology meet the needs of process analytical technology. In 37. Contamination Control Symposium 240, 2006; 97-107.

Castellani, A.; Chalmers, A. J. Manual of Tropical Medicine. 3rd ed. London: Bailliere,; 1919.

Costerton, W.; Lappin-Scott, H. M. Behaviour of bacteria in biofilms. *Am. Soc. Microbiol. News,* 1987; 55, 650-654.

Cotter, J.J.; Maquire, P.; Soberon, F.; Daniels, S.;O'Gara, J.P.; Casey, E.Disinfection of methicillin-resistant *Staphylococcus aureus* and *Staphylococcus epidermidis* biofilms using a remote non-thermal gas plasma. *Journal of Hospital Infection*, 2011; 78, 204-207.

Dolan, A.; Bartlett, M.; McEntee, B.; Creamer, E.; Humphreys, H. Evaluation of different methods to recover methicillin-resistant Staphylococcus aureus from hospital environmental surfaces. *J. Hosp. Infect.*, 2011; 79, 227-230.

Dneker, E. Connecting water quality with air quality with microbial aerosols. Academic dissertion. Columbia University, USA.

Durham, H. E. A simple method for demonstrating the production of gas by bacteria. *Brit. Med. J.*, 1893; 1, 1387.

Ellwood, D. C.; Keevil, C. W.; Marsh, P. D. Brown, C. M.; Wardell, J. N. Surface-associated growth. *Phil. Trans. R. Soc. Lond.*, 1982; B 297, 517-532.

Escherich, T. Die Darmbakterien des Neugeborenen und Säuglings. *Fortschr. Med.,* 1885; 3, 515-522-547-554.

Evliyaoğly, Y.; Kobaner M.; Celebi, H.; Yelsel, K.; Doğan, A. The efficancy of novel antibacterial hydroxyapatite nanoparticle-coated indwelling urinary catheter in preventing biofilm formation and catheter-assosiated urinary tract infection in rabbits. *Urol. Res. Dec.*, 2011; 39, 445-449.

Freter, R., Abrams, G.D. Function of various intestinal bacteria in converting germfree mice to the normal state. *Infect. Immunol.*, 1972; 6, 119-126.

Groopman, J. How Doctors Think. New York Times. New York, USA: Houghton Mifflin Company, 2007.

Hakalehto, E. Syringe for collecting microbiological sweep samples. US Patent 5846209 A, 1998.

Hakalehto, E. Semmelweis' present day follow-up: Updating bacterial sampling and enrichment in clinical hygiene, Review. *Pathophysiology*, 2006; 13, 257-267.

Hakalehto, E. Hygiene monitoring with the Portable Microbe Enrichment Unit (PMEU). 41st R3 -Nordic Symposium. Cleanroom technology, contamination control and cleaning. VTT Publications 266. Espoo, Finland: VTT (State Research Centre of Finland); 2010.

Hakalehto, E. Antibiotic resistance traits of facultative *Enterobacter cloacae* strain studied with the PMEU (Portable Microbe Enrichment Unit). In: Antonio Méndez-Vilas, editor. *Science against microbial pathogens: communicating current research and technological advances.* Badajoz, Spain: Formatex Research Center; 2011a; Microbiology Series 3 (2),. 786-796.

Hakalehto, E. Simulation of enhanced growth and metabolism of intestinal Escherichia coli in the Portable Microbe Enrichment Unit (PMEU). In: Rogers M. C., Peterson N. D., editors. *E. coli infections: causes, treatment and prevention.* New York, USA: Nova Publishers; 2011b; 159-175

Hakalehto, E. Enhanced mycobacterial diagnostics in liquid medium by microaerobic bubble flow in Portable Microbe Enrichment Unit. *Pathophysiology,* 2013; 20, 177-180.

Hakalehto, E. Bacteriological indications of human activities in the ecosystems. In: Armon, R.; Hänninen, O. editors. Environmental indicators. Germany: Springer Verlag; 2014. In Print.

Hakalehto, E.; Heitto, L. Minute microbial levels detection in water samples by Portable Microbe Enrichment Unit Technology. *Environment and Natural Resources Research,* 2012; 2, 80-88.

Hakalehto, E.; Jaakkola, K. Synergistic effect of probiotics and prebiotic flax product on intestinal bacterial balance. *Clinical Nutrition,* 2013; 32, Suppl. 1, S200.

Hakalehto, E.; Hujakka, H.; Airaksinen, S.; Ratilainen, J.; Närvänen, A. Growth-phase limited expression and rapid detection of *Salmonella* type 1 fimbriae. In: Hakalehto, E., editor. *Characterization of Pectinatuscerevisiiphilus and P. frisingiensis surface components. Use of synthetic peptides in the detection of some Gram-negative bacteria.* Kuopio, Finland: Kuopio University Publications C. Natural and Environmental Sciences 112; 2000.

Hakalehto, E.; Humppi, T.; Paakkanen, H. Dualistic acidic and neutral glucose fermentation balance in small intestine: Simulation in vitro. *Pathophysiology,* 2008; 15, 211-220.

Hakalehto, E.; Pesola, J., Heitto, A., Deo, B. B., Rissanen, K., Sankilampi, U., Humppi, T., and Paakkanen, H. (2009). Fast detection of bacterial growth by using Portable Microbe Enrichment Unit (PMEU) and ChemPro100i® gas sensor. *Pathophysiology*, 2009; 16, 57-62.

Hakalehto, E.; Hell, M.; Bernhofer, C.; Heitto, A.; Pesola, J.; Humppi, T.; Paakkanen, H. Growth and gaseous emissions of pure and mixed small intestinal bacterial cultures: Effects of bile and vancomycin. *Pathophysiology,* 2010; 17, 45-53.

Hakalehto, E.; Vilpponen-Salmela, T.; Kinnunen, K.; von Wright, A. Lactic acid bacteria enriched from human gastric biopsies. *ISRN Gastroenterol.*, 2011; 2011, 109183. doi: 10.5402/2011/109183.

Hakalehto, E.; Heitto, A.; Heitto, L.. Fast coliform detection in portable microbe enrichment unit (PMEU) with Colilert® medium and bubbling. *Pathophysiology*, 2013; 20, 257-262.

Hakalehto E, Nyholm O, Kagambèga, A., Bonkoungou, I., Haukka K., Heitto A. Development of microbiological field methodology for water and food-chain hygiene analysis of *Campylobacter* sp. and *Yersinia* sp. in Burkina Faso. *Pathophysiology*, 2014a. In print.

Hakalehto, E.; Heitto, A.; Heitto, L.; Rissanen, K.; Pesola, I.; Pesola, J. Enhanced recovery, enrichment and detection of Mycobacterium marinum with the Portable Microbe Enrichment Unit (PMEU). 2014b, Accepted for publication in Pathophysiology.

Hakalehto, E. Bacteriological indications of human activities in the ecosystems. In (Armon R. and Hänninen O.) Enviromental Bioindicators. Springer Verlag, Germany; 2014.

Heitto, L., Heitto, A., Hakalehto, E. Environmental monitoring using the enrichment of hygienic indicators. In: Hakalehto, E, editor. *Alimentary microbiome - a PMEU approach.* New York, NY, USA: Nova Science Publishers, Inc.; 2012; pp. 215-231.

Hell, M., Bernhofer, C., Huhulescu, S., Indra, A., Allerberger, F., Maass, M., Hakalehto, E. How safe is colonoscope-reprocessing regarding *Clostridium difficile* spores*? The Journal of Hospital Infection* Vol. 76, Supplement 1: Abstracts, 8th International Congress of the Hospital Infection Society, 10-13 October 2010, Liverpool, UK, S21-22.

Hübner, N. O.; Flessa, S.; Haak, J.; Wilke, F.; Hübner C.; Dahms, C.; Hoffman, W.; Kramer, A. Can the Hazard Assessment and Critical Control Points (HACCP) system be used to design process-based hygiene concepts? GMS Krankenhhyg Interdiszip. 2011; 6(1): Doc24. Published online Dec. 15, 2011. doi: 10.3205/dgkh000181

Kramer A.; Assadian O.; Exner M.; Hübner N.; Simon A. Editors. Krankenhaus- und Praxishygiene: Hygienemanagement und Infektionsprävention in medizinischen und sozialen Einrichtungen. 2nd ed. München/Berlin/Kusterdingen: Urban and Fischer Verlag/Elsevier GmbH; 2011.

Laitiomäki, E.; Pesola, J.; Hakalehto, E. *Projected improvement in the fast microbiological analysis of neonatal blood samples; 2014*. Submitted for publication.

Luna, V. A.; King, D. S.; Peak, K. K.; Reeves, F.; Heberlein-Larson, L.; Veguilla, W.; Heller, L.; Duncan, K. E.; Cannons, A. C.; Amuso, P.; Cattani, J. Bacillus anthracis virulent plasmid pX02 genes found in large plasmids of two other Bacillus species. *J. Clin. Microbiol.,* 2006; 44:2367-77.

MacConkey, A. T. Lactose-fermenting bacteria in faeces. *J. Hyg*., 1905; 5, 333.

Makino, S. et al., Does enterohemorrhagic Escherichia coli O157:H7 enter the viable but nonculturable state in salted salmon roe?, *Appl. Environ. Microbiol*., 2000; 66(12): 5536–5539.

Mentu, J. V.; Heitto, L.; Keitel, H. V.; Hakalehto, E. Rapid Microbiological Control of Paper Machines with PMEU Method. *Paperi ja Puu / Paper and Timber*, 2009; 91, 7-8.

Pesola, J.; Hakalehto, E. Enterobacterial microflora in infancy - a case study with enhanced enrichment. *Indian J. Pediatr*., 2011; 78(5),562-8.

Pesola, J.; Paakkanen, H..; Hakalehto, E. Enhanced diagnostics of pyelonephritis – a case study. *Int. J Med. Med. Sci*, 2012; 2, 273-277.

Pitkänen, T.; Miettinen, I. T.; Heitto, A.; Pesola, J.; Hakalehto, E. Enhanced enrichment and detection of thermotolerant Campylobacter species from water using the Portable Microbe Enrichment Unit and real-time PCR. *Can. J. Microbiol*., 2009; 55,849-58. doi: 10.1139/w09-040.

Quinto, E.J.; Arinder, p:; Axelsson, L.; Meir, E.; Holck, J.A.; Lindqvist, R.; Lindblad, M.; Andreou, P.; Lauzon, H.L.; Marteinsson, V.; Pin, C. Predicting and concentration of Verotoxin-producing *Escherichia coli* during processing and storage of fermented raw meat sausages. *Appl. Env.Microbiol.*, 2014; 80, 2715-2727.

Rollins, D. M.; Colwell, R. R. Viable but nonculturable stage of Campylobacter jejuni and its role in survival in the natural aquatic environment. *Appl. Environ. Microbiol*., 1986; 52,531–538.

Rutala, W.A.; Weber, D.J.Surface disinfection: should we do it? *Journal of Hospital Infection*, 2001; 48, Suppl A, S64-S68.

Rutala, W.A.; Weber, D.J. Guideline for disinfection and sterilization in healthcare facilities, 2008. Department of Health & Human Services, USA. 2008.

Sharan, R., Chhibber, S., Reed, R.H. Inactivation and sub-lethal injury of *salmonella* typhi, *salmonella* typhimurium and *vibrio cholera* in copper water storage vessels. *BMC Infect. Dis.*, 2011; 11, 204.

Sileika, T. S.; Kim, H.-D.; Maniak, P.; Messersmith, P. B. Antibacterial performance of polydopamine-modified polymer surfaces containing passive and active components," *ACS Appl. Mater. Interfaces*, 2011; 3, 4602-4610.

Slanetz, L. W.; Bartley, C. H. Numbers of enterococci in water, sewage and fecesdetermined by the membrane filter technique with an improved medium. *J. Bacteriol.*, 1957; 74, 591-595.

Smith, F. R. S. The role of microbial interactions in infectious disease. *Phil. Trans. R. Soc. Lond.,* B 1982; 297, 551-562.

Thomas, Y. O.; Lulves, W. J.; Kraft, A. A. A convenient surface plate method for bacteriological examination of poultry. *Journal of Food Science*, 1981; 46, 1951-1952.

van Belkum, A.; Durand, G.; Peyret, M.; Chatelier, S.; Zambardi, G.; Schrenzel, J.; Shortridge, D.; Engelhardt, A.; Dunne Jr. W. M. Rapid clinical bacteriology and its future impact. *Ann. Lab. Med.*, 2013; 33, 14-27.

Varghese, S.; Elfakhri, S.; Sheel, D. W., Sheel, P.; Bolton, F. J.; Foster, H. A. Novel anti-bacterial silver-silica surface coatings prepared by chemical vapour deposition for infection control. *J. Appl. Microbiol.*, 2013; 115, 1107-1116.

Wells, W. F. Airborne contagion and air hygiene. Publisher for The Commonwealth Fund by Harvard University Press, Cambridge Massachusetts, USA; 1955.

Wingfield, T.; Boccia, D.; Tovar, M.; Gavino, A.; Zevallo, K.; Montoya, R.; Lönnroth, K.; Evans, C. A. Defining catastrophic costs and comparing their importance for adverse tuberculosis outcome with multi-drug resistance: A prostective cohort study. Peru. *PLOS Med.*, 2014 11, doi:10.137/journal.pmed.1001675

Winslow, C. E. A.; Walker, L. T. Note on the fermentation of the B. coli group. *Science,* 1907; 26, 797.

Xu, H. S.; Roberts, N.; Singleton, F.L.; Attwell, R.W.; Grimes, D.J.; Colwell, R.R., Survival and viability of nonculturable *Escherichia coli* and *Vibrio cholerae* in the estuarine and marine environment, *Microb. Ecol.*, 1982; 8,313–323.

In: Microbiological Clinical Hygiene
Editor: Eino Elias Hakalehto
ISBN: 978-1-63463-428-1

Chapter 7

Legionella in Hospitals ("The Hidden Bacterium")

Robert Armon
Faculty of Civil & Environmental Engineering, Technion, Haifa, Israel

Abstract

Legionella spp. are aquatic bacteria colonizing water systems. When present in aerosols reaching the respiratory system of elderly persons the bacterium induces a lung disease resembling pneumonia with a primarily dry cough as one main symptom and in young person a flu like illness called Pontiac fever. Hospitals are excellent environments of *Legionella* infections due to predisposing clinical conditions of many patients. This bacterial pathogen is able to grow successfully in microbial biofilms and also to multiply within protozoa such as amoebae, hence preventing disinfectionefficiency.

1. Introduction

The term legion, a Roman military unit, originates from the Latin word "*legio*" (verb-*legere*) meaning "to choose". However, the unchosen disease Legionellosis originates from the American Legion (a United States' veterans organization of members of the Armed Forces, veterans, and their dependents) 1976' epidemic (Rumer, 1990), as well the bacterium nomenclature *Legionella* (acquired at July 1976 convention and further identified as the etiological agent) (Guthrie et al., 1987). The outbreak of a then-unknown "mystery disease" sickened 221 persons with 34 fatalities. Since then, several major outbreaks had been reported around the world (Table 1). Most of these major outbreaks were linked to: air conditioning, cooling towers and spa. Indeed, these sources have been studied for many years and identified as high risk sources of Legionellosis (Osawa et al., 2014, Graman et al., 1997, Coetzee et al., 2012).

Table 1. Worldwide major Legionellosis cases from 1976 to 2013

Year	City	Venue	Source	Cases	Deaths	Fatality rate	Comments and References
1976	Philadelphia, PA, US	Legionnaires Convention at the Bellevue-Stratford Hotel	Air Conditioning	221	34	15.4 %	First recognized outbreak of legionellosis McDade et al. (1979)
1985	Stafford, England, United Kingdom	**Stafford District Hospital**	Air Conditioning	175	28	16%	Epidemiological investigation traced the source of the infection to the air-conditioning cooling tower on the roof of Stafford District Hospital O'Mahony et al. (1990)
1999	Bovenkarspel, Netherlands	Westfriese Flora flower exhibition in Bovenkarspel	Hot tub	318	24	7.5%	The source of the bacteria was a hot tub in the exhibition area Den Boer et al. (2002)
2000	Melbourne, Australia	Melbourne Aquarium	Cooling tower	125	4	3.2%	Source of the infection traced to the cooling tower at the newly opened aquarium Greig et al. (2004)
2001	Murcia, Spain	**Hospital**	?	800	6	0.8%	The epidemiologic investigation implicated the cooling towers at a city hospital García-Fulgueiras et al. (2003)
2002	Barrow-in-Furness, UK	Barrow-in-Furness town's Forum 28 arts centre	Air conditioning	172	7	4.1%	The air-conditioning unit of a council-owned arts and leisure centre confirmed to be the source of infection Bennett et al. (2013)
2005	Toronto, Canada	Seven Oaks Home for the Aged	Cooling tower	127	21	16.5%	The source of the outbreak was traced to the air-conditioning cooling towers on the nursing home's roof Ng et al. (2009)
2005	Fredrikstad, Norway	Factory	Air scrubber	56	10	17.8%	Bacteria growing in an air scrubber of a nearby factory Olsen et al. (2010)

Year	City	Venue	Source	Cases	Deaths	Fatality rate	Comments and References
2010	Wales, United Kingdom	South Wales Valleys	Cooling towers ?	22	2	9%	Wide geographical distribution. Cooling towers in local industry (?) Keramarou and Evans (2010)
2012	Québec City, Canada	Lower Québec City	Possibly cooling towers	180	13	7.22%	Probably due to contaminated water in industrial cooling towers Anonymous (2012)
2012	Calp, Spain	AR Diamante Beach Hotel	Solar water heating system for spa and domestic hot water	18	3	17%	Anonymous (2012 a, b, c)
2012	Edinburgh, Scotland, UK	South west of Edinburgh	Possibly cooling towers	92	4	4.3%	Anonymous (2012d)
2012	Pittsburgh, Pennsylvania, US	**Veteran's Administration Hospital**	Unknown	22	6	27.3%	Anonymous (2013a)
2013*	Reynoldsburg, Ohio, US	Wesley Ridge Retirement Community	Potable water system	44	6	13.6%	Outbreak still in progress Gillespie (2013)
2013*	Warstein, Germany	Warsteiner Brewery	Air conditioning	165	2	1.2%	Outbreak still in progress Anonymous (2013b)

*Outbreak still in progress.

Note: Venue in bold characters is a hospital.

Historically, the bacterium has been discovered by Tatlock in 1943 that named it: "rickettsia-like organisms" later related to "Pittsburgh pneumonia agent" called TATLOCK and HEBA organisms (Tatlock, 1944, Bozeman et al., 1968). When these organisms were first grown on artificial media, they were shown to have identical cultural, biochemical, and antigenic characteristics. They also have the same cellular fatty-acid composition, and DNA relatedness indicating similar species (Hebert, 1959). Since then, a whole family has been defined: *Legionellaceae* that comprises one genus *Legionella,* 50 species and 70 serogroups (Fields et al., 2002).

From the 50 species 20 species other than *L. pneumophila* have been associated with human infections (Table 2). Today, the bacterium is mainly related to nosocomial infections in hospitals beside some environmental cases related to water contamination. Moreover, *Legionella* is responsible for 10%–50% of hospital-acquired pneumonia when a hospital's water system is colonized by *L. pneumophila* (Sabria and Yu, 2002). This chapter describes hospital Legionellosis, its health problem and reduction approaches based on our recent knowledge on disinfection.

Table 2. *Legionella* species and serogroups associated with human pathogenicity

Species	Number of serogroups associated with human disease
L. pneumophila	16
L. bozermanii	2
L. dumofii	1
L. micdadei	1
L. longbeachae	2
L. jordanis	1
L. wadsworthi	1
L. hackelae	2
L. feelii	2
L. maceachernii	1
L. birmingamensis	2
L. cincinnatiensis	1
L. gormanii	1
L. sainthelensi	2
L. tucsonensis	1
L. anisa	1
L. lansingensis	1
L. erythra	2
L. parisiensis	1
L. oakridgensis	1

2. The Bacterium

Legionellae is a thin gram negative organism (lightly staining with gram staining) pleomorphic (short rods and long filaments when grown on artificial medium, providing a preliminary identification). It is a fastidious microorganism able to grow on BCYE agar (Buffered Charcoal Yeast-Extract) supplemented with L-cysteine, but not without (Feeley et al., 1979). To prevent contamination with other bacteria, *Legionella* are plated onto BCYE with glycine vancomycin polymyxin cyclohexamide (GVPC) agar or MWY (BCYE with glycine, polymxin B, anisomycin and vancomycin) that contains dyes that will colour the target colonies aiding in their identification. Its growth is relatively slow: 3 to 5 days at 36 ± 0.5°C under aerobic conditions sometimes modified with ~5% CO_2 (found to enhance growth). Its fastidiousness is biochemically expressed of not being sugars fermentative (asaccharolytic) and deriving its energy from amino acids metabolism (Pine 1979). Retrospectively, these biochemical characteristics make sense as the main target of this pathogen is the lungs, where the majority of organics are proteins or glycoproteins and much less sugars! Another interesting feature of Legionella is its high membranal content of the phospholipid "phosphatidylcholine", as a major phospholipid. Legionella phosphatidylcholine is also an important virulence determinant and acts through multiple mechanisms. Dipalmitoyl phosphatidylcholine (aka: lecithin) is a major component of pulmonary surfactant and is often used in the L/S ratio to calculate foetal lung maturity. These biochemical overlapping may explain why Legionella has lungs as primary attack target! Non-fermentative and deriving energy from the metabolism of amino acids are other biochemical features of Legionella. Most of the species are motile and catalase and oxidase-positive (weakly), liquefy gelatin, and do not reduce nitrate or hydrolyze urea. From the macroscopic point of view, Legionella colonies show a "ground glass" or "opal" resemblance when illuminated. Another colonial characteristic is the mucoid behaviour when the colony is raised by a microbiological loop. A rapid biochemical test has been reported by Armon et al (1990) that used a biochemical test based on redox reaction of inoculated colonies and colour development producing a characteristic pattern or "metabolic fingerprint" from discrete test reactions performed within a 96 well microplate (Biolog Microbial ID System).

Initially, Legionellae were identified to the serogroups level by using polyclonal or monoclonal antisera (Luck et al., 1991). Currently, *L. pneumophila* serogroup 1 can be divided into a number of subtypes by various molecular techniques (Orsini and Romano-Spica, 2012, Luck et al., 1994, Lawrence et al., 1999). The various techniques include pulsed-field gel electrophoresis (PFGE), arbitrarily primed PCR (AP-PCR), electrophoretic alloenzyme typing, plasmid typing, restriction fragment length polymorphism, ribotyping and amplified fragment length polymorphism. Subtyping is used to match environmental isolates with those of patient isolates, obtained during epidemiological investigations of legionellosis outbreaks.

3. *Legionella* in Water

Legionella is an aquatic microorganism found in a variety of water sources such as: river, drinking water, water on plants in rainforests, groundwater, effluents and seawater (Riffard et al., 2001, Brooks et al., 2004, Ortiz-Roque and Hazen, 1987).

Natural and artificial aquatic environments, e.g., cooling towers, water systems in hotels and hospitals, homes, ships and factories, respiratory therapy equipment, fountains, misting devices and spa pools are the man made source of high risk of Legionella infections! In relation to spa pools, a recent publication reported on the presence and colonization of thermal saline waters used in balneotherapy! (Walczak et al., 2013). Hospitals as health-care facilities can hold the bacterium in its cold and hot-water systems or plumbing systems, cooling towers, bathing pools and dental units. Artificial water containing high sodium concentrations (up to 3%) nearly seawater has been proved to support Legionella survival in spite of early reports on its sensitivity to sodium ions in growth medium (Heller et al., 1998, Feeley et al., 1979). It should be pointed out that survival isn't equivalent to growth, as mentioned by Heller et al. (Heller et al., 1998) that also found sodium ions toxicity at concentrations > 1.2 % at 30-37°C expressed in reduced cell numbers. Water temperature is a crucial factor in Legionella colonization. Legionella can survive under extensive varying conditions, e.g., temperatures of 0°C–63°C, pH of 5.0–8.5 and dissolved oxygen (DO) concentrations as low as 0.2 ppm. Colonization of hot water tanks is more likely to occur if water temperatures are between 35°C and 46°C (95°F–115°F), which are known to be optimal (Fig. 1). At 50°C Legionella is capable to survive, however after 2 hours at this temperature its numbers drop by two orders of magnitude. Above 60°C Legionella is inactivated after 2 minutes (two orders of magnitude) and at > 70°C the inactivation is complete. Legionella can attach to and colonize various materials found in water systems, including plastics, rubber, metals and wood (Armon et al., 1997). Organic and inorganic sediment scales provide bacterium with a surface for attachment and a protective barrier.

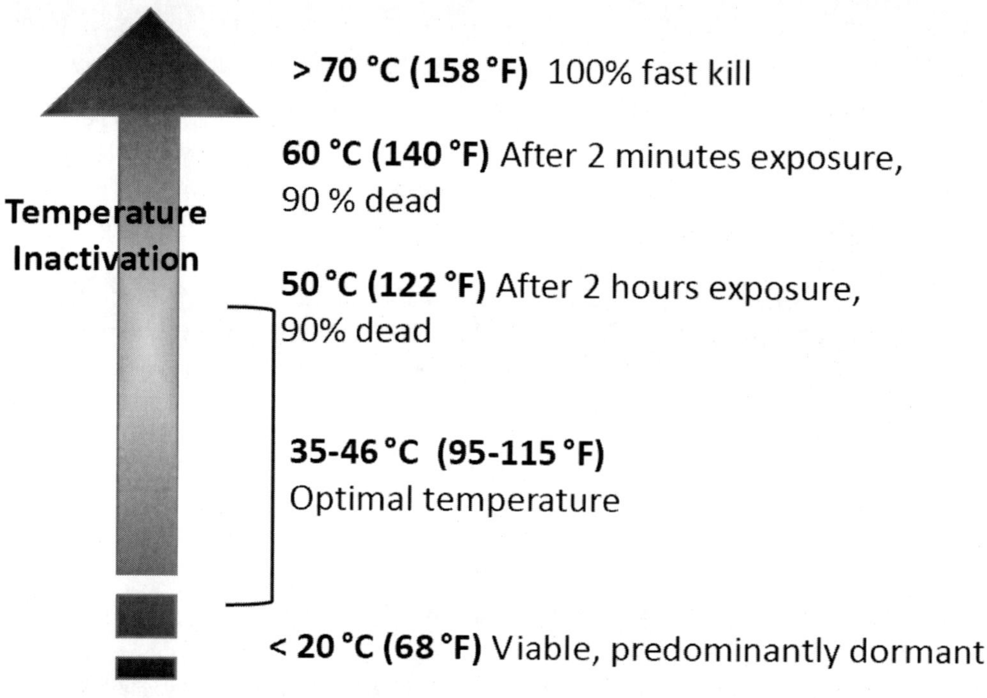

Figure 1. *Legionella* reaction to increasing temperatures.

In spite of its ubiquitous presence in water systems, Legionella bacterium is not contagious and the major infection route is via aspiration of aerosolized contaminated water! (Lin, 2010).

An interesting feature has been reported by Yarom et al (Yarom et al., 2010) on an Israeli survey of Legionella serogroups present in different water sources for a period of five years (2003-2007). The most frequently isolated species was *L. pneumophila* serogroup 3 (prevalence 60.44±5.6) followed by *L. pneumophila* serogroup 1 (26.98±5.2) and other serogroups and unidentified species (12.6±9.8). *L. pneumophila* serogroup 1 is the worldwide prevalent serogroup in water sources while serogroup 3 was only occasionally reported. Previous reports on *L. pneumophila* serogroup 1 as the main causative of respiratory disease in Israel revealed a drop from 52 to 15% in incidence during a 5-year survey, with a rise in the incidence of seropositivity to "other Legionellae", mainly sg. 3. Figure 2 shows the good correlation between waterborne Legionella and hospital cases (Yarom et al., 2010). As antigenuria is the main clinical tool to detect Legionellosis among infected patients; the shift from serogroup 1 to serogroup 3 in water sources will go undetected for obvious reasons. The process of serogroups prevalence shift in water sources is an interesting issue that has to be investigated further in order to advance our understanding of Legionella epidemiology.

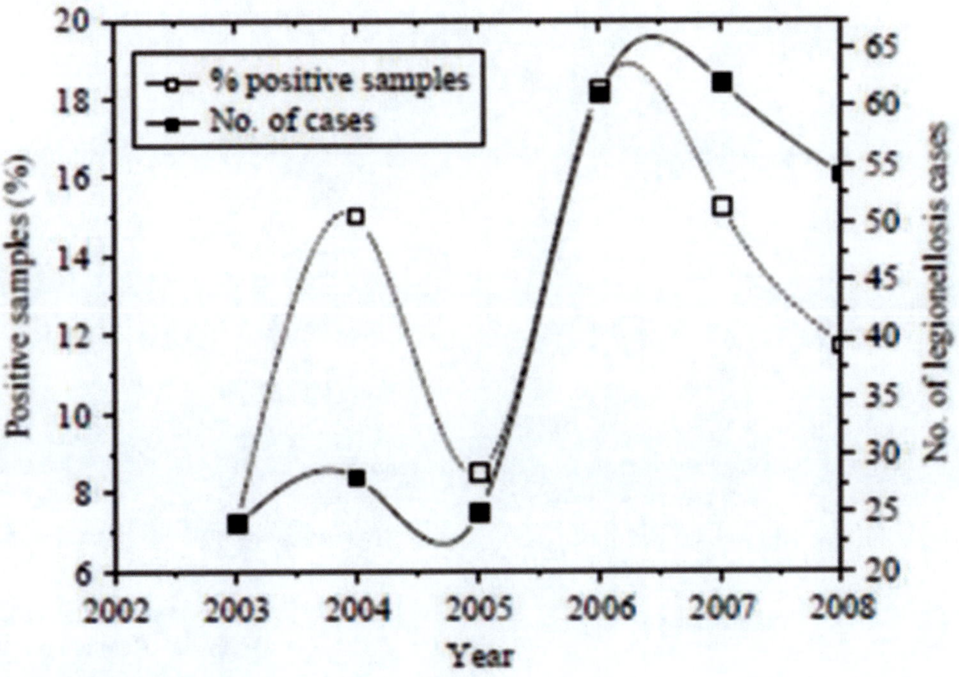

Figure 2. Correlation of Legionellosis cases to positive water samples prevalence (%) in Israel for 2003–2008. Legionellosis cases from 2003 to 2008 were adapted from www.GIDEONonline.com (Anonymous 2009) (Yarom et al., 2010).

4. *Legionella* and Protozoa ("Relatives of Human Macrophages")

Legionella primary infection occurs in lungs through aspiration of contaminated water aerosols. Basically there are two pathways of intracellular trafficking: one that deals with any avirulent bacteria and a second one that deals with virulent strains of *Legionella pneumophila* (Figure 3). An avirulent bacterium is contained by a macrophage cell in its phagosome that moves along the endosomal route to gradually mature into a lysosome (phagosome-lysosome fusion) which inactivates and degrades the bacterium through a series of enzymatic and oxidation processes. A virulent bacterium such as the case of *L. pneumophila* is able to escape the above endo-lysosomal pathway facilitated by its effector proteins that enter the host cell through the Dot/Icm type IV secretion system. Then proteins and transport vesicles are recruited to ***Legionella***-containing vacuole (LCV), which is slowly transformed into a ribosome-studded compartment that mimics host-cell rough endoplasmic reticulum (ER) and supports replication of ***L. pneumophila***. Ultimately, the host cell is lyzed, and ***L. pneumophila*** bacteria are released to infect other macrophages (Figure. 3).

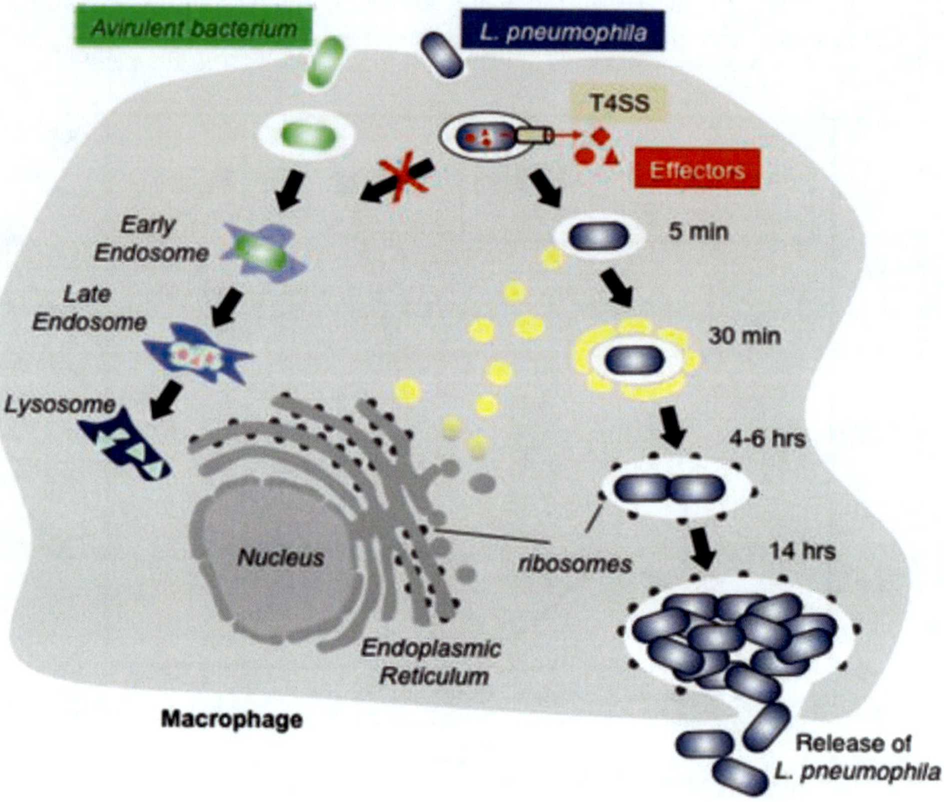

Figure 3. Time scale of a virulent *L.pneumophila* intracellular pathways compared to an avirulent bacterium degraded by a macrophage (Machner, 2011). Effectors (red color); Proteins and transport vesicles (yellow); Ribosomes (dark blue).

A similar infection pathway is followed by virulent *L. pneumophila* in a protozoan infection (Bandyopadhyay et al., 2004). *Legionella* are able to infect different genera of amoebae among which *Hartmanella vermiformis* and *Acanthamoeba* spp. are the most well-known as well to multiply successfully in *Tetrahymena* spp (ciliated protozoa) (Rowbotham, 1980, Lasheras et al., 2006, Kikuhara et al., 1994). Amoebae that form cysts under extreme conditions (thermal, pH or disinfection chemicals) while infected with *Legionella* facilitate protection of this bacterium from those effects (Lasheras et al., 2006, Barker et al., 1992, Storey et al., 2004). Infected amoebic cysts beside biofilms are the main challenge in the disinfection process against *Legionella* in all water sources.

5. *Legionella* and Biofilm

Biofilms are found in many water supply systems where they form an environment in which different bacteria are entrapped for long periods. Besides the aesthetic aspect, biofilm has a major contribution in biocorrosion, disinfection inefficiency and possibly may act as a reservoir for pathogenic and non-pathogenic microorganisms. Biofilms, a multi bacterial aggregation onto surfaces, are one of the *Legionella* protected shelter. Bacterial species that appear to provide *Legionella* with growth-promoting factors include *Pseudomonas* spp., *Acinetobacter* spp., *Flavobacterium*, and *Alcaligenes* spp. (Armon et al., 1997, Stewart et al.,. 2012). On the other hand, some bacteria were found inhibitory to *Legionella* for example

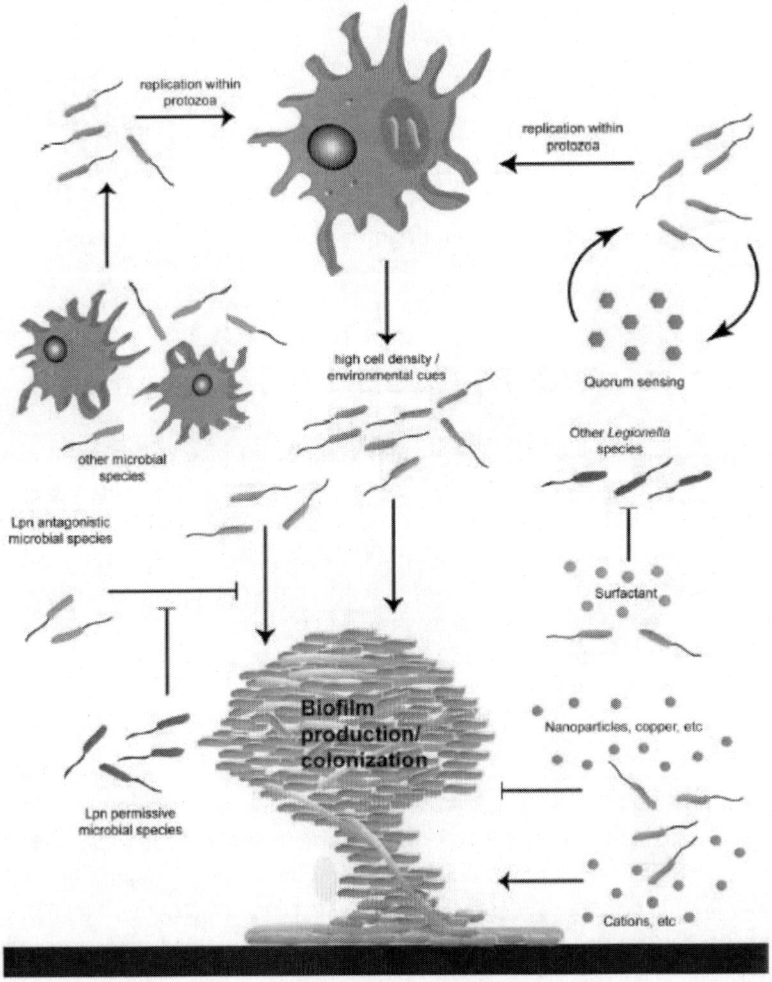

Figure 4. *Legionellapneumophila* colonization and growth in biofilms mediated by other bacterial species and environmental cues. (Reproduced with permission from Abdel-Nour et al., 2013). Orange bacteria (L. pneumophila, Lpn); Blue bacteria (Permissive bacteria e.g., *Klebsiella pneumoniae*); Red bacteria (other *Legionella*spp. inhibited by *L. pneumophila* surfactant secreted by protein TolC)(Stewart et al., 2011); Green dots (Quorum sensing through the autoinducer LAI-1 (3-hydroxypentadecane-4-one) (Schell et al., 2014); Brown bacteria (other bacterial species).

P. aeruginosa while others are permissive, alleviating the inhibition e.g., *K. pneumoniae* (Kimura et al., 2009, Mampel et al., 2006, Stewart et al., 2012). In this context, it should be mentioned that biofilms are composed of various bacterial species, with a definite stratification array creating physiological conditions that may permit *Legionella* colonization in spite of released inhibitors. In this complex environment, amoebae are also present (normally feeding on biofilm biomass) accessible to *Legionella* infection through phagocytosis (Figure 4).

In our laboratory, *Legionella pneumophila* was introduced into a biofilm simulation flow system supplied with sterile and non-sterile tap water. *L. pneumophila* survival into a biofilm formed on glass and PVC coupons at two temperatures (24°C and 36°C) were examined (Armon et al., 1997). On glass supports, under sterile conditions at 36°C, *Legionella pneumophila* sg3 decreased by 6 logs during 40 days of continuous recirculation. Under non-sterile conditions, *L. pneumophila* decreased by only half log after <48 days. At 24°C, *L pneumophila* remained stable for >40 days under sterile conditions, while under non-sterile conditions, *it* dropped by one log for the time interval of 35 days. *L pneumophila* colonizing PVC coupons at 36°C survived better compared with glass support. The experimental reveled that survival of pathogenic microorganisms into biofilms is variable and depends on many factors, making the survival prediction a difficult task. However, the survival results of *L. pneumophila* in time terms should raise important questions on their potential threat in water distribution systems.

6. *Legionella* in Health-Care Facilities

Health-care facilities include hospitals, health centers, hospices, residential care facilities and dialysis units. In these institutions the main problem lays in the presence of immunocompromised people or with so called predisposing risk factors for *Legionella* infections (case–fatality rate up to 50%) (Yu, 2000). For instance, through epidemiological and microbiological investigation the world's biggest outbreak of legionellosis (Murcia, Spain in 2001 with 449 confirmed cases) was shown to be associated with an air-conditioning cooling towers of a city hospital (Garcia-Fulgueiras et al., 2003).

7. Disinfection Efficiency against *Legionella*

There are more than six methods of disinfection against *Legionella*. The following describes methods that have been well documented and the advantages and disadvantages are discussed. It should be remembered that the success is measured in terms of experience gained through practical use of the variety of disinfectants in a variety of health-care institutions.

Copper-Silver Ionization

The process of dissolution of copper and silver through ionization has been in use since Olympic swimmers could not endure the scorching effect of chlorine. Both ions have a bactericidal effect on a variety of water bacteria, independent of water temperature. In hospitals, installation and maintenance of such a devise is easy and does not require special installments. It should be that oral consumption is limited especially for persons with kidney problems; however it has a prolonged efficacy especially because copper and silver ions accumulate in biofilms and water circulation. A copper concentration of 0.2-0.8 ppm and 0.01-0.08 ppm of silver are the recommended concentrations for efficient disinfection; for *Legionella* bacterium a concentration of 0.2-0.4 ppm copper and 0.02-0.04 ppm silver is sufficient. Interference with the process has been reported in such cases where water pH was above 8.5 or phosphates were present in water (Lin et al., 2002, Lin and Vidic, 2006). Another significant issue is the emergence of resistance as reported in few hospitals, several years after system installation, but the resistance prevalence is unknown (Mietzner et al., 2005). In summary, it seems that copper-silver ionization fulfills the standardized evaluation criteria established for disinfection methods and is the less corrosive than all other oxidants employed today in disinfection! (Stout and Yu, 2003). Those criteria are listed below:

1) In vitro efficacy.
2) Reports on practical experience in hospitals.
3) Scientific reports of controlled studies on successful hospital disinfection for prolonged terms (years).
4) Validation step-confirmatory reports from multiple hospitals also for long terms follow-up.

Chlorine Dioxide (ClO_2)

This gas in solution has been used since 1940 in Europe for water treatment. Now is also used for *Legionella* disinfection in USA. It can be generated on site via mix of chemical precursors or electrochemical generation. In contrast to copper-silver ionization, chlorine dioxide is affected by elevated temperatures and reduced concentrations are detected after temperature increases (e.g., in cold water of a New York hospital, the residual chlorine dioxide in cold water was 0.3-0.5 ppm while in hot water it dropped to 0.04 ppm) (Zhang et al., 2007) . In United Kingdom, a hospital positive for *Legionella* in water system required an injection of 3–5 ppm of ClO_2 into the hot water supply to achieve a 0.25–0.5 mg/L free residual concentration at tap (Makin, 1998).

In summary, chlorine dioxide has a superior biofilms' penetration compared to chlorine. It produces by-products such as chlorite and chlorate (not carcinogenic) and still corrosive (reaction with magnetite-Fe3O4 from galvanized pipes) however less than chlorine. It is effective over a wide range of pH-s compared to chlorine and copper-silver ionization, but less effective at higher temperature as already mentioned.

Monochloramine

Monochloramine has been proved to be efficient against *Legionella* in plumbing systems (Donlan et al., 2002). Due to its amine group it has a better biofilm penetration capability and has higher disinfection ability at a wider pH range compared to copper-silver ionization and chlorine. On the disadvantage side, monochloamine installation and production is problematical as hypochlorous acid is injected upstream and ammonia downstream which may result in three components simultaneously present in water system: chlorine, ammonia and monochloramine due to poor mixing! In addition, monochloramine has an unpleasant smell when mixed in water, can cause anemia in patients undergoing hemodialysis, supports the growth of other bacteria (e.g., *Mycobacterium* spp.), presence of nitrogen compounds and increased lead leaching (Pryor et al., 2004, Lin et al., 2000).

Hyperchlorination

By definition, hyperchlorination is the use of chlorine in excess. As such, it was abandoned due to its major disadvantages: high cost, poor biofilm penetration, persistance of *Legionella* in the system and strong corrosive activity damaging the pipes systems (increasing maintenance cost) and formation of carcinogens in water (Muraca et al., 1990).

Ozone

Ozone is a very strong oxidizing chemical with high potential to inactivate *Legionella* as well other water pathogens. However as already mentioned in this chapter, ozone does not have a residual to maintain a certain concentration of disinfectant in water system, e.g., chlorine, chlorine dioxide, etc. Therefore it should be used only in cases were a thorough disinfection is needed or in combination with other residual producing oxidants. Muraca et al. (1987) evaluated ozone in vitro as a *Legionella pneumophila* control method in a plumbing system. Their studies showed effective control at 1-2 ppm residual in water; however they also mentioned that because the rapid decomposition of the ozone it may be limited as a supplemental. In our laboratory, ozone was evaluated on *L. pneumophila* at a Ct value of 1.05 mg min l^{-1} at 12 °C and pH 7, resulted in a 2 logs reduction of viable cells, in comparison to *E. coli* that under same condition required a Ct of 0.009 mg min l^{-1} and has been reduced by 4 logs (personal communication). In a recent study, ozone has been applied at low levels at various pH-s and 40°C (simulating bathtub water) (Nakamura et al., 2012). These authors reported that the dissolved ozone concentration decreased rapidly when phosphate was present in the high pH range. However, in the absence of phosphate at an ozone concentration of 0.026 ppm after 3 minutes, *L. pneumophila* was completely inactivated at 40°C and at a pH range of 5.8-9.5.

Heat Shock Treatment

Heat shock treatment is perhaps the most well-known disinfection process against *Legionella* in hospitals. It is easy to perform as the thermostat can be controlled to reach 60-70°C and kept at these temperatures to flush the hot water systems including taps. However it needs special care to prevent patients' burns and accidents along the process. It is also costly because of energy investment and in large hospitals it requires prolonged time to reach these elevated temperatures. In a recent publication, Farhat et al. (2010) evaluated thermal inactivation at pilot scale unit for *Legionella* elimination from biofilm in a hot water network. Their results revealed that thermal inactivation ended up in a rapid recolonization of the system as well uncompleted biofilm destruction. In addition, they showed that following a second heat shock treatment *Legionella* developed thermo-acclimation! The final conclusion was "Thermal disinfection does not seem to be efficient enough to eliminate *Legionella* when it is used as a curative treatment". Regarding amoeba cysts inactivation by thermal shock, Cervero-Aragó et al. (Cervero-Aragó et al., 2013) showed effectiveness of thermal treatments at 60 and 70°C that was higher for both life stages (throphozoites and cysts) of *Hartmannella vermiformis* strains in comparison with *Acanthamoeba* strains, where *Acanthamoeba* cysts proved to be the most resistant.

Point-of-Use Filtration

Filtration is perhaps the best method to remove bacteria from water systems without chemical addition, although it has a major bottle neck: water should be free of particulate matter otherwise the filter is rapidly clogged. Filters with 0.2 μm pore size is expected to remove all known bacteria by size exclusion and could be used to prevent nosocomial infections in high-risk units such as: transplant and intensive care.

The main advantage beside complete bacteria exclusion is its cost-effectiveness and good tolerance by patients. Due to the small pore size, it prones to fast clogging and is limited to relatively small volumes of water (best in small specialized hospital units).

UV Light

UV irradiation has the same advantage as point-of-use filtration as no chemicals are added to water. Its efficiency is dependent on the input water quality (no particulate matter) and reduced biofilms presence as UV light point-of-entry assemble does not allow distal eradication of *Legionella* within biofilm. UV is more effective when combined with another chemical disinfectant such as chlorine dioxide or else. One of the main requirements from a disinfectant is to have residual and this is not the case with UV that is an effective disinfectant of surfaces only (Franzin et al., 2002).

Table 3. Various parameters of disinfection methods used to eradicate *Legionella* in hospital (Lin et al., 2011)

Method	Concentration (ppm)	Advantage	Disadvantage	Hospital size	Cost ($)
Copper-silver ionization	Copper :0.20–0.80 mg/L Silver: 0.01–0.08 mg/L	Easy installation & maintenance	Interference with high pHs (> 8.5)	250 beds 1200 beds	$40,000–$50,000 for a hot water recirculating line and $80,000–$100,000 for both hot and cold water treatment. $200,000
Chlorine dioxide	3-5 mg/L to achieve 0.25–0.5 mg/L residual in hot water	Biofilm good penetration; biocidal activity along a wide range of pHs	Maintenance of an effective residual chlorine; formation of chlorate and chlorite	438 beds	$34,000 per year for 2 units maintenance; ClO_2, chlorite and chlorite monitoring ~$ 40,000
Monochloramine	Free chlorine concentration of 0.39-0.38 mg/L and an ammonia concentration of 0.045 mg/L	Stable residual and good biofilm penetration; wider pH range of activity	On site generation complex; nitrogen compounds generation	-	-
Hyperchlorination	2048–4096 ppm	Highly active against planktonic bacteria	Corrosion; increase in THMs; poor biofilm penetration; recolonization	-	Very expensive
Ozone	1-2ppm free residual	Strong oxidant; effective for shock inactivation	No residual; phosphate interference	-	Expensive
Heat shock treatment	60-70°C	Effective for short term against planktonic bacteria	Thermo-acclimation of Legionella	-	Expensive
Point -of use filtration	0.2 mm filters	Very effective in removal of planktonic bacteria	Limited use for special units only; fast clogging	-	Cost effective
UV	289 to 860 μW sec/cm^2 low-pressure mercury-vapor discharge lamp	Effective at very low UVGI dosage	No residual; does not allow distal eradication; particulate matter interference	-	~$100.000 to $150.000 For a high volume continuous device

Conclusion

Table 3 summarizes the disinfection methods tested on site or at laboratory scale to eradicate *Legionella* bacterium. In relation to hospitals where the health priority is very high and nosocomial infections are to be limited to a minimum, it seems that a holistic approach such as chlorine dioxide and chlorine (as bleach or obtained by electro-chlorination) are the most effective treatments where chlorine dioxide shows a longer residual activity (Loret et al., 2005). In Israel, the company C.Q.M. developed an electro-chlorination and electro-oxidation device for warm and hot water disinfection called SRBL. According to their results and claims, the system consistently delivers zero *Legionella* and bacteria count in the mandated periodic water tests conducted in Israeli hospitals. SRBL effectively eliminates bacteria and *Legionella* at returning water temperatures of 35-50°C, providing significant energy savings by reducing heated water temperature from the recommended 60°C.

References

Abdel-Nour, M; Duncan, C; Low, DE; Guyard, C. Biofilms: the stronghold of *Legionella pneumophila*. *Int J Mol Sci*, 2013; 14(11), 21660-21675.

Anonymous. (2013a) Report: Healthcare Inspection Legionnaires' Disease at the VA Pittsburgh Healthcare System Pittsburgh, Pennsylvania. Department of Veterans Affairs Office of Inspector General. 2013a. 2013-04-23. pp 36. http://www.va.gov/oig / pubs/VAOIG-13-00994-180.pdf

Anonymous. (2013b) Legionnaires bacteria found at leading brewery.. *Retrived 2014-06-11.* http://www.thelocal.de/20130912/51877.

Anonymous. DRSP - Direction régionale de santé publique de la Capitale-Nationale. (in French) 2012a. Retrieved 2013-08-25.

Anonymous. GIDEON—the Global Infectious Disease Epidemiology Network. 2009. http://www.gideononline.com

Anonymous. Legionnaires' Disease outbreak: Third death reported. 2012c. 2012-07-03. Retrieved 2012-07-03. http://www.bbc.com/news/uk-scotland-18693873

Anonymous. Outbreak of *Legionella*in South West Edinburgh. 2012d. 2012-07-18. http://www.nhslothian.scot.nhs.uk/MediaCentre/PressReleases/2012/Pages/*Legionella*SouthWestEdinburgh.aspx

Anonymous. Three British pensioners die after Legionnaires' Disease outbreak 'at Spanish beach hotel. *The Daily Mail.* 2012b. 2012-02-04. Retrieved 2012-02-07. http://www.dailymail.co.uk/news/article-2095709/Legionnaires-outbreak-3-British-pensioners-die-disease-AR-Diamante-Beach-Hotel-Spain.html

Armon, R, I. Potasman, I, Green, M. Biochemical fingerprints of Legionellae spp. by the BIOLOG system: presumptive identification of clinical and environmental isolates. *Lett Appl Microbiol,* 1990; 11, 290 – 292,

Armon, R; Starosvetzky, J; Arbel, T; Green, M. Survival of *Legionella pneumophila* and *Salmonella typhimurium* in biofilm systems. *Water Sci Technol,* 1997; 35 (11–12), 293–300.

Bandyopadhyay, P; Xiao, H; Coleman, HA; Price-Whelan A; Steinman, HM. Icm/Dot-Independent Entry of *Legionella pneumophila* into Amoeba and Macrophage Hosts. *Infect Immun*, 2004; 72(8), 4541–4551.

Barker, J; Brown, MR; Collier, PJ; Farrell, I; Gilbert, P. Relationship between *Legionella pneumophila* and acanthamoeba polyphaga: Physiological status and susceptibility to chemical inactivation. *Appl Environ Microbiol,* 1992; 58, 2420–2425.

Bennett, E; Ashton, M; Calvert, N; Chaloner, J; Cheesebrough, J; Egan, J; Farrell, I; Hall, I; Harrison, TG; Naik, FC; Partridge, S; Syed, Q; Gent, RN. Barrow-in-Furness: a large community legionellosis outbreak in the UK. *Epidemiol Infect,*2013; 11, 1-15.

Bozeman, FM; Humphries, JW; Campbell, JM. A new group of rickettsia- like agents recovered from guinea pigs. *Acta Virol (Praha),* 1968; 12, 87-93.

Brooks, T; Osicki, R; Springthorpe, V; Sattar S; Filion, L; Abrial, D; Riffard, S. Detection and identification of *Legionella* species from groundwaters. *J Toxicol Environ Health,* 2004; Part A, 67, 1845–1859.

Cervero-Aragó, S; Rodríguez-Martínez, S; Canals, O; Salvadó, H; Araujo, RM. Effect of thermal treatment on free-living amoeba inactivation. *J Appl Microbiol,* 2013; 116, 728-736.

Coetzee, N; Duggal, H; Hawker, J; Ibbotson, S; Harrison, TG; Phin, N; Laza-Stanca, V; Johnston, R; Iqbal, Z; Rehman, Y; Knapper, E; Robinson, S; Aigbogun, N. An outbreak of Legionnaires' disease associated with a display spa pool in retail premises, Stoke-on-Trent, United Kingdom, July 2012. *Euro Surveillance*, 2012; 17 (37).

Den Boer, JW; Yzerman, EPF; Schellekens, J; Lettinga, KD; Boshuizen, HC; Van Steenbergen, JE; Bosman, A; Van den Hof, S; Van Vilet, HA; Peeters, MF; Van Ketel, RJ; Speelman, P; Kool, JL; Conyn-Van Spaendonck, MA. A Large Outbreak of Legionnaires' Disease at a Flower Show, the Netherlands, 1999. *Emerging Infect Dis,* 2002; 8(1), 37-43.

Donlan, R; Murga, R; Carpenter, J; Brown, E; Besser, R; Fiedis, Barry. Monochloramine disinfection of biofilm-associated *Legionella pneumophila* in a potable water model system. In: Marre R, Abu Kwaik Y, Bartlett C, Cianciotto NP, Fields BS, Frosch M, Hacker J, Lück PC editors. *Legionella*. Washington, DC: American Society for Microbiology; 2002; 406–410.

Farhat, M; Trouilhé, M-C; Briand, E; Moletta-Denat M; Robine, E; Frère, J. Development of a pilot-scale 1 for *Legionella* elimination in biofilm in hot water network: heat shock treatment evaluation. *Journal of Applied Microbiology,* 2010; 108, 1073–1082.

Feeley, JC; Gibson, RJ; Gorman, GW; Langford, NC; Rasheed, JK; Mackel DC; Baine, WB. Charcoal yeast-extract agar: a primary isolation medium for *Legionella pneumophila. J Clin Microbiol*, 1979; 10, 437-441.

Fields, BS; Benson, RF; Besser, RE. *Legionella* and Legionnaires' disease: 25 years of investigations. *Clin Microb Rev,* 2002; 15, 506-526.

Franzin, L; Cabodi, D; Fantino, C. Evaluation of the efficacy of ultraviolet radiation for disinfection of hospital water contaminated by *Legionella. J Hosp Infect,* 2002; 51, 269–274.

García-Fulgueiras, A; Navarro, C; Fenoll, D; García, J; González-Diego, P; Jiménez-Buñuales, T; Rodriquez, M; Lopez, R; Pacheco, F; Ruiz, J; Segovia, M; Balandrón, B; Pelaz, C. Legionnaires' Disease Outbreak in Murcia, Spain. *Emerging Infect Dis*, 2003; 9(8), 915-921.

Gillespie C. Legionnaires' Outbreaks In Wisconsin and Ohio. Food Poisoning Bulletin, 2013. Retrived 2014-07-05. http://foodpoisoningbulletin.com/2013/legionnaires-outbreaks-in-wisconsin-and-ohio/

Graman, PS; Quinlan, GA; Rank, JA. Nosocomial legionellosis traced to a contaminated ice machine. *Infection Control and Hospital Epidemiology*, 1997; 18 (9): 637–40.

Greig, JE; Carnie, JA; Tallis, GF; Ryan, NJ; Tan, Ag; Gordon, IR; Zwolak, B; Leydon, JA; Guest, CS; Hart, WG. An outbreak of Legionnaires' disease at the Melbourne Aquarium, April 2000: investigation and case–control studies. *Med J Aust,* 2004; 180 (11), 566-572.

Guthrie, PJ; Silberg, SL; Lawrence, CH. *Legionella pneumophila* infections in Oklahoma: prevalence among VA hospital patients prior to the 1976 Philadelphia outbreak. *J Okla State Med Assoc*, 1987; 80(8), 585-588.

Hébert, GA; Moss, CW; McDougal, LK; Bozeman, FM; McKinney, RM; Brenner, DJ. The rickettsia-like organisms TATLOCK (1943) and HEBA (1959): bacteria phenotypically similar to but genetically distinct from *Legionella* pneumophila and the WIGA bacterium. *Ann Intern Med*, 1959; 92, 45-52.

Heller, R; Höller, C; Süssmuth, R; Gundermann, KO. Effect of salt concentration and temperature on survival of *Legionella pneumophila. Lett Appl Microbiol,* 1998; 26(1), 64-68.

Keramarou, M; Evans, MR. A community outbreak of Legionnaires' disease in South Wales, August–September 2010. *Eurosurveillance*, 2010; 15(42), 1-4.

Kikuhara, H; Ogawa, M; Miyamoto, H; Nikaido, Y; Yosihada, S. Intracellular multiplication of *Legionella pneumophila* in *Tetrahymena thermophile*. *J UOEH.,* 1994 16, 263–275.

Kimura, S; Tateda, K; Ishii, Y; Horikawa, M; Miyari, S; Gotoh, N; Ishiquro, M; Yamaquchi, K. *Pseudomonas aeruginosa* Las quorum sensing autoinducer suppresses growth and biofilm production in *Legionella* species. *Microbiol,* 2009; 155(Pt 6), 1934-1939.

Lasheras, A; Boulestreau, H; Rogues, AM; Ohayon-Courtes, C; Labadie, JC; Gachie, JP. Influence of amoebae and physical and chemical characteristics of water on presence and proliferation of *Legionella*species in hospital water systems. *Am J Infect Control,* 2006; 34, 520–525.

Lawrence, C; Ronco, E; Dubrou, S; Leclercq, R; Nauciel, C; Matsiota-Bernard, P. Molecular typing of *Legionella pneumophila* serogroup 1 isolates from patients and the nosocomial environment by arbitrarily primed PCR and pulsed-field gel electrophoresis. *J Med Microbiol,* 1999; 48(4), 327-333.

Lin, YE. *Legionella* in water systems. In: Amjad Z, editor. *The Science and Technology of Industrial Water Treatment*. Boca Raton, FL, USA: *CRC Press*; 2010; 411-420.

Lin, YE; Janet, E; Stout, JE; Yu, VL. Controlling *Legionella* in Hospital Drinking Water: An Evidence-Based Review of Disinfection Methods. *Infect Control Hosp Epidemiol,* 2011; 32(2), 166-173.

Lin, YE; Vidic, RD. Possible phosphate interference with copper-silver ionization for *Legionella* control. *J Hosp Infect,* 2006; 62, 119.

Lin, YE; Yu, VL; Vidic, RD; States, SJ. Discussion of monochloramine and Legionnaires' disease. *J Am Water Works Assoc*, 2000; 92, 88–90.

Lin, YS; Vidic, RD; Stout, JE; Yu, VL. Negative effect of high pH on biocidal efficacy of copper and silver ions in controlling *Legionella pneumophila*. *Appl Environ Microbiol,* 2002; 68, 2711–2715.

Loret, JF; Robert, S; Thomas, V; Cooper, AJ; McCoy, WF; Lévi, Y. Comparison of disinfectants for biofilm, protozoa and *Legionella* control. *J Water Health*, 2005; 3(4), 423-433.

Luck, PC; Bender, L; Ott, M; Helbig, JH; Hacker, J. Analysis of *Legionella* pneumophila Serogroup 6 Strains Isolated from a Hospital Warm Water Supply over a Three-Year Period by Using Genomic Long-Range Mapping Techniques and Monoclonal Antibodies. *Appl Environ Microbiol,* 1991; 57(11), 3226-3231.

Luck, PC; Dinger, E; Helbig, JH; Thurm, V; Keuchel, H; Presch, C; Ott, M. Analysis of *Legionella pneumophila* strains associated with nosocomial pneumonia in a neonatal intensive care unit. *Eur J Clin Microbiol Infect Dis,* 1994; 13(7), 565-571.

Machner, MP; *The Machner Lab: Unit on Microbial Pathogenesis*. Eunice Kennedy Shriver National Institute of Child Health and Human Development. 2011. Last accessed on May 2014. https://science.nichd.nih.gov.

Makin,T. Control of *Legionella* in domestic water systems and potential energy savings resulting from the control of *Legionella*e with chlorine dioxide. In: Program and abstracts of the 15th IFHE Congress; 1998; Edinburgh, Scotland.

Mampel, J; Spirig, T; Weber, SS; Haagensen, JA; Molin, S; Hilbi, H. Planktonic replication is essential for biofilm formation by *Legionella* pneumophila in a complex medium under static and dynamic flow conditions. *Appl Environ Microbiol,* 2006; 72(4), 2885-2895.

McDade, JE; Brenner, DJ; Boeman, FM. Legionnaires' disease bacterium isolated in 1947. *Ann Intern Med,* 1979; 90, 659-661.

Mietzner, M; Hangard, A; Stout, JE; Rohr, U; Pedro-Botet, ML; Samore, MH; Yu, VL. Reduced susceptibility of *Legionella pneumophila* to the antimicrobial effects of copper and silver ions. 45th Interscience Conference on Antimicrobial Agents and Chemotherapy, December 16–19, 2005; Washington, DC.

Muraca, P; Stout, J; Yu, V. Comparative assessment of chlorine, heat, ozone, and UV light for killing *Legionella pneumophila* within a model plumbing system. *Appl Environ Microbiol,* 1987; 53(2), 447-453.

Muraca, PW; Yu, VL; Goetz, A. Disinfection of water distribution systems for *Legionella*: a review of application procedures and methodologies. *Infect Control Hosp Epidemiol,* 1990; 11, 79–88.

Nakamura, K; Doi, H; Hizuika, T; Edagawa, A. Disinfection efficacy of low levels of dissolved ozone against *Legionella pneumophila* at various pHs and 40°C. *Bokin Bobai,* 2012; 40(2), 75-79 (In Japanese).

Ng V, Tang P, Jamieson F, Guyard C et al (2009) Laboratory-based evaluation of legionellosis epidemiology in Ontario, Canada, 1978 to 2006. *BMC Infect Dis,* 9:68 doi:10.1186/1471-2334-9-68.

Olsen, JS; Aarskaug, T; Thrane, I; Pourcel, C; Ask, E; Johansen, G; Waagen, V; Blatny, JM. Alternative routes for dissemination of *Legionella* pneumophila causing three outbreaks in Norway. *Environ Sci Technol*, 2010; 44(22), 8712-8717.

O'Mahony, MC; Stanwell-Smith, RE; Tillett, HE; Harper, D; Hutchinson, DN; Lee, JV; Dennis, PJ; Duggal, HV; Scully, JA; Denne, C. The Stafford outbreak of Legionnaires' disease. *Epidemiol Infect*, 1990; 104(3), 361-80.

Orsini, M; Romano-Spica, V. A rapid PFGE protocol for typing Legionella isolates from fresh or frozen samples. *J Infect Chemother,* 2012; 18(5), 747-752.

Ortiz-Roque, CM; Hazen, TC. Abundance and distribution of *Legionellaceae* in Puerto Rican waters. *Appl Environ Microbiol*, 1987; 53, 2231–2236.

Osawa, K; Shigemura, K; Abe, Y; Jukimoto, T; Yoshida, H; Fujisawa, M; Arakawa, S. A case of nosocomial *Legionella* pneumonia associated with a contaminated hospital cooling tower. *Journal of Infection and Chemotherapy,* 2014; 20 (1), 68–70.

Pine, L; George, JR; Reeves, MW; Harrel, WK. The development of a chemically defined liquid medium for the growth of *Legionella pneumophila. J Clin Microbiol,* 1979 9, 615-626.

Pryor, M; Springthorpe, S; Riffard, S; Brooks, T; Huo, Y; Davis, G; Sattar, SA. Investigation of opportunistic pathogens in municipal drinking water under different supply and treatment regimes. *Water Sci Technol,* 2004; 50, 83–90.

Riffard, S; Douglass, S; Brooks, T; Springthorpe, S; Filion, LG; Sattar, SA. Occurrence of *Legionella* in groundwater: an ecological study. *Water Sci Technol,* 2001; 43, 99–102.

Rowbotham, TJ. Preliminary report on the pathogenicity of *Legionella pneumophila* for freshwater and soil amoebae. *J Clin Pathol*, 1980; 33, 1179-1183.

Rumer, TA. The American Legion: An Official History, 1919-1989. New York: *M. Evans;* 1990.

Sabria, M; Yu, VL. Hospital-acquired legionellosis: Solutions for a preventable infection. *Lancet Infect Dis,* 2002; 2, 368–373.

Schell, U; Kessler, A; Hilbi, H. Phosphorylation signalling through the *Legionella* quorum sensing histidine kinases LqsS and LqsT converges on the response regulator LqsR. *Mol Microbiol*, 2014 92(5), 1039-1055.

Stewart, CR; Burnside, DM; Cianciotto, NP. The surfactant of *Legionella*pneumophila Is secreted in a TolC-dependent manner and is antagonistic toward other *Legionella* species. *J Bacteriol,* 2011; 193(21), 5971-5984.

Stewart, CR; Muthye, V; Cianciotto, NP. *Legionella pneumophila* persists within biofilms formed by *Klebsiella pneumoniae, Flavobacterium sp*., and *Pseudomonas fluorescens* under dynamic flow conditions. *PLoS ONE,* 2012; 7(11), e50560.

Storey, MV; Ashbolt, J; Stenstrom, TA. Biofilms, thermophilic amoebae and *Legionella pneumophila*–a quantitative risk assessment for distributed water. *Water Sci Technol,* 2004; 50, 77–82.

Stout, JE; Yu, VL. Experiences of the first 16 hospitals using copper-silver ionization for *Legionella* control: implications for the evaluation of other disinfection modalities. *Infect Control Hosp Epidemiol,* 2003 24, 563–568.

Tatlock, H. A rickettsia-like organism recovered from guinea pigs. *Proc Soc Exp Biol Med.*, 1944; 57, 95-99.

Walczak, M; Krawiec, A; Lalke-Porczyk, E. *Legionella pneumophila* bacteria in thermal saline bath. *Ann Agric Environ Med,* 2013; 20(4), 649-652.

Yarom, R; Sheinman, R; Armon, R. Legionella pneumophila serogroup 3 prevalence in drinking water survey in Israel (2003–2007). *Water Sci Technol,* 2010; 10(5),744-752.

Yu, VL. Legionella pneumophila (Legionnaires' disease). In: Mandell GL, Bennett JE, Dolin R editors. *Principles and practice of infectious diseases.* Philadelphia: Churchill Livingston; 2000; 2424–2435.

Zhang, Z; McCann, C; Stout, JE; Piesczynski, S; Hawks, R; Vidic, R; Yu, VL. Safety and efficacy of chlorine dioxide for *Legionella* control in a hospital water system. *Infect Control Hosp Epidemiol*, 2007; 28, 1009–1012.

Many are losing their health, or ability to work, as a consequence of intruding microbes (or the strains derived from within the patient's own body system, see above). In the best case, the recovery from the operation is delayed. Nevertheless, the human body is opened for the admission of outside microbes during many demanding operations (Figure 2).

With respect to infectious spine diseases, some severe conditions may be caused by unsuccessful operations, for instance. Such disease is pyogenic spondylodiscitis, for instance (Skaf et al., 2010). The major causative agents include *S. aureus* in 57% of the cases and coagulase negative staphylococci 3.4% (Sapico and Montgomerie, 1979). *Escherichia coli* nd other facultative or aerobic gram-negatives count for more than 25% of the cases, hereas strict anaerobes only for 3% (*Propionibacterium* sp. strains 2%). The latter ones are e most difficult ones to cultivate, and their proposition in the lumbar, neural or other such nditions could be higher than it is possible to get determined. In the review article by Skaf l co-workers (2010) there is an interesting postulation regarding the origins of the sative agent from preceding infection:

- Skin infection – *S. aureus*
- IVDA (intravenous drug abuse) – *Pseudomonas aeruginosa*
- Genitourinary tract infection – *E. coli* / *Proteus* sp.
- Respiratory tract infection – *Streptococcus* sp.
- Alcoholism - *Klebsiella pneumoniae*
- Acute endocarditis – *S. aureus*
- Subacute endocarditis – *Streptococcus* sp.

factors for surgical infections can be divided as three different steps, preoperative, ative and postoperative phases. Several factors affecting these period can be detected t infection complications.

erative risks:

derlying diseases; diabetes, pulmonary diseases, malignant diseases, smoking, gienia status of the skin, obesity, use of alcohol, chronic diseases affecting nunological deficiency

ing the skin hairs too early before the operation (should not be done for hygienic ns whenever possible)
nt depending risks: some immunological deficiencies;
trition (meaning mainly overweight in industrialized countries)

ive risks:

-contamination by unsterile "things"
ed operation time
ienced operation theatre team
lity of instrumentation care and sterilization unit

In: Microbiological Clinical Hygiene
Editor: Eino Elias Hakalehto
ISBN: 978-1-63463-428-1

Chapter 8

Microbiological Protection in Operations

Urho Väätäinen[1], Markus Hell[2] and Elias Hakalehto[3]
[1]Ite Lasaretti, Kuopio, Finland
[2]Zentrum für Krankenhaushygiene und Infektionskontrolle der SALK, Universitätsklinikum Salzburg, Salzburg, Austria
[3]Department of Environmental Sciences, University of Eastern Finland, Kuopio, Finland

Abstract

Surgical operations include a risk factor related to the dissemination of microbial contamination. Any invasive treatment may provoke an infection of the object tissue, or also other potential sites in the body system. In order to eliminate the routes of contamination, the following should be paid extra attention to: patient hygiene, correct action and high motivation of the personnel, proper device clean up, as well as maintaining environmental safety in the clinical milieu. In this chapter the risks with respect to operation rooms and their potential avoidance are introduced. It is important that acuta and prolonged microbiological consequences of surgical treatments are charted, and their prevention is effectively worked out.

1. Introduction to Infections and Surgical Operations – Surgical Site Infections (SSI's)

When a patient is received at the hospital for surgical operation, his or her safety needs to be safeguarded also from the hygienic point of view. The practical precautions have been taught since the days of the Austrian-Hungarian physician, Ignaz Philipp Semmelweis (1818-1865) (Wyklicky and Skopec, 1983; Hakalehto, 2006). Modern surgical techniques (so called minimal invasive techniques), such as endoscopic (Figure 1), laser operations have offered less invasive options for many demanding operations. However, continuous alertedness and preparedness for microbiological risks have to be maintained. This requires understanding on the behavior of the microbes in the clinical setting.

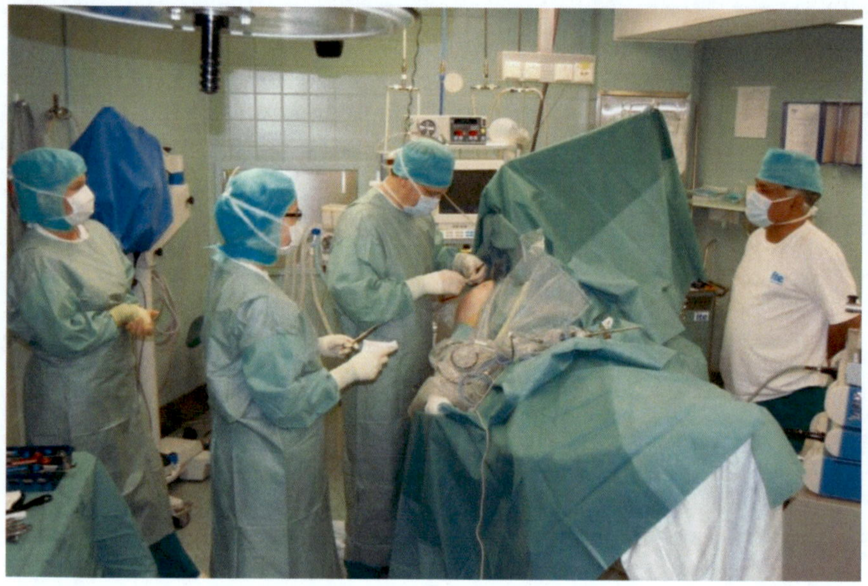

Figure 1. Arthroscopic operation of humeral joint. Arthroscopy is performed through short (approx. 4mm) incisions, when the risk for bacterial exposure is considerably smaller than during open surgery.

2. Microbiological Routes for Infection

In the hospital the acquired bacteriological or other microbiological infection may originate from

a. an environmental contamination from the equipment, hospital rooms, water etc.,
b. a man-to-man contagion from other patients, personnel, visitors etc., and
c. an endogenous infection from the patient own microbiota.

Since all these are relevant risks, the long-lasting debate and questions risen up from it (e.g., in the Meeting of Hospital Infection Society in Liverpool 2010) whether it is more important to keep the hygienic standards by washing and disinfecting hands, or by cleaning up the patient surroundings, could be answered that both ways should be elaborated. See also Appendix II "Hand Hygiene in Healthcare and Nursing".

Additionally, in the era of emerging personalized medicine approach, we should try to map the risks caused by the normal flora of any particular patient. This latter issue is more or less a futuristic ideal in many cases, but should be striven for when developing the hospital microbiology further on. Consequently, we have to understand also the endogenous risks caused by the normal flora, regardless of whether it is considered as a physiological or transiently colonizing one.

3. What Is Surgical Site Infection?

Generally, infections in hospitals, are graded according to Centers of Disease C (CDC) (Garner et al., 1988). For surgical site infections more defined classification is d Horan et al. (1993), as well as by Howard and Lee (1994).

Infections in the surgical wounds vary according to the locations and types o from a few percent up to 10-13.

Typical microbes causing wound infections and infections on surgical area are negative stafylococcus, *Staphylococcus aureus*, *Staphylococcus epidermidis*, *E* sp., *Pseudomonas aeruginosa*, *Escherichia coli*, difteroid bacteria, alfa streptococci, *Bacteroides* sp., gramnegative rods and the antibiotic-resistan MRSA, MRSE, and antibiotic resistant coliformic bacteria (e.g., ESBL-produc low virulent organism like propionic acid bacteria or coryneformic bacteria with implantation of diverse foreign bodies (e.g., total hip endoprosthesis).

Even if we wish to omit any scandalous statements, one has to admit th hygiene there is a need for well-focused attention, and novel precau developed with the idea that still about 20 to 30% of these infections ar their exogenous origin. Many protocols, as like the hospital HACPP, guidelines for the personnel to cope with the most prominent risks inside h

However, since the overall picture of infections and their origins has complex, we need to develop our understanding on this matter, togeth individual touch into the patient care with this respect.

Annually, there are about 50.000 hospital infection in Finland wounds varies from nearly zero up to 20% depending on the site They are causing losses of billions of euros annually.

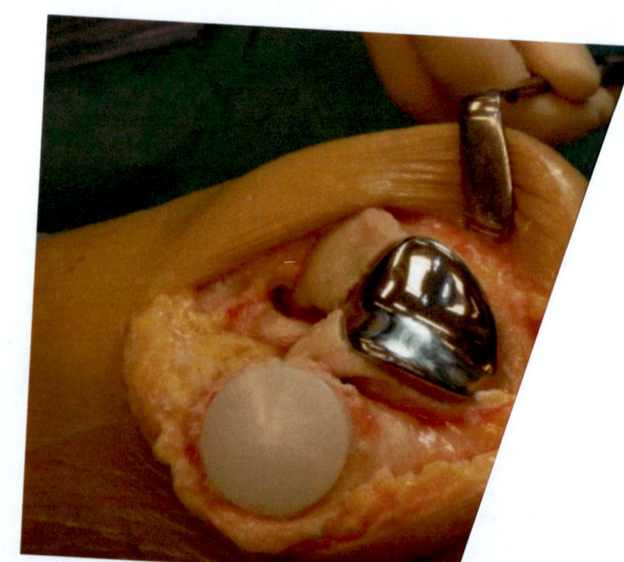

Figure 2. Arthroplasty of patellofemoral joint has been per procedure typically large surfaces of tissues are at risk of

- poor air condition of operation room (OR); too warm conditions increase the risk of infection
- poor temperature economy of the patient during the operation; temperature under 36°C increases infection risk
- glucose balance over 11 mmol/l increases risk of infection
- poor surgical technique; leaving the dead space at the operation area,
- broken gloves (depending on the quality of gloves there are very often invisible micro-lesions of gloves)
- too many persons in operation theatre
- too much traffic through the OR doors during operation, unorganized work at OR.
- open surgery (versus endoscopic-minimal invasive technique)
- too many flat surfaces in OR
- emergency operations
- use of NSAIDs
- late and also too early administration of perioperative antibiotic prophylaxis (Patzakis and Wilkins, 1989)
- use of blood anticoagulants and similar drug like specimens
- poor health condition of OR personal (either chronic skin wounds, allergy or acute viral or bacterial infections, for example)
- unsufficient maintenance of laminar air flow and other technical systems
- pre-existing wounds
- surgery in contaminated and/or already infected tissues/organs
- operating room to small, assisting staff and anesthesiologist cannot keep the necessary distance to sterile areas
- prosthesis and any kind of artificial material remaining in the patient

Preoperative skin-preparation of the patient includes the use of disinfectants. This chemical disinfection is required for the equipment and operation theatres as well. According to Gould and Brooker (2008) the main factors determining the effectiveness of chemical disinfectants include the following:

- Satisfactory contact
  - Disinfection requires complete contact with all surfaces
  - Air bubbles can disturb penetration
  - Sometimes gaseous disinfectant can be used
- Avoiding neutralization
  - Impurities or detergents, as well as some materials (plastic, rubber etc.) may disturb the effect
- Concentration
  - Correct concentrations for complete effect need to be evaluated
- Stability
  - Check the expiry date
- Speed of action
  - Hypochlorites and alcohols are rapid

  - Glutaraldehyde acts slowly
- Range of action
  - Chemical disinfectants have different effects on different target microbes
  - Method of choice has to be selected
- Cost

Postoperative risk factors:

- immediate postoperative care; poor wound protection and unsufficient tissue oxygen saturation.
- use of strong, central nervous system affecting pain killers diminish tissue oxygen penetration
- postoperative stress
- hyperglycemia
- prolonged hospital stay
- large units
- poor instructions to the patients
- wound drains, stomata, surgeon decided not to close the wound at all

Other risk factors for infections related to operations are hematomas and need for repeated surgeries. This could be needed because e.g., of technical problems related to the operation or complications, or when second look is needed in order to find the explanation for prolonged symptoms, for example, in case of acute abdominal pains.

In all these phases, microbes are present. The amount of microbes and the pathogenic ability of dominant microbial populations will set the degree and the type of infection. Infections in surgery are harmful, unexpected and expensive.

They often destroy benefits of surgery and may result to permanent handicap. Infections are multifactorial and Surgical Care Improvement Program (SCIP) has promoted guidelines to prevent postoperative and potentially preventable complications (Poggio, 2013).

Many factors and procedures have been shown to reduce surgical infections: Nasal decolonization, antibiotic prophylaxis, preoperative showers, preoperative oxygen supplementation, antimicrobial sutures, proper hand hygiene, surgical safety checklist. Shower for cleaning is used, but there is an ongoing discussion if it would be better to be done in the evening before – dry skin after washing or bathing is prone to release even more skin microbes (same reason why hand washing and preoperative hand disinfection should be separated. Hand hygiene is advised to be carried out according to EN 1500 directive in general nursing, and according to EN 12791 in surgical situation.

See also Appendix II "Hand Hygiene in Healthcare and Nursing". However, surgical infections are still present although all those steps are important means for avoiding them, as well as the good practices maintained in the surgical units and during recovery (Spruce, 2014).

In order to add safety, more microbiological research and understanding thereof need to be established.

4. What Is the Future?

Risks of supermicrobes (e.g., panresistant bacteria) are increasing because of the wide use of the antibiotics. Also, virulence and other infective properties of microbes may change, and they can develop resistance for antimicrobial therapies. Mixed infections with several causative agents form a problem often difficult to handle in due time. Continuously increasing globalization makes transmission all the time easier for the tedious and harmful micro-organisms.

Better understanding on microbial interactions with each other and with the human host tissues may help us to balance human life in cohabitation with some opportunistic and emerging pathogens and with the entire microbiota.

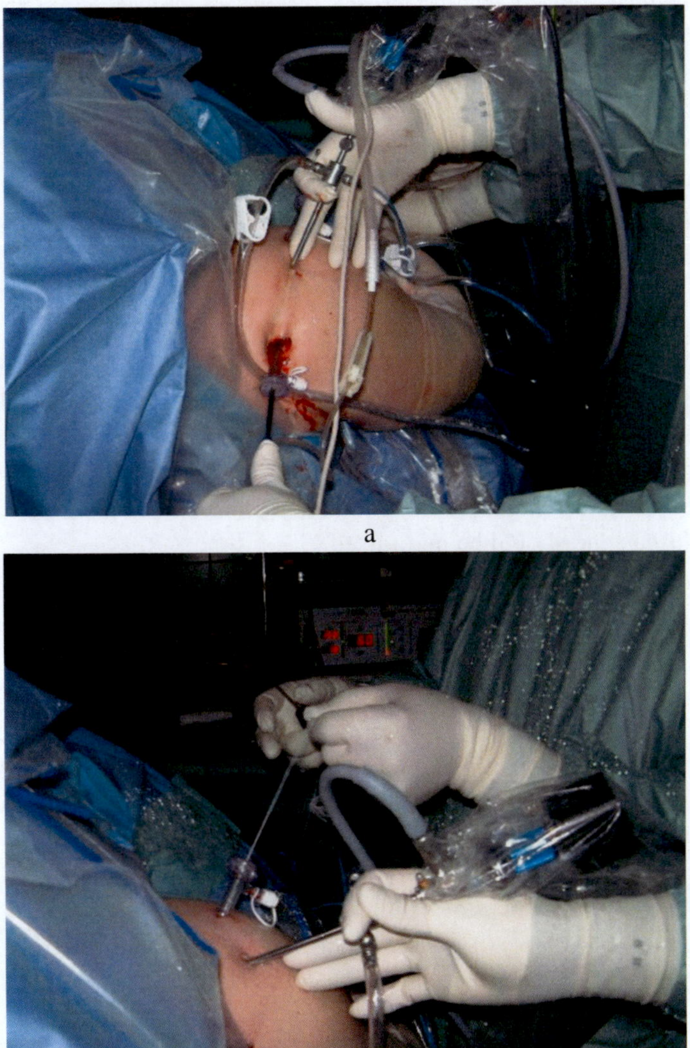

a

b

Figure 3. (a-b) Advanced arthroscopic techniques, like rotator cuff tendon repair, have markedly reduced the risk of infection.

After all, the pathogenicity of a particular organism, such as *Klebsiella pneumonia* could often be subject to other parameters related to the other microflora or host defenses, or both (Hakalehto, 2013). For example, 3% of individuals are carriers of salmonellas in their gut without any symptoms occurring on the personal level. More attention should also be paid on surgical material technology, resistance of materials against microbial action etc., meanwhile also more hygienic surgical techniques are developed (Figure 3a-b). It should be taken into consideration that microbial growth could occur in operating theatre as well as in surgical implants, equipment and devices.

In western hemisphere as well in many other countries, the mean age has increased rapidly. It means also huge demands to threat even old and very old patients with invasive operations. This is a potential threat, causing increasing risks for the development of antibiotic resistant or multi-resistant superbacteria and prolonged infections.

Also, the "medical tourism" will increase the risks of distributing tedious microbial strains (Laupland and Fisman, 2010; Poirel et al., 2011 Zanger, 2014).

It is very crucial to identify every surgical infection and try to understand all the possible factors behind the contamination, or contagion process. Registering the infection helps to follow the rates of various infections, to identify the type of infections and to react to the developments swiftly, and to recognize those steps, which should or could be improved.

Conclusion

Major purpose of surgical operations is to 1. help in improving patient's health status, and 2. aim for optimal recovery from invasive treatments. In order to maintain both objectives, good knowledge on microbiological threats is required, as well as correct preventive measures. Different instructions are to be implemented for normal and exceptional conditions. The latter include epidemics, increased travelling, and crisis situations. If proper preparedness is maintained, risks can and should be minimized.

References

Garner, J. S., Jarvis, W. R., Emori, T. G., Horan, T. C., Hughes, J. M. CDC definitions for nosocomial infections. *J. Infect. Control*, 1988; 16, 128-140.

Gould, D., Brooker, C. *Infection prevention and control. Applied microbiology for health care*. 2nd edition. Basingstoke, UK: Palgrave McMillan; 2008.

Hakalehto, E. Semmelweis' present day follow-up: Updating bacterial sampling and enrichment in clinical hygiene. *Pathophysiology,* 2006; 13, 257-267.

Hakalehto, E. Interactions of *Klebsiella* sp. with other intestinal flora. In: Pereira, L. A., Santos, A., Editors. *Klebsiella infections: Epidemiology, pathogenesis and clinical outcomes*. 1st edition. New York; US: Nova Science Publishers, Inc.;2013; 1-33.

Horan, T. C., Culver, D. H., Gaynes, R. P., Jarvis, W. R., Edwards, J. R., Reid, C. R. Nosocomial infections in surgical patients in the United States, January 1986-June 1992. The national nosocomial infections surveillance system (NNIS). *Infect. Control Hosp. Epidemiol.*, 1993; 14, 73-80.

Howard, R. J., Lee, J. T. Surgical wound infection: epidemiology, surveillance, and clinical management. In: Howard, R. J., Simmons, R. L., editors. *Surgical infections.* Norwalk, Connecticut: Appleton and Lange; 1994; 401-411.

Laupland, K. B., Fisman, D. N. The accidental medical tourist. *Can. J. Infect. Dis. Med. Microbial*, 2010; 21, 155-156.

Patzakis, M. J., Wilkins, J. Factors influencing infection rate in open fracture wounds. *Clin. Orthop. Relat. Res.,* 1989; 243, 36-40.

Poggio, J. L. Perioperative strategies to prevent surgical-site infection. *Clin. Colon Rectal Surg.,* 2013; 26, 168-173.

Poirel, L., Schrenzel, J., Cherkaoui, A., Bernabeu, S., Renzi, G., Nordmann, P. Molecular analysis of NDM-1-producing isolates from Geneva, Switzerland. *J. Antimicrob. Agents Chemother.*, 2011; 66, 1730-1733.

Sapico, F. L., Montgomerie, J. Z. Pyogenic vertebral osteomyelitis: report of nine cases and review of the literature. *Rev. Infect. Dis.,* 1979; 1, 754-776.

Skaf, G. S., Domiloj, N. T., Fehlings, M. G., Bouclaous, C. H., Sabbagh, A. S., Kanafani, Z. A., Kanj, S. S. Pyogenic spondylodiscitis: An overview. *J. Infect. Public Health*, 2010; 3, 5-16.

Spruce, L. Back to basics: preventing surgical site infections. *AORN J.*, 2014 99, 600-611.

Wyklicky, H., Skopec, M. Ignaz Philipp Semmelweis, the prophet of bacteriology. *Infect. Control,* 1983; 4, 367-370.

Zanger, P. Methicillin-resistant *Staphylococcus aureus* and intercontinental travel – "Bad bugs on the move!". *Journal of Travel Medicine*, 2014; 21, 225-227.

In: Microbiological Clinical Hygiene
Editor: Eino Elias Hakalehto
ISBN: 978-1-63463-428-1

Chapter 9

Mycobacterial Detection Views

Elias Hakalehto
Department of Environmental Sciences,
University of Eastern Finland, Kuopio, Finland

Abstract

Besides of the potential side-effects of the tuberculosis vaccinations, they are nowadays given in Finland only to newborns belonging to a certain risk group. In practical clinical care, the leading principle is the isolation of the patients being staining-positive (acid resistant rods in the sputum). In a global perspective the situation is very different with almost 1,5 M lethal cases annually. With emerging and increasing antibiotic resistant strains, and because of especially the increasing multi-resistance (MDR, XDR, TDR), *Mycobacterium tuberculosis* is forming a significant global risk from which no country can escape. In order to overcome this horrifying disease, the worst killer of its kind in human history, determined international action is warranted. An essential part of the strategy for eradicating tuberculosis in the first phase should be, besides the vaccinations, the development of effective diagnostic measures. In order to define the infections caused by mycobacterial strains in time, and more specifically for finding the correct treatment for each patient, fast, broad and deep reaching diagnostic arsenal has to be developed. With positive personal medicine approach, a simulation of optimal care methods could be performed in such devices as the PMEU (Portable Microbe Enrichment Unit), where the medicines and treatment practices for serious mycobacterial infections could get solved in a relatively rapid fashion.

1. Introduction

Mycobacterium tuberculosis has been estimated to have killed more humans than any other infectious disease in human history. This could correspond to a billion lives in the past two hundred years (Lehrman, 2013; Paulson, 2013). It has been estimated that over 1/3 of the global population are carriers of M. tuberculosis, predominantly as latent infection (Dye and William, 2010; Fung, 2013). It is a very slow growing bacterium, but recent experiments with some environmental mycobacteria have given us hope that the laboratory incubation times of *M. tuberculosis* and other slow-growing mycobacteria could be shortened by several days, or even by weeks (Hakalehto, 2013a, 2014; Hakalehto et al., 2014).

The PMEU technique is a field capable stand-alone type of device. This could be an important attribute in the prevention of epidemics.

The general views on the tuberculosis (TB) epidemics worldwide are causing increasing concern. Total tuberculosis mortality rate has come down 41% since 1990 but an increasing proportion of the new cases are caused by antibiotic resistant strains (Mahr, 2013). Morover, 4% of new TB patients have multi-resistant strains (MDR) causing the infection globally. Among the patients who had been treated for TB before, about 20% have MDR-TB according to the World Health Organization (WHO). About 1,4 million persons were killed because of tuberculosis in 2011. More than 2 million new cases of MDR tuberculosis will come up between 2011 and 2015. Only 10% of all MDR patients get proper treatment. A person with active tuberculosis can infect 15 others in a year. In India only,2 million persons get the disease annually, which is comprising 25% of total cases in global scale.

Therefore, Indian government has initiated “Operation ASHA”, which aims for proper handling and eradication of tuberculosis in long term.

In Pakistan, the mean age of tuberculosis patients was 32.5 years, and the proportion of male patients 54.4% (Ejaz et al., 2010). With respect to the efforts for achieving tuberculosis recovery target of 85% in Saudi-Arabia, the first step in improving the control is to unify the standards of diagnostic services and laboratories responsible for tuberculosis (Al-Hajoj, 2010). Currently, there are several diagnostic tests in the pipeline worldwide, but they must be shown to be effective in all areas, applicable to the local conditions (de Lange, 2013).

The treatment for tuberculosis is consisting of several medications, which normally take about 6 months (Mahr, 2013). The medication process starts with a 2 month intensive treatment and continues with 4 month period of extended care. In case of MDR tuberculosis more second line drugs are used. They can be highly toxic for the patient and total period for treatment in case of MDR is 2 years. Therefore, it is not recommendable to start the latter kind of heavy treatment without certain evidence for MDR-TB. “We are on the brink of another epidemic, and it has no treatment.” If totally drug-resistant TDR-TB spreads, we will go back to “the Dark Ages” (Dr. Shellybatra, President of Operation ASHA, India – Time Magazine March 4, 2013). The first TDR cases were detected in late 2011. If the MDR or TDR cases could be detected in time, and treated as required, the survival rates could be increased and contagious processes decreased. More than 60% of the TB patients In India are in the private sector. In many countries, such as Russia and Britain, drug-resistant TB is spreading in prisons. Global loss in the productivity is 12 billion dollars per year due to TB, half of which is resulting from the spreading of this disease in India and China. Lack of adequate susceptibility testing, insensitivity of current diagnosis methods and delayed tuberculosis testing cause problems in many countries (Dye and William, 2010).

Many novel applications have been developed for diagnosing TB. One new device is called GeneXpert, which is claimed to detect drug-resistant TB in hours instead of weeks (Scott, 2014). This is, however, requiring preceding cultivation of the strain into a pure culture. Enhanced enrichment with the PMEU technology has been developed for fast cultivation and detection of mycobacteria (Hakalehto, 2013a, 2014; Hakalehto et al., 2014). PMEU Spectrion® is using optical light, IR or UV for detection. It can be used also for finding out the correct choices for the medication by simulating the antibiotic effects in short time. In case of urgent and demanding patient condition it is possible to try different variations of medications bedside. In case of *Mycobacterium marinum* with 1 million colony forming units per ml, no remarkable growth occurred in 4 days in stagnate cultures, whereas in the PMEU cultivation the mycobacterial concentration multiplied to several tens of millions of cells or colony forming units in the same time (Hakalehto et al., 2014). This kind of relatively rapid growth of normally slow-growing mycobacterial species could indicate potential for the fast detection of *M. tuberculosis*, too. This kind of enrichment approach could be used for the fast treatment of slime samples. Bwanga et al. (2009) have stated: "Even though liquid-based indirect susceptibility tests have improved the turn-around time, they are still not rapid enough to allow timely decisions on patient management in case of MDR-TB. More rapid TB susceptibility tests are needed, particularly in TB high burden countries. Recently, the focus has shifted to rapid direct tests in which decontaminated respiratory samples are directly inoculated in drug-free and drug-containing medium or amplified for detection of MDR-TB".

It is of crucial importance to maintain high standards of air hygiene in order to prevent this spread of *Mycobacterium tuberculosis*. It has been said by O'Hara (1943) that "a silent partner" of medicine has contributed to a similar decline in other "problematic infections" during the last century. In here with "the silent partner" it is referred to an increased consideration on the air hygiene which is a consequence of a better standard of living. Therefore, improved hygienic level is often associated with better quality of life in general. We would like to turn this consideration the other way around. This means that if we pay attention to improving the measures of hygienic control, it can eventually lead to improved standard of living.

2. Novel Treatments and Diagnostics

Besides the investigations on the detection methods for mycobacterial species (Hakalehto 2013a, 2014; Hakalehto et al., 2014) there has been an intense search going on for finding novel antimicrobial compounds against these hazardous pathogens e.g., in Japan by the group of Prof. Hiroshi Tomoda and others at the Kitasato University. These include a fungal metabolite calpinactam, which is a hexapeptide with a caprolactam ring at its C-terminal (Koyama et al., 2010a, b). This molecule was found to be selectively active against mycobacterial strains among other bacteria. It is also a first novel antibiotic substance developed against tuberculosis for many decades. This kind of explorative work is of high importance during the era of emerging multidrug-resistant infections (see also chapter19).

Other anti-mycobacterial peptides were also identified by the researchers of Kitasato University and other Japanese institutes, namely the lariatins (Iwatsuki et al., 2007). Further studies on the specific activities are warranted. The combined effect of various medicines and treatments on the microflora could be studied with simulation tools for personalized medicine, such as the PMEU (Hakalehto, 2012, 2013a, b).

The antibacterial effect of magainin peptides were, in fact, studied with the PMEU, with clear demonstration of the effect (Samgina et al., 2012).

In our recent tests with the PMEU (Portable Microbe Enrichment Unit) a fast-growing species *Mycobacterium fortuitum* was grown onto detectable levels in the PMEU in 10-11 hours (Hakalehto et al., 2013; Hakalehto, 2014). In case of culturing *M. marinum* we achieved detection times of even 2-4 days in minimum for this slow-growing species (Hakalehto, 2013a, Hakalehto et al., 2014) (Figure 1).

In the literature, enrichment of this water-borne organism is supposed to take weeks at optimal conditions (Levinson, 2010).

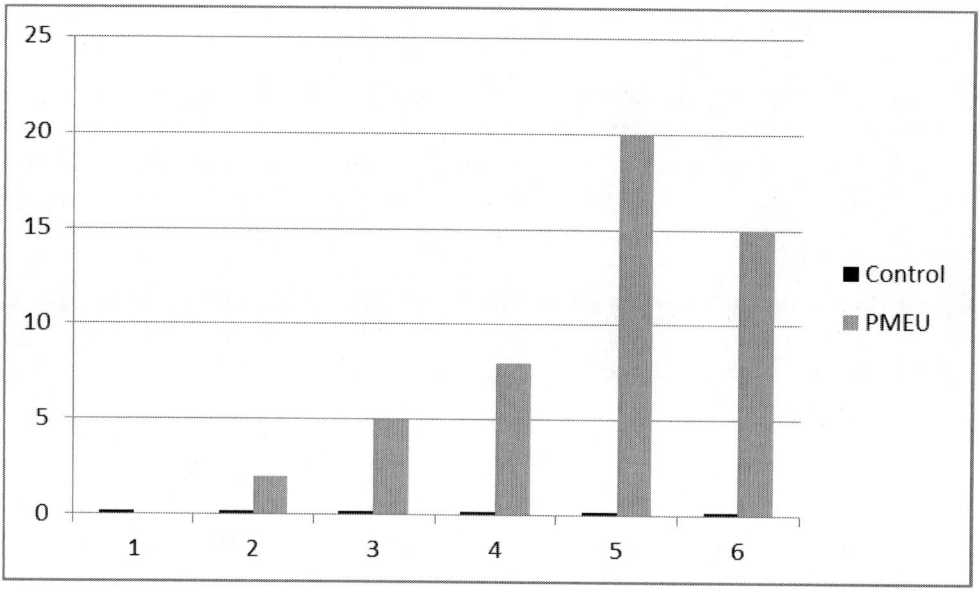

Figure 1. Schematic presentation of approximated growth of *Mycobacterium marinum* environmental isolate (ATCC 927) on the M7H9 broth with Middlebrook ADC Enrichment Supplement (Becton Dickinson, US) (Hakalehto et al., 2014). The growth of the a. in the stagnant control tubes and b. in the PMEU Spectrion® (illustrated with grey columns). Propositional decrease in the IR-transparency in percentages is presented here. Experiments with M. tuberculosis will probably produce results in line with the current findings, when the tests in a safety level 3 laboratory are completed. In case of *M. marinum* with an inoculation of 100.000-1.000.000 cfu*s per ml no growth occurred during four days in stagnant test tube cultures, whereas in the PMEU the mycobacterial concentration multiplical to tens of millions during this period of time.

The slow mode of growth of *M. marinum* is visualized in Figure 2. This emphasizes the applicability and potential of the PMEU principle in detecting hazardous mycobacterial infections, including MDR and TDR-TB. Further validation is warranted for giving this tool into everyday use of the healthcare units.

The mode of *M. tuberculosis* invading the pulmonary alveoli and then being ingested by the macrophages is partially a cause for the long maturing period of the tuberculosis *in vivo*. In the Portable Microbe Enrichment Unit (PMEU) a suitable gas atmosphere is directed as a bubble flow into the liquid medium with clear enhancement of the growth speed of the bacteria.

3. Tuberculosis Background

Major tuberculosis lineages are divided into four "ancient" ones:

1 West African 1
2 West African 2
3 Indo-Oceanian
4 [Hypothesized common ancestor (in Africa)] Horn of Africa

and into three "modern" ones:

5 Euro-American
6 East-African Indian
7 East Asian

The typing is based on DNA fingerprinting, and this kind of division was first hypothesized in 1991 in the San Francisco area, where immigrants from various locations in Africa, Latin America, Europe, and Asia were demographically mixed.

In 1998 it came up then a surprise finding that the outbreaks in New York in the 1980s and 1990s fell within the East Asian "Beijing" type instead of the American-European type otherwise dominatingin the area. This is an example of bacterial typing used for verifying, or at least for speculations on the origins of epidemics, or on the routes of dissemination.

In practical clinical considerations many factors have been found to correlate with the prevalence of tuberculosis, see Table 1.

On the level of host pathogen axis combined actions of three factors have been reported (Lienhardt et al., 2002):

1 infectivity in the source depending on the microbial virulence and density in the sputum
2 intensity and function of exposure
3 susceptibility of the patient to the infection

A particular challenge for the healthcare system is the multidrug-resistant tuberculosis (MDR-TB) (Fung, 2013). In 2009, around 100.000 cases were estimated in India and China, and 10.000 – 40.000 cases in Pakistan, Russia, Nigeria and South Africa. The major cause is suspected to be an incomplete and inadequate treatment of active disease.

An extreme form of the MDR, extensively drug-resistant tuberculosis (XDR-TB) was reported in 65 countries. On cellular level, *M. tuberculosis* can grow intracellularly, which can hamper its eradication (Kuijl et al., 2007).

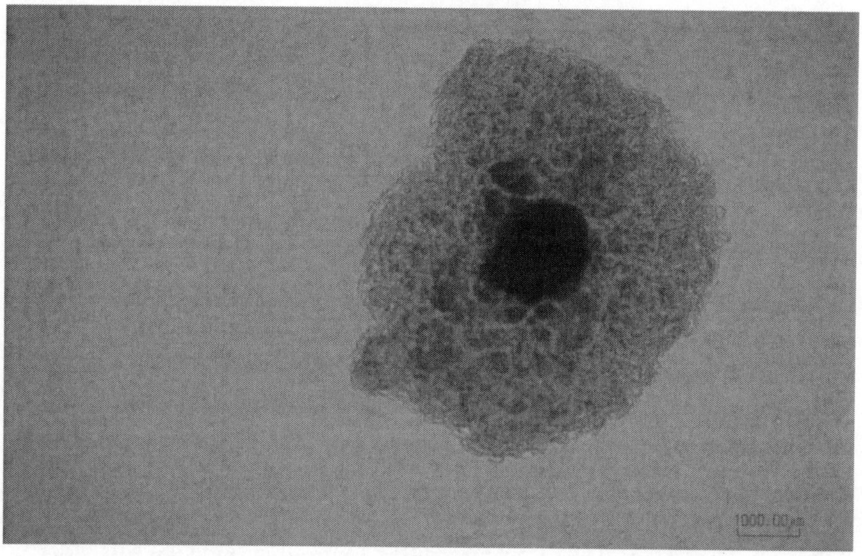

Figure 2. Views on microscopic images of *Mycobacterium marinum* colony growth and cells are presented after pre-enrichment in PMEU Spectrion®.

Table 1. Risk factors for acquiring tuberculosis according to Bisen and Raghuvanski (2013)

Factor	Positive correlation
Age	childhood
	old age (males)
	reproductive age (females)
Sex	female
Ethnic background	isolated populations
Occupation	joint effects (e.g., silica industry workers)
Concomitant diseases and drugs	diabetes mellitus, hypothyroidism, HIV, end-stage malignant diseases, diseases that reduce immunity, mental stress, alcoholism, treatment with immunosuppressive drugs (corticosteroids, anticancer drugs)
Nutrition	shortage of food, non-pasteurized milk
Population density	crowded areas

Besides *M. tuberculosis*, Also Another Mycobacterial Species Can Be Serious Pathogens

Being a potent contaminant of raw milk, and milk and meat products MAP (*Mycobacterium avium* ssp. *paratuberculosis*) has also been suggested as a possible cause of Crohn's disease (CD) (Chamberlin et al., 2001; Hermon-Taylor and Bull, 2002).

Many severe mycobacterial pathogens can be distributed via waterways (Chiao et al., 2014). They are usually highly resistant to purification methods and chemicals, which could produce unforeseeable infections.

A test protocol for *Mycobacterium marinum* about 24 hours (Hakalehto, 2013a; Hakalehto et al., 2014).

- *M. marinum* was transferred from a plate originally obtained from the Finnish Institute of Health and Welfare (Environmental Section)
- Cultivation carried out in the PMEU Scentrion® with 15ml of medium (see above) in each syringe
- Temperature + 33-35 °C
- Larger syringes (60 ml) were used because of foaming of the culture, and bubble formation
- Autoclaved Colilert-Antifoam was added to the syringes (2 drops/ 100ml)
- Five identical enrichment syringes were prepared: into autoclaved (M7H9 +supplement, see above) medium bottle with antifoam substance, and after cooling inoculated with the loopful of the inoculant (from plate culture into 1ml of medium, which suspension was used for inoculating the bottle, from which the inoculated medium was sucked into five PMEU syringes with a sterilized tube
- Sterile-filtered air or gas was directed to the the enrichment syringes. Microaerobic gas mixture with 5% of oxygen and 10% of carbon dioxide into syringes was applied for the tests, as in the cultivation of the *Campylobacteria* (Pitkänen et al., 2009; Hakalehto et al., 2014.
- Growth was detected to be commencing in 24 hours

Conclusion

The global risk of spreading of the tuberculosis infections, including potential epidemics caused by the antibiotic resistant strains, has risen up wide international concern. In a recent meeting with the heads of state of the Scandinavian and Baltic countries, US president and his colleagues named tuberculosis as one of the most serious threats to global health, which should be combatted against by joint international action. In India, concentrated efforts have been initiated in a nationwide governmental ASHA project. Besides novel medications, such efforts could largely benefit from new screening methods, such as PMEU application developed for enhanced enrichment and detection of *M. tuberculosis* and other hazardous mycobacteria.

References

Al-Hajoj, S. A. Tuberculosis in Saudi Arabia: Can we change the way we deal with the disease? *Journal of Infection and Public Health*, 2010; 3, 17-24.

Bisen, P. S., Raghuvanski, R. *Emerging Epidemics – Management and Control*. New Jersey, US: Wiley Blackwell. John Wiley and Sons Inc., 2013.

Bwanga, F., Hoffner, S., Haile, M., Joloba, M. L. Direct susceptibility testing for multi drug resistant tuberculosis: A meta-analysis. *BMC Infectious Diseases*, 2009; 9, 67-81.

Chamberlin, W., Graham, D. Y., Hulten, K., El-Zimaity, H. M., Schwartz, M. R., Naser, S., Shafran, I., El-Zaatari, F. A. Review article: Mycobacterium avium subsp. paratuberculosis as one cause of Crohn's disease. *Aliment. Pharmacol. Ther.*, 2001; 15, 337-346.

Chiao, T. H., Clancy, T. M., Pinto, A., Xi, C., Raskin, L. Differential resistance of drinking water bacterial populations to monochloramine disinfection. *Environ. Sci. Technol.*, 2014; 48, 4038-4047.

De Lange, C. Waiting for results. *Nature*, 2013; 502, S10-S12.

Dye, C., William, B. G. The population dynamics and control of tuberculosis. *Science,* 2010; 328, 856-861.

Ejaz, M., Siddiqui, A. R., Rafiq, Y., Malik, F., Channa, A., MAngi, R., Habib, F., Hasan, R. Prevelance of multi-drug resistant tuberculosis in Karachi, Pakistan: identification of at risk groups. *Transactions of the Royal Society of tropical Medicine and Hygiene*, 2010; 104, 511-517.

Fung, I. W. Multidrug-resistant tuberculosis: A global challenge. In: Fong, I., editor. *Challenges in Infectious Diseases*. New York, US: Springer, 2013.

Hakalehto, E. (Ed.). *Alimentary microbiome - a PMEU approach*. New York, NY, US: Nova Science Publishers, Inc.; 2012.

Hakalehto, E. Enhanced mycobacterial diagnostics in liquid medium by microaerobic bubble flow in Portable Microbe Enrichment Unit. *Pathophysiology*, 2013a; 20, 177-180.

Hakalehto, E. Interactions of *Klebsiella* sp. with other intestinal flora. In: Pereira, L. A., Santos, A. editors. *Klebsiella infections: Epidemiology, pathogenesis and clinical outcomes*. New York, US: Nova Science Publishers, Inc., 2013b.

Hakalehto, E. Bacteriological indications of human activities in the ecosystems. In: Armon, R., Hänninen, O., editors. *Environmental Bioindicators*. Germany: Springer Verlag, 2014.

Hakalehto, E., Heitto, A., Heitto, L., Rissanen, K., Pesola, I., Pesola, J. Enhanced recovery, enrichment and detection of *Mycobacterium marinum* with the Portable Microbe Enrichment Unit (PMEU). 2014 http://dx.doi.org/10.1016/j.pathophys.2014.07.005.

Hermon-Taylor, J., Bull, T. Crohn's disease caused by *Mycobacterium avium subspecies paratuberculosis*: a public health tragedy whose resolution is long overdue. *J. Med. Microbiol.*, 2002; 51, 3-6.

Iwatsuki, M., Uchida, R., Takakusagi, Y., Matsumoto, A., Jiang, C.-L., Takahashi, Y., Arai, M., Kobayashi, S., Matsumoto, M., Inokoshi, J., Tomoda, H., Õmura, S. Lariatins, novel anti-mycobacterial peptides with lasso structure, produced by *Rhodococcus jostii* K01-B0171. *J. Antibiot.*, 2007; 60, 357-363.

Koyama, N., Kojima, S., Fukuda, T., Nagamitsu, T., Yasuhara, T., Õmura, S., Tomoda, H. Structure and total synthesis of fungal calpinactam, a new antimycobacterial agent. *Org. Lett.*, 2010a; 12, 432-435.

Koyama, N., Kojima, S., Nonaka, K., Masuma, R., Matsumoto, M., Õmura, S., Tomoda, H. Calpinactam, a new anti-mycobacterial agent, produced by *Mortierella alpina* FKI-4905. *J. Antibiot.* (Tokyo), 2010b; 63, 183-186.

Kuijl, C., Savage, N. D. L., Marsman, M., Tuin, A. W., Janssen, J., Egan, D. A., Ketema, M., van den Nieuwendijk, R., van den Eeden, S. J. F., Geluk, A., Poot, A., van der Marel, G., Beijersbergen, R. L., Overkleeft, H., Ottenhoff, T. H. M., Neefjes, J. Intracellular bacterial growth is controlled by a kinase network around PKB/AKT1. *Nature Letters*, 2007; 450, 725-730.

Lehrmann, S. "The Diabolical Genius of an Ancient Scourge" – Tuberculosis seems to be evolving in unexpected ways that outsmart humans. *Scientific American*, 2013; July, 69-73.

Levinson, W. *Review of Medical Microbiology and Immunology*. Eleventh Edition. The McGraw-Hill Medical Companies, Inc. by Appleton and Lange, US, 2010.

Lienhardt, C., Bennett, S., Del Prete, G., Bah-Sow, O., Newport, M., Gustafson, P., Manneh, K., Gomes, V., Hill, A., McAdam, K. Investigation of environmental and host-related risk factors for tuberculosis in Africa. I. Methodological aspects of a combined design. *Am. J. Epidemiol.* 2002; 155, 1066-1073.

Mahr, K. The drugs don't work. *Time*, 2013; 181, 28-36.

O'Hara, D. *Air-borne infections: some observations on its decline*. New York, US: Commonwealth Fund, 1943.

Paulson, T. Epidemiology: A mortal foe. *Nature,* 2013; 502, 2-3.

Pitkänen, T., Bräcker, J., Miettinen, I., Heitto, A., Pesola, J., Hakalehto, E. Enhanced enrichment and detection of thermotolerant *Campylobacter* species from water using the Portable Microbe Enrichment Unit (PMEU) and realtime PCR. *Can. J. Microbiol.,* 2009; 55, 849-858.

Samgina, T., Vorontsov, E., Gorshkov, V., Hakalehto, E., Hänninen, O., Zubarev, R., Lebedev, A. Composition and antimicrobial activity of the skin peptidome of Russian brown frog *Rana temporaria*. *J. Proteome Res.*, 2012; 11, 6213-6222.

Scott, L. E. Method for identifying bacteria in a sample. *US Patent 8709712 B2;* 2014.

In: Microbiological Clinical Hygiene
Editor: Eino Elias Hakalehto

ISBN: 978-1-63463-428-1

Chapter 10

Infections during Invasive Treatments and Chronic Pain Management

Hannu Kokki
Anesthesia and Operative Services,
Kuopio University Hospital, Kuopio, Finland

Abstract

In modern treatments of hospitalized patients, especially central venous catheters and subcutaneous venous access devices are associated with elevated infection risks. Infections can arise due to contamination during catheter implantation, or later during the use and maintenance of the venous access devices. Central venous catheter–associated infections are a reason for concern, because those catheters are causing one of the most costly health-care associated infection problems. All openings into the skin are adding the risks of spreading infections into the bloodstream and underlying tissues and spaces. In this chapter intravenous treatment methods and strategies, as well as the infectious risk management, are introduced.

1. Introduction

The use of opioids in the treatment of chronic pain is widespread and in many pain conditions they are highly effective. In some pain patients and in some pains, such as neuropathic pain, the efficacy of opioid analgesics is not always sufficient, and thus other treatment modalities are required. Moreover, opioids are associated with significant adverse effects. Long-term use of higher doses of opioids is assumed to compromise immunofunction and, thus, increase the infection risks in chronic pain patients. A growing body of experimental data indicates that microbes *per se*, e.g., *Staphylococcus aureus*, may directly activate nociceptors, emphasizing proper aseptic approach in pain patients when any kind of invasive treatments are provided.

Different types of injections and infusion techniques are increasingly used in the diagnosis and management of both acute and chronic pain conditions. Implanted devices, medicine pumps and electrotherapy devices are often highly effective in the treatment of different types of medical conditions resistant to conventional therapies. Infusion pumps and electrotherapy may also be used in patients where the use of other treatment modalities is limited by decreased efficacy or untoward adverse effects. Deep brain stimulation is highly effective in Parkinson's disease patients were symptoms are not optimally controlled with medications. Peripheral nerve stimulation is used increasingly. Occipital nerve stimulation can be used in cluster headaches in patients with severe debilitating symptoms who have failed standard treatments. Because infusion pumps and electrotherapy devices are implanted for long term therapies, strict aseptic conditions are necessary during implantation and manipulation, and prompt recognition of early signs and symptoms of infections is important to avoid any persistent harms.

Implanted devices are needed also for accurate vascular access in pain management, but the main indications for these devices are infusions of medicines, antibiotic treatments, cytostatics and parenteral nutrition solutions. Central venous catheters and subcutaneous venous access devices are associated with significant infection risk. Infections can arise early due to catheter contamination during implantation, or later during the use and maintenance of the venous access device. As a foreign material to body venous catheters are prone to bloodstream infections. Short-term catheters are often removed as soon as a suspicion of infection is raised. However, with devices aimed for long-term use, diagnostic and treatment strategies should be considered carefully. Central venous catheter–associated infections are a concern because they are the most costly health-care associated infection.

2. Tunneled Venous Catheters and Implantable Venous Access Ports

Feasible, accurate and safe long-term venous access is a core requisite in modern infusion therapy. Venous lines are needed for parenteral medicine and nutrition administration, and for renal replacement therapy. Many compounds cause venous irritation and are thus, incompatible and contraindicated for peripheral administration. Infusion extravasation may cause serious adverse events, and long-term and repeated anti-infective and cytostatic infusions are associated with a high risk of thrombophlebitis. In many patients peripheral veins are not always available and in these cases central venous access is needed also for administration of fluids and medicines appropriate for peripheral administration. In some patient groups, such as pediatric patients, repeated indwelling venous cannulations or blood tests can be frightening experiences, and thus, in pediatric oncology long-term venous access is established as soon as a diagnosis is ascertained. However, infection complications associated with these devices are common. Most chronic illness where long-term venous access is needed impair body's immunopathogen defense. Thus, an aseptic technique should be followed for the placement, use and handling of these devices. Infection complications are common with these devices.

The first long-term central venous catheter was used for parenteral nutrition in early 1970s (Broviac et al., 1973) and a few years later, in 1979, a long-term venous access device was used for the first time for chemotherapy (Hickman et al., 1979). Implantable venous access ports were introduced for clinical practices thirty years ago. Initially they were used for both arterial and venous access (Niederhuber et al., 1982). Since then the use of arterial ports has diminished and nowadays totally implantable ports are used mainly for venous access. Venous ports are used for the administration of chemotherapy, antibiotics, other medications, fluids, blood products and parenteral nutrition. Blood samples can also be collected through a port. Totally implanted ports are associated with a lower infection rates than percutaneous long-term intravenous catheters, and are more comfort for the patients. Ports are preferred when parenteral treatment is less active while tunneled catheter are used in indications when accurate venous access is needed daily. Totally implanted ports were introduced also for hemodialysis patients but were not feasible for that indication and tunneled catheters are used universally for long-term renal replacement therapy.

3. Central Venous Catheters Complications

The most common complications of central venous catheter are infection, mechanical dysfunction, thrombosis, and catheter occlusion. These complications increase morbidity, interrupt treatment, require catheter removal and are associated with significant increase in healthcare-costs (Ramanathan et al., 2007).

Central venous catheter–associated infections are the third most common nosocomial infections, surgical site infections and catheter-associated urinary tract infection being more commonly reported. Two-third of the sepsis patients has a central line and central venous catheter–associated bloodstream infections are the most costly health-care associated infections. It is estimated that a single catheter-related bloodstream infection results in a mean cost of 31 000-65 000 USD per hospitalization (Zimlichman et al., 2013). Up to two-thirds of the central venous catheter–associated infections are preventable with simple interventions (Umscheid et al., 2011). Implementation of these readily available strategies is not only cost-effective but should have a significant impact on the patient safety.

Device-related bacteremia is the most frequent complication in patients with indwelling central venous catheter. Catheter-related infections results in a significant increase in morbidity, mortality, hospitalization and the overall cost of health care. Infection complications include those associated with the procedure *per se* as well as later arising problems. Procedural complications are due to extraluminal colonization of the devices during the insertion and later infections associated with the use and care of device. However, infection due to colonization during the insertion may appear only later during the course of treatment. A fibrin sheath forms around catheter within the first hours after their insertion and pathogens from the skin adhere to the surface of the catheter and may emergence as an infection only after a delay (Hoshal et al. 1971).

Insertion site affects the incidence of mechanical dysfunction. Right jugular internal vein is preferable site for catheter insertion because it is associated with fewer complications than other sites. Mechanical complications are rare also with femoral vein, but this site is not feasible for long-term venous catheterization (Parienti et al., 2010). When left jugular internal vein is used a risk for catheter malposition, kinking and catheter tip blocked by the vessel wall is relatively high. In subclavian approach a special risk is pinch-off syndrome described by Aitken and Minton (1984). They note that the small gap between the first rib and the clavicle may lead to mechanical compression and shearing forces acting on the catheter. Especially soft, silicone catheters are in increased risk for pinch-off syndrome and several cases of catheter fractures have been reported.

In order to avoid these potentially dangerous infectious adverse events, a strict aseptic technique should be maintained always for the insertion and use of these devices. If the catheter is colonized during insertion, bacteria can adhere and form biofilm and subsequently disperse into the bloodstream. To decrease these risks, the operator inserting a central venous catheter should wear cap, mask, and sterile gown and gloves, and the patient should be covered with sterile drapes. For the skin disinfection of the cannulation area a mixture of chlorhexidine 0.5-2% in alcohol is recommended. If there are contraindications to chlorhexidine alcohol 70% or povidone-iodine in alcohol can be used for antisepsis (Maki et al., 1991). Antiseptics should be allowed to dry before any skin puncture or palpation of the port area.

The presence of a central venous catheter is an independent risk factor for venous thromboembolism. This is a concern because thromboembolism is associated with an increased risk of infection (Eastman et al., 2001). Up to 50% of central venous catheters are complicated by intraluminal clot or venous thrombosis. Frequent flushes with saline may reduce the frequency of intraluminal clots but do not reduce the rate of venous thrombosis in the catheterized blood vessel.

Such a simple reasons as a tight suture or a clamp left in the closed position on an external catheter are easily recognized explanations for catheter malfunction. A non-thrombotic internal occlusion can occur due to precipitation of medications or parenteral nutrition constituents.

Flushing with normal saline seems to be as effective as heparin in maintaining patency of central venous catheter. Mechanical central venous occlusions need cause-specific treatment, whereas thrombotic occlusions usually resolve with thrombolytic treatment.

4. Pathogenesis of Catheter-Associated Infections

Long-term central venous catheter- and implantable venous-access port-related infections can be classified as: (i) catheter colonization, (ii) exit-site infection, (iii) tunnel/pocket infection and (iv) bloodstream infection. Bloodstream infections can be further classified as infusate- and catheter-associated infections. Patients with exit-site and tunnel/pocket infection are commonly classified as having catheter-related bloodstream infection if they have a positive blood culture.

The two main pathways for catheter colonization that precedes manifest infections are by the extra-and intraluminal routes. Central venous catheters may contaminate due to migration of skin organisms at the insertion site into the cutaneous catheter tract and along the surface of the catheter.

Extraluminal colonization is common with short-term catheters. In tunneled catheters an attachable subcutaneous cuff, as soon as growth in surrounding tissues, inhibits micro-organisms migration and thus, catheter colonization by this mechanism is rare with tunneled cuffed catheters. In totally implantable ports extraluminal colonization is unlikely, and these devices are least prone to catheter-related blood-stream infections.

Central line maintenance practices are crucial in preventing infections. Risk of infections can be reduced by careful and strict antiseptic care of the catheter and the infusion systems. Appropriate hand hygiene should be performed before manipulating the catheter, palpating port site, inserting port needle or replacing dressing at the injection site. Use of topical antibiotic ointment on insertion sites has been attempted to prevent extraluminal colonization but not recommended because there is a potential for increased risk of fungal infections and antimicrobial resistance.

Intraluminal colonization constitutes the most frequent way of pathogenesis of infection in tunneled central venous catheters and implanted ports. Direct contamination of the catheter hub during manipulations by contact with hands, contaminated syringes or other devices is a risk with any central venous access. Hubs and stopcocks represent a potential portal of entry for microorganisms into catheters and bloodstream. Closed catheter access systems are supposed to be associated with less risk of colonization and fewer catheter related infections. Two decades ago different types of needleless connectors were introduced in order to decrease the infection risk. Initial results were encouraging but recently in some reports the mechanical valve connectors have been associated with two-times higher incidence of catheter related infections than split septum connectors (Field et al., 2007). Routinely use of needleless connectors with mechanical valves is not recommended before the risks and benefits of these devices have been established. However, whatever devices are used appropriate disinfectants must be used for cleaning of central lines hubs and connectors to prevent transmission of microbes.

The catheter colonization undergoes through several phases. In the first phase contaminated microbes adhered on the catheter surface. In the second phase microbes may break their contacts with the catheter surface or attach more tightly to the catheter. In the later case, microbes adhere irreversibly with a polymer-coat. When a firm attachment with the surface has developed, the bacteria start to produce a biofilm. Electron microscopy scanning has shown that virtually all indwelling central venous catheters are colonized by microorganisms embedded in a biofilm matrix (Caldwell et al., 1992). However, clinical signs of local infection are often unnoticeable during this phase, but micro-organisms embedded in a biofilm matrix can subsequently disperse into the bloodstream and lead to a catheter-related infection.

The organisms most commonly associated with biofilm formation are *Staphylococcus aureus*, *Staphylococcus epidermidis*, *Candida albicans*, *Pseudomonas aeruginosa*, *Klebsiella pneumoniae* and *Enterococcus faecalis*. *Staphylococcus aureus* and *Candida* biofilms are highly resistant to the action of antibiotics and antifungal agents. It is often impossible to clean catheters with antibiotics once their lumen is coated with a biofilm. Microbes growing in biofilms are protected from host defense mechanisms and antibacterial and –fungal agents. Ultimately the only way to treat the infection is to remove the catheter.

As a foreign material in body central venous catheters are prone to bloodstream infections, and hematogenic extraluminal colonization may occur also. If a patient has bacteremia catheters might become hematogenously seeded with these micro-organisms from a distant infection.

5. Microbiology of the Intruding Pathogens

The incidence of central venous line associated infections has decreased during the last decade after adaptation the guidelines for the insertion and maintenance of these devices. Totally implanted ports are associated with a lower infection rates than indwelling catheters, a no such an evident decrease in the infection rates has been noticed. It is estimated that two-thirds of catheter-related infections originate from the skin flora and one third from the contaminated hubs, and only 5% through other pathways. Thus, the rate of catheter related infections should be possible to reduce even further with appropriate infection control measures. During the last decade the reduction in catheter related infections has been greatest for *Staphylococcus aureus* infections but significant for gram-negative pathogens; *Klebsiella pneumoniae*, *Escherichia coli*, *Acinetobacter baumannii*, *Pseudomonas aeuriginosa*, *Candida albicans* and *Enterococcus* species also (Srinivasan et al., 2011).

The microbes that colonize catheter hubs and the skin surrounding the insertion site are the source of most catheter related infections, and the microbiology of infections pathogens seems to have a time-based trend. *Staphylococcus aureus* and *Candida albicans* are more common in early occurring infections while there is an increasing trend for *Pseudomonas aeruginosa* and *Enterococcus species* in infections over time.

As coagulase-negative staphylococci including *Staphylococcus epidermidis* adhere to polymer surfaces more readily than other pathogens they are the most common microbes in catheter related infections, their incidence rate being 22-57 %. *Staphylococcus aureus* can be isolated in 7-39% of cases. E*nterobacteriaceae*, 10-27%, such as *Escherichia coli* and *Klebsiella pneumonia, Enterococcus* species can be isolated in 2-5% of cases. *Pseudomonas aeruginosa* is the most commonly aerobic gram-negative rod, 8-27%. *Candida albicans* is the most common yeast, 3-23%, but it has a relatively high colonization-to-infection rate (Lebeaux et al., 2012).

6. Clinical Diagnosis

In general tunneled central venous catheter- and implantable venous access port-related infection should be suspected if a patient exhibits local signs of infection at the subcutaneous tunnel or implantation site, such as purulence, oozing or redness. However, catheter-associated infections can be difficult to diagnose because the clinical condition in patient's having central venous catheter often fluctuate and can mimic characteristics of infection, or immunocompromised patients with neutropenia may not develop other signs or symptoms of infection than cardiovascular alterations. Common clinical findings of infection, such as fever and chills, have poor specificity for intravascular device-related infection. Physicians caring for patients with indwelling central venous catheter or implantable venous access port need to have a high index of suspicion in order to make a timely diagnosis of catheter-related infection.

Accurate and prompt diagnosis to validate that the catheter is the source of bacteremia is essential to guide the management of catheter-related infections. Half of the patients having *Staphylococcus aureus* infection in the central venous line may develop hematogenous complications such as infective endocarditis, deep-tissue abscesses, septic thrombosis or pulmonary emboli, septic arthritis or osteomyelitis. When a patient has a high suspicion of infection, non-tunneled catheter intended for short term use is often removed and tip segment of the catheter is sent for culture of micro-organisms. With tunneled catheters subcutaneous venous ports catheter-sparing diagnostic methods should be applied.

Diagnostic approach to catheter-related infection is based on clinical evaluation and microbiological evidence based on blood cultures taken from both peripheral vein and central venous catheter. Proper sampling technique is important to differentiate between contaminations versus colonization. The catheter infections are usually caused by same organisms that can be culture from the skin's normal flora and thus, it is important to avoid contamination during specimen collection. Catheter colonization can be established only after the catheter has been removed. With catheters in place colonization is judged when at least fifteen colony forming units exhibit on roll-plate method described by Maki et al. (1977).

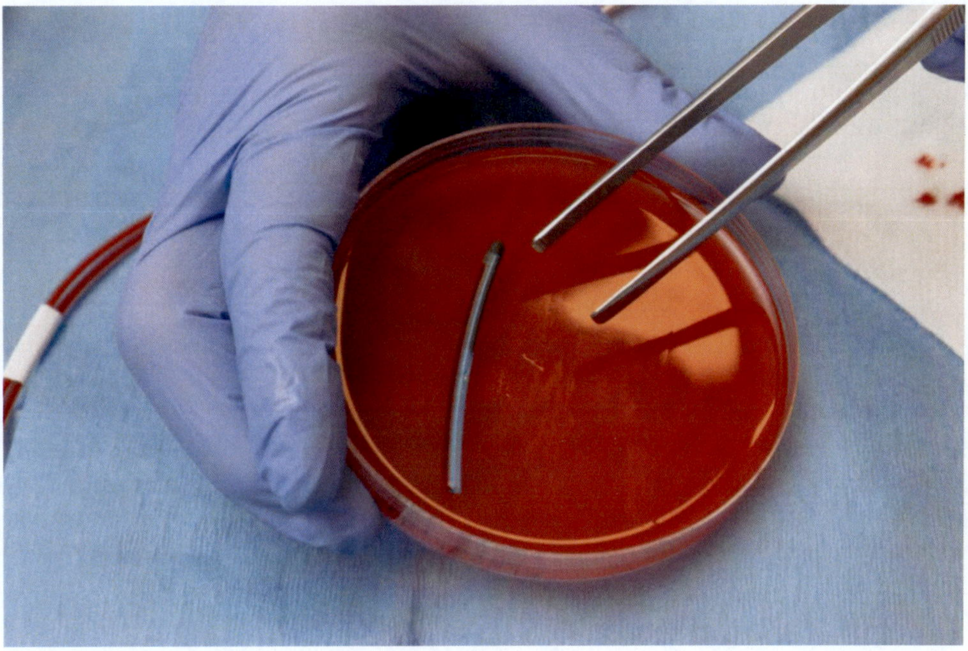

Figure 1. The roll-plate method described by Maki et al. in 1977in NEJM is commonly used semiquantitative culture technic for identifying infection due to intravenous catheters because of its simplicity. A 5-cm catheter tip segment is rolled over a blood agar plate, and colony forming units are counted after incubation overnight.

Two techniques are used to obtain paired blood cultures: simultaneous quantitative blood culture and differential time to positivity technique. In the first method paired blood cultures are drawn at the same time from the central venous catheter and the peripheral vein. If the colony count in the blood culture drawn through the central line is at least three- or five-fold higher than that from the peripheral vein, this is highly predictive for catheter related infection. The second, differential time to positivity is a qualitative test. Blood cultures are drawn through the central venous catheter and a peripheral vein, and a diagnosis of catheter related infection is established when the blood culture drawn from the central line becomes positive at least 2 hour earlier than the peripheral blood culture.

Simultaneous quantitative blood culture is highly accurate test for catheter related infection diagnosis, for long-term catheters sensitivity is > 90% and specificity almost 100%, respectively. Differential time to positivity technique has a similar sensitivity, 90%, but the specificity is lower, for long-term catheters 72% (Safdar et al., 2005).

Peripheral venous blood samples cannot be always obtained. In these cases a single quantitative blood culture can be drawn through the central line. However, this method is not optimal. The interpretation of the result could be compromised in cases of high-grade bacteremia, e.g., in immunocompromised patients who have sepsis. If antibiotics have been given through the catheter colonized catheters may show falsely negative result. However, blood cultures that are positive for *Staphylococcus aureus*, coagulase-negative staphylococci or *Candida* species, are highly predictive for catheter-related infections.

7. Opioid Induced Immunosuppression

Higher doses and long-term use of opioids may alter immunofunction. Both experimental and human data indicates that opioids have intrinsic immunosuppressive activity. This is a concern because opioids are commonly used in different pain conditions in patients who may have already acute or persistent alterations in their immunofunction such as surgical and cancer patients. Moreover, other analgesics may be contraindicated, such as non-steroidal anti-inflammatory analgesics, or induce undesired adverse effects, e.g., dizziness with gabapentinoids, that opioids could be preferred options.

There is no convincing evidence whether opioids *per se* increase the rate of infections in all patient categories. However, elderly are supposed to be a risk group for opioid-induced immunosuppression. Immunofunction declines in the elderly, they have more diseases, more pain conditions, more other medicine that may alter immunofunction, and they have more often contra-indications and are more prone to adverse effects of other analgesics. Opioid abusers have also increased risk for infections. They are known to have high prevalence of opportunistic bacterial infections such as pneumonia, hepatitis, tuberculosis and vertebral osteomyelitis.

Chronic opioid use, either medical or abuse use affects both innate and adaptive immunity. Opioid use contributes to increased susceptibility to microbial pathogens. *Staphylococcus aureus*, *Streptococcus*, and *Pseudomonas* are examples of bacterial infections that seem to correlate with long-term opioid use. In addition to bacterial infections, opioid abusers have an increased risk of viral and fungal infections. Morphine upregulates HIV entry into immune cell, and enhances activation and viral replication. Opioids modulate also HIV associated neuropathogenesis. Experimental data indicates that long-term opioid use may modulate the immune responses to fungal and parasite infections.

There seems to be distinct differences between opioids in their immunomodulating effects. Morphine and fentanyl are the two most immunosuppressive opioids. Moreover, experimental data indicates that immunosuppression induced by fentanyl is dose-related. Some other opioid analgesics do not have substantial effects on immune system. Oxycodone, hydromorphone, and in especially buprenorphine have been reported to be less immunosuppressive than morphine and fentanyl. Opioid antagonist naloxone may increase immune responses. Thus, it should be interesting to know how the recently launched oxycodone-naloxone combination product may perform. In the combination product naloxone is added to counteract opioid-induced constipation by blocking the action of oxycodone at opioid receptors locally in the gut. Whether the product may also have advantageous effects from the point of immunofunction has not been evaluated (Pergolizzi et al., 2008).

Not only the long-term morphine use but also morphine withdrawal may induce immunosuppression. Thus appropriate attention should be paid on decision whether there is medical indication for opioid analgesic and, if, on the selection of most appropriate compound. Those compounds known to affect immunofunction, morphine, fentanyl, methadone and codeine, should not be the first choices at least in immunocompromised patients or in patients known to have clinical condition or concomitant medication that may alter immunofunction. At this time buprenorphine and oxycodone seems to be more rational choices from the perspective of immunofunction.

Although some potential mechanism has been known for over a century, such as that morphine inhibit phagocytosis, it has not been established why some opioids adversely affect the immune system while the effect of others is less obvious. Kappa-opioid- and non-classical and naloxone insensitive-receptor antagonism, and differences on central nervous system penetration are among proposed pharmacokinetic mechanisms. Activation of sympathetic nervous system and hypothalamic-pituitary-adrenal axis has potential to depress immune response. Released glucocorticoid and norepinephrine modulates leukocytes function, depress natural killer cell activity, and suppress lymphocyte proliferation mechanisms and function. In addition to indirect action, morphine alters immune cells function also by direct binding into immune cells' opioid receptors. Several mechanisms seem to be involved and further researches are needed to better understand the effects of opioids on the immune system.

On the other hand, severe pain is a stressor to body and physiological effects can lead to immunosuppression. Pain relief is obviously beneficial for the immune function (Eisenstein, 2011; Al-Hashimi et al., 2013).

8. Risks of Infections in Invasive Pain Management and Their Avoidance

Perineural and intrathecal infusions are highly effective in management of both acute and persistent pain states. As an indwelling catheter is needed for drug administration the infection risk are similar as with central venous catheters. Local anesthetics are the main components in the infusion. Local anesthetics are bacteriostatic best shown with racemic bupivacaine and lidocaine. Antimicrobial capacity of these two compounds seems to be greater than that of ropivacaine and levobupivacaine levo-enantiomeric amino-amides increasingly used in infusions were higher doses of anesthetics are needed.

The most common indication for peripheral perineural catheters is prolonging of intraoperative surgical anesthesia and early postoperative analgesia after surgery where the typical duration of infusion is 48-72 hours. Perineural catheters are used also in trauma patients during transportations and awaiting surgical procedures. As regional blocks are often highly effective, the need for other analgesics is minimal. Use of opioid analgesics can be reduced and, thus, the adverse effects of opioids such as nausea and vomiting, respiratory depression and decreased level of consciousness are avoided, important safety issue in trauma patients. Local anesthetics infusions can be induce also for sympathectomy and vasodilation to alleviate vasospasm and to improve blood flow to the affected extremity. In trauma patients continuous local anesthetic infusions are used also for the treatment of complex regional pain syndrome and intractable phantom limb pain.

Reported incidences of perineural catheter bacterial colonization are relatively high, 6%–57%, but because the catheters are often removed within the first 48-72 hours, the incidence of local or systemic infection is low, most reports less than <1% rate of infections. Insertion site may affect the infection risk; it seems to be increased with axillary and femoral catheters. Other potential risk factors are the patient's need for an intensive care unit stay, duration of catheter use for longer than 48 h, absence of antibiotic prophylaxis during the catheter insertion and frequent catheter dressing changes (Ilfeld, 2011).

However, strict aseptic principles should be followed during the catheter insertion. There is some evidence that subcutaneous catheter tunneling may decrease the risk of bacterial colonization and infection risk significantly. When the insertion site is prepared with alcohol-clorhexidine, sterile drapes are used and the physician has a cap, gown, facemask and sterile gloves during the insertion, the colonization rare of the catheters at 48 hours was 6% and no cases of infections were noted. Coagulase-negative staphylococci were the most common pathogens in the catheter tip cultures accounting 72 % of all microbes (Compere et al., 2009). If long-term use is anticipated, the catheter should be tunneled to reduce the risk of infection. The insertion site should be checked daily and if there is any sign of superficial infection, the catheter should be removed.

Single-injection peripheral nerve blocks are supposed to have a lower risk of infection when compared with continuous catheter techniques. However, devastating complications have been reported with single-injection techniques as well. When infections occur they are generally related to the patients' underlying health status, such as diabetes mellitus. Moreover, in pain clinics in peripheral nerve blocks local anesthetics are often injected with steroids. Although infectious complications from these interventions are rare appropriate precautions should be applied.

Epidural drug delivery can be made either by single or repeated injections, or an epidural catheter can be advanced to the level of painful dermatomes for continuous infusion analgesic admixture.

Epidural injection, corticosteroid, local anesthetic and other compounds, is one of the most common procedures performed for chronic pain management. The most common indication is low back pain and radiculopathy to lower extremities. With epidural injection local anesthetic and corticosteroid are targeted to be delivered to the segmental area of corresponding spinal nerve roots and the injection can be performed at any level depending on the indication and patient's pain state. In low back, lumbosacral, pelvic and lower extremities pain injection is often performed via sacral epidural space. Caudal approach to the epidural space is used also in patients who have had lumbar surgery or who have severe degenerative changes, which could make lumbar approaches difficult. Important consideration especially in immunocompromised patients is that infection, although rare, can be a higher risk with caudal approach given the needles entry site close to the anus.

Not only aseptic preparation of the injection area and injection technique but also the proper preparation of the injectate is critical in infection control. Fungal infections are rare complications of single-shot injections. However, recently Smith et al. describe epidemiologic data from an outbreak of fungal infections associated with injection of contaminated corticosteroid preparation. A total of 749 patients developed injection-associated with corticosteroid infections, and 61 patients died. The most common infections were spinal and paraspinal reported in 476 patients and meningitis reported in 384 patients (Smith et al., 2013).

Epidural analgesia is given most often with a continuous epidural catheter. The catheter tip is advanced to the middle of the most painful segmental area, e.g., lower thoracic level in abdominal and pelvic pain conditions and upper thoracic interspace in thoracic pain. Epidural catheters are often tunneled if expected used is longer than few hours. Tunneling may decrease the infection risk and prevent unintended dislodge of the catheter. In long-term treatment epidural catheters are attached to subcutaneous ports which provide greater protection from infection.

The greatest concerns with epidural pain management are risk of spinal hematoma and epidural abscess because of their potentially devastating squeal, e.g., meningitis and paralysis. The prognosis of epidural hematoma is poor even when diagnosed and operated early, while that of epidural abscess can be more favorable with prompt recognition of suggestive signs and symptoms and early initiation of appropriate treatment, i.e., removal of suspected catheter and systemic antibiotic treatment. Earlier data indicated that the frequency of severe infection complications is low, estimated risk of 1 to 40 000 or 100 000 intrathecal block. Recent data indicates that the incidence of infective complications could be significantly higher in perioperative use, between 1 to 2 000 and 1 to 4 000 epidural catheterization. However, patients who develop epidural abscesses are frequently immunocompromised having diabetes mellitus, malnutrition, cancer or steroid therapy as a risk factors for infection. *Staphylococcus aureus* is the predominant pathogen reported in epidural abscesses. Proper skin preparation with alcohol based disinfectant should be applied before insertion, and it is important to remember that the patients could develop signs and symptoms of epidural abscess or meningitis only after few days after epidural catheter removal (Hebl and Niesen, 2011).

On to contrary what could be expected, but then compared to epidurally placed catheters, intraspinal catheters are associated with lower rates of infectious complications. Implanted intrathecal drug-delivery systems delivering an opioid with or without an adjunctive medication are also used in selected patient who have failed more conservative options and/or have developed unacceptable adverse effects from other administration routes. The intraspinal drug delivery systems are highly effective also in the treatment of spasticity in patients with failure with per oral medication. Implantable pumps are assumed to provide even greater protection against infection. However, infection is always a potential complication with any of the intraspinal techniques used. Thus, a strict aseptic technique should be a standard practice, proper preparation of infusate solutions is needed, and catheter/port/pump pocket site must be checked regularly, and patient's signs and symptoms suggestive for any infective complications should be monitored closely in order to avoid any permanent harms (Prager, 2002).

Since the first spinal cord stimulator was implanted in 1967 (Sealy et al., 1967) this technique has become a popular for the management of wide range of chronic pain states. Main indications have been failed back surgery and other conditions resulting radicular pain on extremities. As the clinical evidence with spinal cord stimulators had grown it has been applied for a wide range medical indications, including intractable angina, peripheral vascular disease, chronic pancreatitis, chronic pelvic pain as well as bladder and bowel dysfunction. As no infusate is given, the infection risk is less than that of intraspinal medication pumps.

Deep infection rates of 0.1 % have been found associated with spinal cord stimulation and a total infection rates is between 2 and 4 %.

However, appropriate aseptic technique should be used in implantation because the device and lead colonization may result skin or epidural abscess, meningitis, and osteomyelitis. These patients have often been on high doses of opioids, received epidural corticosteroid injection and have concomitant diseases that may compromise immunofunction, and are, thus, in higher risk for infections.

Neuromodulation techniques are used also for peripheral nerves. In peripheral nerve stimulation is the direct electrical stimulation is given for named nerves outside of the neuraxis while in peripheral nerve field stimulation a subcutaneous lead is placed to a provide superficial stimulation of small nerves in the vicinity of pain. Occipital nerve stimulation is an example of new, highly effective treatment modality for treating intractable headaches. Peripheral nerve stimulation has been used also for complex regional pain syndrome and other neuropathic pains associated with a distribution of single nerve(s). With peripheral neuromodulation the risks of infections are less severe than those with more deep stimulators implanted in adjunct to central nervous system. However, implantation of these devices requires meticulous sterile preparation and handling (Weiner and Reed, 1999).

In more difficult pain conditions deep brain stimulation has been used in selected patients with central pain with encouraging experience. As the target for deep brain stimulation leads is deep sensory nuclei of thalamus and periaqueductal and periventricular gray areas in brain these devices are implanted only in most sterile environment. This because, if developed, the consequences of infections can be devastating.

In addition to stimulation of deep cerebral structures the stimulation of the contralateral motor cortex has given promising results in selected patients with chronic neuropathic pain. Cerebral neuromodulation is used also in the treatment of refractory movement disorders, such as Parkinson disease, essential tremor, and dystonia. In these indications stimulation electrodes are placed in thalamic nuclei or basal ganglia. Deep infections are rare, but stimulator pocket infection may occur in up to 3–13 % of cases (Levy et al., 2010).

Although the incidence of infection complications with these implanted devices is relatively low, the outcome after infection could be poor. Thus, catheter, lead, pump and generator colonization risk during implantation and handling should be minimized. In addition, constant surveillance for infection, and counseling and education of the patient regarding signs and symptoms of infection is import in order to provide timely diagnostic and treatment.

9. Management and Care of Infections

The management of infections associated with short-term central venous catheters includes catheter removal and often also the initiation of systemic antibiotic treatment. However, it is not always possible to prove that the central line is the source of infection, and an alternative vascular access must be available before catheter is removed. Before removing the device it should be confirm that the patient has a true catheter-related bloodstream infection and no skin contamination, simple catheter colonization, or infection from another source. Thus, with tunneled central venous catheter- and implantable venous-access port-related infections in non-septic patients the initial attempt is catheter salvage with appropriate antimicrobial treatment.

Indications for catheter and port system removal are persisting sepsis and bacteremia or relapse of infection after antibiotic treatment. Signs of port or catheter tunnel infection in unstable patient and in those with systemic complications prompt the catheter removal. Certain micro-organisms such as *Staphylococcus aureus* and *Candida* species are associated with low response rate for conservative treatment and because these organisms are often present in early infections, catheter removal is often indicated in these patients (Raad et al., 2007). If the catheter is decided to retain, the patient should be monitored closely for any symptom and signs of spreading infection, and repeat blood cultures should be collected accordingly. Persistent bacteremia beyond 72 hours is a highly predictive for complicated outcome and higher relapse rate, and is, thus, often an indication for catheter removal.

Only identical bacterial strains isolated from both the peripheral vein and blood sample obtained through the catheter provide evidence for catheter related blood stream infection. However, when there is a high suspicion of central venous catheter-related infection decision should be made how to manage with the catheter, e.g., removal, guide-wire-assisted exchange or an attempt to salvage. Antibiotic therapy is often initiated with empiric therapy followed by subsequent tailoring to culture and sensitivity data.

Catheter salvage may be attempted in uncomplicated infections of long-term catheters and venous access ports. The type of suspected pathogen is important for guiding decision. If the catheter-related infection is supposed to be caused by *Staphylococcus aureus, Pseudomonas* and *Candida species* the success rate without catheter removal is low. Moreover *Staphylococcus aureus* infections are one of those associated with a high risk of hematogenous complications, e.g., infective endocarditis, septic arthritis and vertebral osteomyelitis. Thus, the success of the treatment outcome should be evaluated at 72 hours after initiation of the antimicrobial therapy by obtaining paired blood samples, and by recording patient's signs and symptoms.

Catheter removal is not necessary for hemodynamically stable patients with unexplained fever in the absence of documented bloodstream infection. Catheter removal is warranted in cases of persistent bacteremia after 72 hours of antimicrobial therapy. If the patient has a severe sepsis, is hemodynamically instable, has endocarditis or metastatic infection, erythema or suppurative thrombophlebitis catheter should also be removed. For circumstances in which catheter removal is necessary and risk for complications during catheter reinsertion is high, guide-wire exchange of the catheter may be appropriate.

When catheter salvage is attempted empiric antibiotic therapy should include activity against methicillin resistant *Staphylococcus aureus*; vancomycin is often a reasonable agent. Patients with neutropenia or sepsis should also receive empiric antibiotic therapy for gram-negative organisms including *Pseudomonas* such as third- or fourth-generation cephalosporin. Patients, known to be colonized with drug resistant organisms, should receive empiric antibiotic therapy selected accordingly. Fluconazole should be considered for empirical treatment when fungemia is suspected. Following initiation of empiric treatment, antibiotic therapy should be tailored to culture and susceptibility results as needed once microbiological data are available.

If salvage is attempted, both systemic and antimicrobial lock therapy may be administered through the colonized catheter for the duration of therapy. In patients having multilumen catheter, administration of antimicrobial infusion should be rotated between lumens. The efficacy of antibiotic lock-therapy, e.g., installing the catheter lumen with a highly concentrated antibiotic solution or other antimicrobial compound, is uncertain and concerns have been raised about the emergence of antimicrobial resistance and fungal superinfection and potential toxic effects of exposure to high concentrations of antibiotics and other compounds. The optimal antimicrobial dosing for lock therapy is also uncertain. Lock therapy is not use in the management of catheter infection for devices in place for less than two weeks; because these are usually extraluminal infections.

Antibiotic therapy is not required in patients having positive catheter tip culture without clinical signs of infection and positive blood cultures obtained through a catheter with no microbial growth in peripheral vein cultures, because the positive results are most likely contamination. In cases of localized phlebitis the risk of blood spread infection is also unlikely, and in general antimicrobial therapy is not necessary.

Management of exit site and pocket site infections depends on the nature of the infection (Lebeaux et al., 2012).

Conclusion

In clinical setting it can be difficult to distinguish central venous catheter- and venous access port-related infection signs and symptoms from other infections casing bacteremia/fungemia. In order to provide timely management a high level of suspicion is needed in these patients. There seems to be decreasing trend on tunneled central venous line-associated infection congruently with a more widespread adoption of strict aseptic principles of inserting and management of the catheters. Venous access ports are associated with lower risk of infections but no such a positive change has been found in the port associated infective complications.

Prevention is better than cure. Invasive devices are a significant risk-factor for nosocomial infections. Catheter-related infections can be serious and costly. Better adherence to simple infection prevention practices is required from all health care workers to avoid contamination of these devices. Proper aseptic techniques should result in a low incidence of catheter-related infections.

References

Aitken, DR; Minton, JP. The 'pinch-off sign': a warning of impending problems with permanent subclavian catheters. *Am J Surg* 1984; 148, 633–636.

Al-Hashimi, M; Scott, SW; Thompson, JP; Lambert, DG. Opioids and immune modulation: more questions than answers. *Br J Anaesth.* 2013 Jul;111(1), 80-88.

Broviac, JW; Cole, JJ; Scribner, BH. A silicone rubber atrial catheter for prolonged parenteral alimentation. *Surg Gynecol Obstet* 1973;136(4), 602-606.

Caldwell, DE; Korber, DR; Lawrence, JR. Imaging of bacterial cells by fluorescence exclusion using scanning confocal laser microscopy. *J Microbiol Meth* 1992; 15, 249–261.

Chopra, V; Anand, S; Hickner, A; Buist, M; Rogers, MA; Saint, S; Flanders, SA. Risk of venous thromboembolism associated with peripherally inserted central catheters: a systematic review and meta-analysis. *Lancet.* 2013 Jul 27;382(9889), 311-325.

Compère, V; Legrand, JF; Guitard, PG; Azougagh, K; Baert, O; Ouennich, A; Fourdrinier, V; Frebourg, N; Dureuil, B. Bacterial colonization after tunneling in 402 perineural catheters: a prospective study. *Anesth Analg.* 2009 Apr;108(4), 1326-1330.

Eisenstein, TK. Opioids and the immune system: what is their mechanism of action? *Br J Pharmacol.* 2011 Dec;164(7), 1826-1828.

Field, K; McFarlane, C; Cheng, AC. Incidence of catheter-related bloodstream infection among patients with a needleless, mechanical valve–based intravenous connector in an Australian hematology-oncology unit. *Infect Control Hosp Epidemiol* 2007; 28, 610-613.

Hebl, JR; Niesen, AD. Infectious complications of regional anesthesia. *Curr Opin Anaesthesiol.* 2011 Oct;24(5), 573-580.

Hickman, RO; Buckner, CD; Clift, RA. A modified right atrial catheter for access to the venous system in marrow transplant recipient. *Surg Gynecol Obstet* 1979;148, 871-875.

Hoshal, VL Jr; Ause, RG; Hoskins, PA. Fibrin sleeve formation on indwelling subclavian central venous catheters. 1971; *Arch Surg* 102(4), 353–358.

Ilfeld, BM. Continuous peripheral nerve blocks: a review of the published evidence. *Anesth Analg.* 2011 Oct;113(4), 904-925.

Lebeaux, D; Larroque, B; Gellen-Dautremer, J; Leflon-Guibout, V; Dreyer, C; Bialek, S; Froissart, A; Hentic, O; Tessier, C; Ruimy, R; Pelletier, AL; Crestani, B; Fournier, M; Papo, T; Barry, B; Zarrouk, V; Fantin, B. Clinical outcome after a totally implantable venous access port-related infection in cancer patients: a prospective study and review of the literature. *Medicine (Baltimore).* 2012 Nov;91(6), 309-318.

Levy, R; Deer, TR; Henderson, J. Intracranial neurostimulation for pain control: a review. *Pain Physician.* 2010;13, 157–165.

Maki, DG; Weise, CE; Sarafin, HW. A semiquantitative culture method for identifying intravenous-catheter-related infection. *N Engl J Med.* 1977 Jun 9;296(23), 1305-1309.

Niederhuber, JE; Ensminger, W; Gyves, JW; Liepman, M; Doan, K; Cozzi, E. Totally implanted venous and arterial access system to replace external catheters in cancer treatment. *Surgery.* 1982; 92, 706–712.

Parienti, JJ; Megarbane, B; Fischer, MO. Catheter dysfunction and dialysis performance according to vascular access among 736 critically ill adults requiring renal replacement therapy: a randomized controlled study. *Crit Care Med* 2010; 38: 1118–1125.

Pergolizzi, J; Böger, RH; Budd, K; Dahan, A; Erdine, S; Hans, G; Kress, HG; Langford, R; Likar, R; Raffa, RB; Sacerdote, P. Opioids and the management of chronic severe pain in the elderly: consensus statement of an international expert panel with focus on the six clinically most often used World Health Organization Step III opioids (buprenorphine, fentanyl, hydromorphone, methadone, morphine, oxycodone). *Pain Pract.* 2008;8(4), 287–313.

Prager, JP. Neuraxial medication delivery the development and maturity of a concept for treating chronic pain of spinal origin. *Spine.* 2002;27(22), 2593–2605.

Raad, I; Hanna, H; Maki, D. Intravascular catheter-related infections: advances in diagnosis, prevention, and management. *Lancet Infect Dis.* 2007 Oct;7(10), 645-657.

Ramanathan, V; Chiu, EJ; Thomas, JT; Khan, A; Dolson, GM; Darouiche, RO. Healthcare costs associated with hemodialysis catheter-related infections: a single-center experience. *Infect Control Hosp Epidemiol,* 28 (2007), 606–609.

Safdar, N; Fine, JP; Maki, DG. Meta-analysis: methods for diagnosing intravascular device-related bloodstream infection. *Ann Intern Med.* 2005 Mar 15;142(6), 451-466.

Sealy, CN; Mortimer, JT; Reswick, KB. Electrical inhibition of pain by stimulation of dorsal column: preliminary clinical reports. *Anesth Analg.* 1967;4, 489–491.

Shivakumar, SP; Anderson, DR; Couban, S. Catheter-associated thrombosis in patients with malignancy. *J Clin Oncol* 2009;27, 4858-4864.

Smith, RM; Schaefer, MK; Kainer, MA; Wise, M; Finks, J; Duwve, J; Fontaine, E; Chu, A; Carothers, B; Reilly, A; Fiedler, J; Wiese, AD; Feaster, C; Gibson, L; Griese, S; Purfield, A; Cleveland, AA; Benedict, K; Harris, JR; Brandt, ME; Blau, D; Jernigan, J; Weber, JT; Park, BJ. Multistate Fungal Infection Outbreak Response Team. Fungal infections associated with contaminated methylprednisolone injections. *N Engl J Med.* 2013 Oct 24;369(17), 1598-1609.

Srinivasan, A; Wise, M; Bell, M. Centers for Disease Control and Prevention (CDC). Vital signs: central line-associated blood stream infections—United States, 2001, 2008, and 2009. MMWR *Morb Mortal Wkly Rep.* 2011;60(8), 243-248.

Umscheid, CA; Mitchell, MD; Doshi, JA; Agarwal, R; Williams, K; Brennan, PJ. Estimating the proportion of healthcare-associated infections that are reasonably preventable and the related mortality and costs. *Infect Control Hosp Epidemiol.* 2011;32(2), 101-114.

Weiner, RL; Reed, KL. Peripheral neurostimulation for control of intractable occipital neuralgia. *Neuromodulation.* 1999;2(3), 217–221.

Zimlichman, E; Henderson, D; Tamir, O; Franz, C; Song, P; Yamin, CK; Keohane, C; Denham, CR; Bates, DW. Health care-associated infections: a meta-analysis of costs and financial impact on the US health care system. JAMA Intern Med. 2013 Dec 9-23;173(22):2039-2046.

In: Microbiological Clinical Hygiene
Editor: Eino Elias Hakalehto
ISBN: 978-1-63463-428-1

Chapter 11

Oral Mucosa and Microbial Threats

Ilkka Pesola[1], Jouni Pesola[2], Hannu Kokki[3] and Elias Hakalehto[4]
[1]Dental Clinic, Kuopio, Finland
[2]Clinic of Children and Adolescents,
Kuopio University Hospital, Kuopio, Finland
[3]Anesthesia and Operative Services,
Kuopio University Hospital, Kuopio, Finland
[4]Department of Environmental Sciences,
University of Eastern Finland, Kuopio, Finland

Abstract

For better understanding on the complex interactions in the oral cavity and their impacts on the entire body, there is an increasing need for improved tools for research and diagnostics. Novel methods are needed to assess the function and consistence of oral microbial community.

When the first patients with AIDS were treated at dentistry clinics some 30 years ago, the hygienic precautions of the field changed abruptly. Former methods of dental hygiene had to get reformed completely - up to a such extremes that protective coverings with plastic materials during the treatments were introduced to the clinics. This development brought along also many effective and useful advantages into the overall practical dental hygiene.

Oral focuses are attaining growing interest because major infections could cause problems in any part of the human body, especially in heart, endoprostheses and kidneys. Bacteria from oral surfaces may easily pass into bloodstream through gingival pockets, lingual crypts or mucosal and periapical infections. It has been shown that even tooth brushing of healthy gingiva can cause local microcircular bacteremia..

For many decades cardiologists and specialists of infection medicine have had an on-going debate, if the use of prophylactic antibiotics is recommendable, and should it be associated with oral procedures with bleeding. If oral focuses cause general bacteremia or severe infections for example in heart, it may cause catastrophic consequences for an individual patient. Oral cariogenic bacteria (e.g., *Streptococcus mutans*) are not usually highly pathogenic ones in the systematic sense, unlike many less cariogenic bacteria such as *Streptococcus viridans* strains, which more easily can turn pathogenic elsewhere in the body system.

1. Bacterial Flora of Healthy Mouth

Over 700 bacterial species have been detected from the human oral tract. More than half of them have not been cultivable so far. In general, high bacterial diversity and independent distribution of target sites have been found in healthy mouth (Aas et al., 2005). However, there are areas in mouth where different types of biofilms dominate depending on the local circumstances. Lingual dorsum, buccal mucosa, tonsillar crypts or dental hard tissues are typical bases for different biofilm formation. Interestingly, *Candida albicans* yeast and commensal oral streptococci may display a synergistic interaction during oral biofilm formation (Diaz et al., 2012).

Recent studies have introduced new possibilities for producing multi-species oral biofilms, which resemble naturally occurring oral biofilms. (Nance et al., 2013). They mimic oral circumstances where the host body system and the microbes communicate together. Some photographs on the physical formations of dense bacterial cultures and biofilm-like layers are visualized in the chapter 2 of this book.

The oral biofilms produce enzymes and liberate cells, which then are distributed into the entire GI tract, and elsewhere to the entire body system. Since Langerhans' finding on stellate dendritic like cells in 1889 it is questioned what is the role of dendritic cells in bacterial invasions (Shale and Ghosh, 2009). Recent studies have indicated that intestinal mucosa contain many dendritic cells that can even be in contact with the intestinal lumen. This may be one of the potential routes for bacterial cells to pass the mucosal barrier and invade into deeper tissue structures and finally into the bloodstream.

2. Oral Defenses

On oral epithelia similar mechanisms for host protection as elsewhere in the body system are actively protecting us against infections. These defensive host functions include the mucosal antibodies (Feller et al., 2013), defensins (Beck-Broichsitter et al., 2014), ciliary movements (Braun, 2014), enzymatic action (Craitoiu et al., 2011), and several others. Interestingly, the upper human respiratory tract is designed in such a way that microbes present in the inhaled air mostly end up attached onto the outer surface of the pharynx.

Cilial protrudements return inhaled or swallowed cells from the lower epithelial surfaces toward the mouth. The above-mentioned "anatomical design" is exploited in air sampling with impinger devices for instance (Li, 2011). Consequently, many host defenses for the protection of lower respiratory tract, and the GI tract locate in oropharyngeal areas. The task of the cilia is to transport the mucus on cell surfaces and particles attached to it upwards into the pharynx (Aiello and Sleigh, 1977). Cilia move 12 to 14 times per second in which case mucus moves 100 micrometers per second (6 mm/minute). The liquid envelope capsuling the epithelial cells is indispensable to the efficient activity of cilia.

One key issue in human defences is the oral resistance against microbial influences. Many reasons can cause the lowering of this resistance and make the diseased individual more prone to infections and illnesses. These include mechanical trauma, for example tooth brushing, which can assist microbes in entering via gingival pockets to deeper structures (Figure 1).

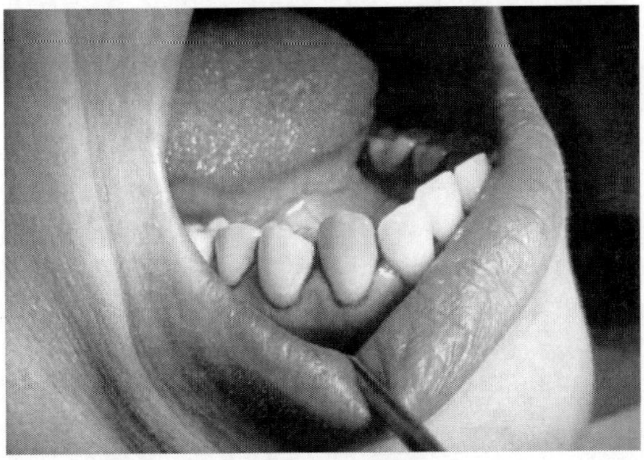

Figure 1. Gingivitis and bleeding after calculus scaling on lower jaw.

Saliva has a major role in maintaining balance in oral mucosa. Therefore, if salivary flow has for some reason decreased, various microbiological problems are eventually. Some medicines, or diseases (for example rheumatoid arthritis, Morbus Sjögren), sytostatic drugs and salivary gland radiation damage are causes for decreases in the saliva flow and changing consistence of the saliva. Consequently, persons with hyposalivation or xerostomia can get help for the mucosal discomfort by artificial saliva products that mimic human saliva and its mucous functions. Unfortunately, those products do not contain the antimicrobial or protective substances, which are present in saliva itself.

The important oral pathogens and principal actions in mouth are listed in Table 1.

Table 1. Oral pathogenic bacteria and infections

Cultivation finding	Importance / detection point
Streptococcus viridans spp.	Endocarditis
Streptococcus mutans	Dental caries
Streptococcus salivarius	Dental biofilm
Streptococcus sanguis	Tongue
Streptococcus mitis	Oral mucosa
Streptococcus milleri	Parodontal abscess
Streptococcus anginosus spp.	Serious odontogenic infections
Lactobacillus spp.	Caries indicators
Aggregatibacter actinomycetemcomitans	Parodontal pathogen
Porphyromonas gingivalis	-- " --
Prevotella intermedia	-- " --
Tannerella forsythia	-- " --
Peptostreptococcus micros	-- " --
Treponema denticola	-- " --
Fusobacterium spp.	Odontogenic abscesses
Bacteroides melaninogenicus spp.	-- " --
Actinomyces spp.	-- " --
Candida albicans	Infection of oral mucosa

3. General Picture of Oral Infections

Biofilms cover all surfaces in various oral cavities; both hard tissues and soft tissues. It is a widely known fact that on different surfaces there are different compositions of microbial flora observed. Therefore, in every situation with tissue traumas or pathogenic invasions, these basically harmless biofilm microbes enter mucosal microvascular veins. It has been shown that every tooth brushing is followed by minor microbial contamination of the veins. For example, in case of immunodeficient patients with cytostatic therapy there is a potential risk of spreading the infections caused by otherwise rather harmless apathogenic bacteria.

Several possible routes exist inside mouth, trough which the infective agents can penetrate the oral mucosa into deeper tissues and into the blood stream (Figure 2). Perhaps the most important routes for intrusion are the gingival pockets surrounding the teeth. Around each tooth there is from 2 mm to several mm deep pocket. Different individuals have quite individual types of microbial population in the biofilms. This relevance of gingival pockets to general health of the body is often underestimated. Even in mild infective circumstances with increased gingival bleeding, mucosal redness and sore mouth are related to health elevated risk status. In such cases microbes have quite an easy route to pass mucosal barriers. Sometimes, if the situation can continue too long even gingival abscesses and deeper parodontal problems can be caused by originally rather harmless inflammation.

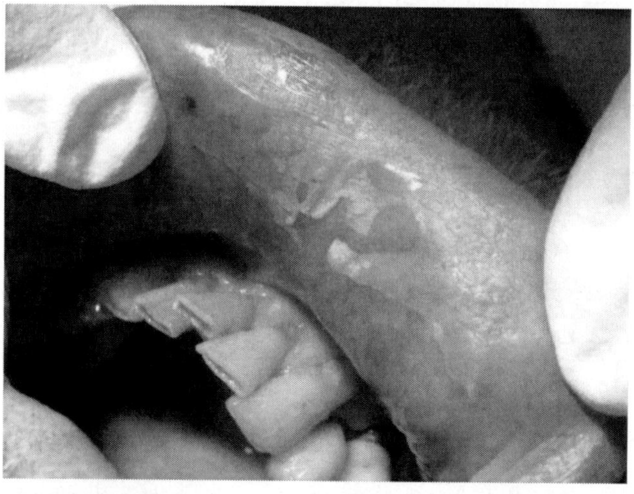

Figure 2. Lesion of leucoplacia on lower lip.

Grooves of lingual mucosa are often suitable locuses to biofilm accumulation. Especially lingual upper surface and buccal mucosa may form a favorable platform for *Candida* growth and infection (Figure 3). Manufacturers of dental devices have developed lingual brushes and circulation spatulas to eliminate microbial load of dorsal lingual mucosa.

Tooth itself may also offer a route for bacterial spreading into the blood circulation. If caries lesions can spread freely deeper into dental pulp the risks are increasing. Pulp inside the dental grown contains arterioles, venulies and nervous fibers. It is quite obvious, that if cariogenic, otherwise quite harmless, bacteria enter pulpal tissue, they can create pulpal inflammation and infection. Then the early symptoms are pain, tenderness to warm liquids and sensitivity to biting forces. If dental caries lesions are not repaired timely enough, infection usually continues as wider pulpal infection with pus and perhaps swelling of the buccal or sublingual tissues. Also the nerve channels may offer a route for the distribution of the pathogens. Mixed strain infections and pathological microbial successions can often take place if proper treatments are delayed. Such generalized infection is severing the health with fever and deeper abscesses associated with numerous acute symptoms. Intravenous antibiotics with drainage are urgently needed in such cases.

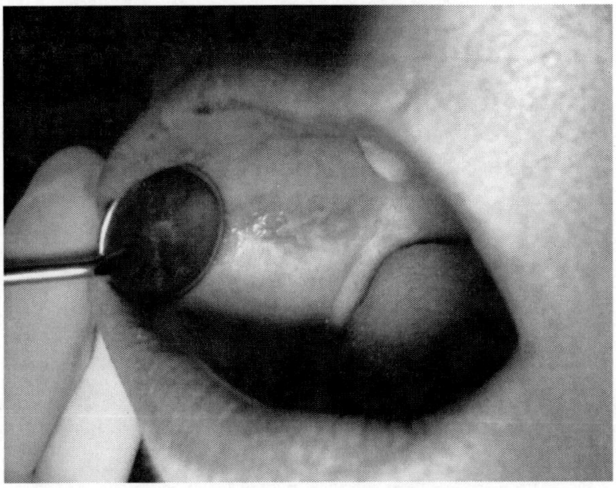

Figure 3. Candidosis of buccal mucosa.

Pro-inflammatory expression and proteolytic activation has been reported in *Porphyromonas gingivalis* provoked gingival infection (Holzhausen, 2010). IL-1α, IL-6, IL-8 and TNF-α expressions are connected with local gingival infection. They are also simultaneous with protease-activated receptor-2, PAR(2) expression. As a clinical result, gingival symptoms like redness, swelling, bleeding, and if continued, bone loss, are caused.

In chronic periodontitis and in periodontal pockets contained infectious *P. gingivalis*, an upregulation of PAR(2) gene expression can occur. At the same time a higher pro-inflammatory profile is associated with advanced clinical parodontal tissue destruction (Fagundes, 2011).

In a Finnish hospital study with 394 patient cases of oral and pharyngeal neck infections, it was found out that bacteriological root cause for even 45 % of the severe deep infections were the microbes originating from the normal flora of the patient (Rajasuo et al., 2014). It is obvious that poor oral hygiene can be associated with a high percentage of relatively harmless flora, but that almost a half of the bacterial infections are caused by the normal flora, brings up many questions, and is also a big issue to be further elucidated.

Why normal flora is that prominent also in infectious situations? Are the bacteriological results from the abscess samples giving a true picture? What is the reason for harmless bacteria inducing life threatening infections? Which is more important, the amount of bacterial load in submucosal tissues or the spectrum of species, or the biofilm composition that colonise certain focuses? Can it be possible that some hazardous pathogens remain hiding during pathogenesis? Green tea and nutrient with rich omega-3 has been found to improve the health of marginal gingival tissues (Hattarki et al., 2013).

Mucosal diseases cause routes for microbes to invade mucosal barriers. Lingual fissures or angular cheilitis, perilabial rhagades, disturb the balance of host and his or her microbes. Normal skin bacteria or fungi may cause harmful lesions to one or both labial commissures (Rabb and Ledher, 1995). Antifungal or antimicrobial local medication is required to improve the situation, and often also a local corticosteroid therapy is needed (Figure 4).

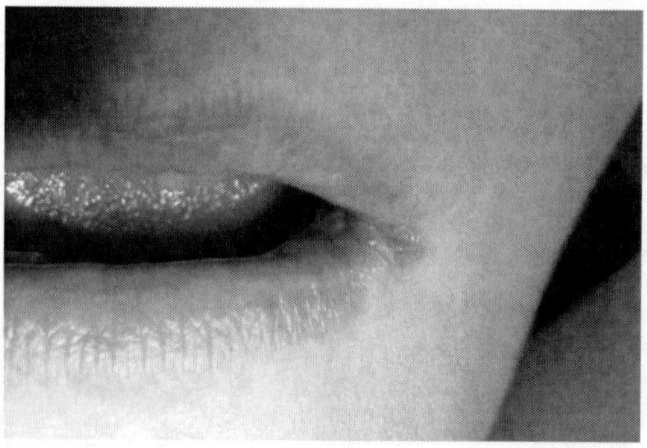

Figure 4. Angular cheilitis with mild skin ulcer.

Patients with HIV are good examples for oral mucosa being highly important for protection against invading pathogens. Many HIV-patients have problems not only with their low ability to resist infections but also with dry mouth, hyposalivation and *Candida* load. Oral mucosa and gingival bleeding can pass easily also other than viral infections. Consequently HIV patients need plenty of careful dental follow up and care. This is the case with all patients suffering from various immunodeficiencies.

High risk for hazardous infections in case of severely sick or other immuno-compromised patients indicates the importance of developing more effective and accurate methods for patient and hygiene monitoring in hospitals (Hakalehto, 2006). The improved level of early-warning techniques is proposed to have a life-saving effect (Hakalehto, 2010).

4. Invasion at Mucosal Level

Bloody marginal gingiva is a suitable target for an inflammatory process. In some conditions the risk of gingival invasion caused by various bacteria is increased. Smoking, diabetes mellitus and some general blood disease like leukemia and lymphoma alter blood circulation in gingival tissue. Circulation in microvessels is limited in smoker's mouth. Diabetic oral mucosa is changed especially when blood sugar is elevated on a continuous basis. Sugar rich gingival crevicular fluid is a very favorable medium for parodontal bacteria. It has been said that one can see the blood sugar balance by observing the color of the marginal gingiva. The higher blood sugar level is, the more reddish is the gingival margin. Typical symptoms are besides the red colour, easy bleeding in brushing and sometimes mild soreness. The elevated sugar levels in the mouth can cause an increase in rapidly growing enterobacterial species normally more abundant in the duodenum (Hakalehto et al., 2008).

Both smoking and diabetes weaken the resistance against parodontogenic bacteria. Long-term prognosis is poor when diabetic patient is also a smoker. The present data suggest that crevicular IL-1β, IL-6 and IL-8 reflect the activity of periodontal destruction, whereas IL-4 shows an inverse correlation to it (Giannopoulou et al., 2003). The enhanced production of inflammatory cytokines in the presence of smoking and stress may have clinical consequences. Certain general blood diseases like acute leukemia may also cause gingival swelling and tissue hyperplastic growth. These can be caused also by some medications. It is known that gingival hyperplasia is caused by the use of hydantoin drug in epilepsia. Similarly some patients have gingival overgrowth, when cyclosporin is used for treatment.

Chronic gingivitis and parodontitis are result from the inflammatory processes in the gingival tissue. The inflammation is caused mainly by the bacterial plaque. The immune response against these processes is regulated in part by different cytokines (Giannopoulou, 2003). These above-mentioned conditions may increase the microbial invasion trough gingival margin and gingival pocket. Many local cytokine chains such as IL-1β, IL-8, IL-18, IL-11, IL-12, TNFα, IL-4, IL-17, IL-1α and IL-6 are found in saliva and crevicular fluid. IL-1β in the saliva and/or crevicular fluid of patients with gingivitis take part to that inflammatory load in gingiva at cell level. Especially in saliva or/and crevicular fluid IL-1β can be used as a marker of gingival inflammation (Boronat-Catala et al., 2014).

Cytokines are strong local inflammatory mediators. Epithelial chemokine (CCL28), interleukin-8 (IL-8), interleukin-1β (IL-1β) and tumor necrosis factor-alpha (TNF-α) are the most important cytokines in the periodontal inflammatory disease. They play a key role in the host response to inflammation. The inflammation in periodontal diseases may be important in prognosis and in understanding the periodontal diseases. (Ertugrul, 2013). It has been found out that IL-6 increase the amount of immature DCs in the chronic parodontitis. IL-2, TNF-α, IFN-γ, IL-10, and IL-17A cytokine levels were higher vs. normal gingiva chronic parodontitis (Souto, 2014).

Mostly Gram-negative bacteria colonize the gingival pockets. As periodontitis is an immune-inflammatory disease of gingival tissues, it is important to understand that immune responses in these tissues have both protective and destructive roles.

Although the cytokines, proteases and prostaglandins struggle at the same time against microbial burden and load, these molecules also promote connective tissue loss and alveolar bone resorption and destruction. Major changes can be seen histopathologically and as destruction of periodontal ligament, with deepening of periodontal pockets. This phenomenon causes bone loss around teeth, which can get converged to attain tooth loss (Trindade, 2014).

5. Dental Clinic at Risk of Infection in Blood Contact and by Dissemination of Mouth Infection

Dentists are almost during every patient visit in contact with the patient`s oral environment and blood. Most dental procedures cause some kind of bleeding or at least contact with blood. Tooth extraction, oral surgical operations, calculus elimination and quite often tooth fillings may cause bleeding and micro-invasion of oral bacteria in and out of biofilms. Local contamination is mostly quite harmless because of good oral tolerance against foreign invaders. In any case, proper mouth hygiene is needed for protecting the patients and other people against transmission.

Also the various oral infections need to be contained. It has been shown that even in 3-4 days oral gingival mucosa can start to develop inflammation around teeth if tooth brushing is neglected. - Why is it like that? Biofilms around teeth, or on gingival epithelia grow rapidly and join together with mucins and many kinds of adhesives. In a few days gingival infection appears with swelling, redness and tenderness – even with visible plague. Biofilms have capacity to form acids and initiate changes in mucosal epithelial cells. Some bacteria have also a capacity to intrude deeper into surface epithelium and start an inflammation process in there.

Even minor traumas with tooth pick or toothbrush can create a passageway trough mucosa (Hupp, 1993). Local inflammation starts immediately. Pain and redness are the signs of leucocytes are gathering to trauma site. At the same time mucosal IgA, salivary hormones and antibacterial agents are introduced to limit the initiation of gingival infection.

Severe gingivitis is often a cource of *Aggregatibacter actinomycetemcomitans* or *Porphyromonas gingivalis* –infections. Mild infection is possible to be treated easily with intensifical tooth brushing and by using chlorhexidin gel or mouth wash.

Most of oral infections including caries, gingivitis, parodontitis or even deeper subepithelial infections are endogenic and contain many pathogenic microbes. In some cases also exogenic bacteria may cause oral infections, for example when skin bacteria contaminate oral surgical wounds. Oral endogenic opportunistic pathogens may also cause diseases elsewhere in the body e.g., cardiac endocarditis.

It is an interesting observation that exogenic bacteria quite seldom can cause severe infections in oral tissues. Oral biofilms on different surfaces effectively hinder intruding strain and saliva has protective effects with similar results. It is a generally recognized fact that bacterial balance in oral biofilms is an exceptional effective protective factor. Saliva has many potential components that limit antigen materials from intruding oral mucosa.

For the development of oral mucosal defense system, one of the most important steps is the onset of s-IgA antibody secretion. Children who get plenty of saliva contacts with their mother early in life have significantly more IgG–class antibodies e.g., against *S. mutans* than children with less salivary contacts to adults (Tenovuo and Aaltonen, 1991).

Secretory IgA (s-IgA) and IgG are the two most important antibodies in the saliva. Secretory antibodies develop in major and minor salivary glands and in their plasma cells, while IgG is mostly derived from the serum (Reynolds, 1999). From salivary glands secretory antibodies flow to salivary ducts transforming simultaneously from monomers into dimeric and polymeric forms. The flow of salivary s-IgA maturates at the school age and after that the amount of s-IgA in saliva secretions is quite stable throughout the entire lifespan.

Secretory IgA has several protective functions in the gastrointestinal mucosa. It has been observed *in vitro* in tissue culture experiments on intestinal epithelial cells (Bollinger et al., 2003). It is supposed that s-IgA may be involved not only in host defense alone, but it may also interact with the gut mucosa and limit local inflammation induced by bacteria. s-IgA may also promote the adhesion of non-pathogenic biofilm to the gut mucosa with mucins, and may have a defensive activity produced by this mechanism. Whether it is the case also on the oral mucosa should be evaluated in future studies (Fagarasan and Honjo, 2004). In passive immunization, egg yolk IgY has been used for oral mucosal protection (Hakalehto and Kuronen, 1998).

Infection of the oral mucosal surfaces often contain specific microbes. Mucosal stomatitis (infection of oral mucosa) can be caused by *Staphylococcus aureus,* and glossitis (infection of lingual mucosa) by haemolytic streptococci, and mucositis (infection of mucosa, in general) by enterococci, and the local or more general mucosal infections can be caused by various intestinal bacteria (*E. coli* and *Enterococcus*, *Klebsiella*, *Proteus* or *Candida* spp.) (Dahlen and Frandsen, 2002).

6. Infection in Deeper Tissues

Most common infective disease in mouth is the tooth caries. If cariogenic microbial process with acid formation continues, the infection goes eventually into deeper structures, and via dentinal tubules into pulpal tissue and periapical bone.

Oral mucosa faces bacterial, viral and fungal microbial loads. Gingival infections and more severe parodontal infections with calculus are almost as usual infections as caries in teeth. In elderly patients parodontitis causes most cases of tooth loss and edentulous jaws. The attention of oral professionals has already for many decades been directed toward investigations on parodontal microbes and into processes inside gingival mucosa and parodontal pockets. Parodontopathogens are seemingly well documented. Other mucosal diseases inside mouth are often viral or fungal, the latter most often being caused by *Candida* sp.

Oral mucosa is a very suitable platform for biofilms to fasten and grow. Saliva and its components regulate in many ways, how much and what kind of microbes can join together into mixed biofilm populations. With oral mouth rinses and local medicines or antibiotics it is possible to change biofilm formation, but as in other bodily mucosal tissues, original biofilm structure and construction will usually return in a few weeks or months.

Even minor mucosal infections may develop deeper infections if the general health of the patient is compromised. Especially patients on cytostatic medications having low amounts of leucocytes may easily develop abscesses and swelling in oral surroundings. Therefore, it is recommendable that if the amount of neutrophils is less than 0,5-1, tooth extractions should be delayed. And if the amount of neutrophils is less than 0,5 it is contraindicated for tooth extraction or other oral surgical therapies.

Streptococcus intermedius belongs to *Streptococcus anginosus* group. It is a part of the common oral microbial flora. Despite being regarded as a harmless apathogenic commensal organism, *S. intermedius* has been documented to also cause severe abscesses in different parts of the body (Leishman et al., 2013).

Deeper oral mucosal infections such as periapical abscesses, dental periconitis, osteomyelitis of jaws or alveolitis may be caused by many anaerobic becteria (*Streptococcus* spp., *Veillonella* spp., *Prevotella oralis / buccae*, *Porphyromonas* spp., *Fusobacterium nucleatum*, *Treponema denticola* etc.). Intravenous antibiotics are usually needed in case of large incision wounds or tooth extractions when deeper infections have penetrated oral tissues.

Serious oral infections appear roughly in the following propositions: ostitis periapicalis 70 %, parodontitis and pericoronitis 15-20%, others 10-15%. All these infections can create harmful symptoms and adverse effects also to the general health, if microbes transfer to blood circulation. General symptoms of infection are for example local swelling, pain and fever. On the basis of laboratory parameters leucocytosis and increase in CRP are commonly detected.

7. Caries and Dental Acidic Milieu

Caries develops when oral bacteria convert sucrose, glucose and fructose into acids, mainly lactic acid, through fermentation in a glycolytic process (Holloway and Moore, 1983).

Enamel demineralization is dependent on the acidity on tooth surface, especially on plaque biofilm. Saliva is a potent natural substance to neutralize the acidic effect. If bacterial acid production is high and long-lasting enough, the balance turns toward demineralization and microscopic defects can be seen on enamel surfaces. After this progress, damages can still be recovered, if only acidic influence decreases and salivary remineralization can be achieved. In this situation fluoric toothpaste or mouth rinse or xylitol supplements are influencing positively. In case of minor defects, the enamel can then be healed.

The oral bacteria being most responsible for dental caries are the strains belonging to *Streptococcus mutans* group, species of oral streptococci and lactobacilli. Especially *S. mutans* and *S. sobrinus* can cause deleterious caries (Hardie, 1982). These microbes produce high levels of lactic acid by fermentation of sugars from the daily diet.

Various parts of teeth differ in their sensitivity to cariogenesis quite remarkably. Cementum of root surfaces demineralize easier than coronal enamel surfaces (Rogers, 2008). Even wider spectrum of bacteria effect the root caries than enamel caries; including *Lactobacillus acidophilus*, *S. mutans*, *Nocardia* spp. and *Actinomyces* spp.

Caries of dental enamel is mainly caused by *S. mutans* or *S. sobrinus*; dentinal caries by lactobacilli and caries on root surface by *S. mutans*, lactobacilli, *Actinomyces* sp., and others (Dahlen, 2002).

8. History of Antibiotic Profylaxis in Oral Hygiene

Antibiotic prophylaxis has been under scientific debate already for many decades with respect to the treatments of oral bacterial diseases. There are controversial studies resulting in recommendations toward the use of prophylactic antibiotics and against it prior to oral surgery. Northrop and Crowley (1943) published a paper of 138 patients with infective endocarditis (IE) treated already more than 70 years ago. They indicated that bacteremia in blood was reduced after dental extraction from 12.8 % to 4 % by using sulfathiatzole. They concluded: ”In patients with valvular disease, the possibility of ensuing subacute bacterial endocarditis is greatly diminished by premedication with sulfathiazole” (Morris, 2001).

Bacterial load in bloodstream after tooth extraction or gingival surgery varies between 82 and 88 %. After tooth brushing it is about 40% (Bisno et al., 1989; Lockhart et al., 2008).

About ten years after the finding the Northrop and Crowley (in 1955) AHA (American Heart Association) made the first recommendation on the prophylactic use of antibiotics. Although it`s controversial whether prophylaxis produces any benefits or not, dental personnel in western countries have been usually motivated to use antibiotic prophylaxis prior to intraoral operations with blood exposition (Wilson et al., 2008). A number of practitioners of inner medicine are against regular prophylactic use of antibiotics mainly because some severe and especially allergenic side effects. Even one dose of amoxicillin (2 g) can cause an anaphylactic reaction with larynx-oedema and a life threating progressive situation.

Nowadays recommendation in Finland is that about one hour prior to surgical oral procedures with bleeding 2 g of amoxicillin, or in case of allergy clindamycin 600 mg or cefalexin 2 g, azithromycin 500 mg, clarithromycin 500 mg or roxithromycin 300 mg, is given to the patient. Finnish dentists are well motivated to use prophylactic antibiotic medication because severe consequences may follow even in small oral procedures without it. Side-effects like anaphylactic reactions after oral antibiotic medication are relatively rare.

The future of prophylactic use needs more studies on causal-relation between oral harmless biofilms and endocardial or endoprosthetic infections. Intestinal side-effects with altered microbial balance after even one dose of prophylactic antibiotic medication gives new light to discussion if systematic prophylactic use is recommended or not. The balance of intestinal flora seems to be important in many inflammatory processes and mild infections of human body. The use of probiotics for the maintenance of both oral and GI microbial is recommended (Hakalehto, 2012, Hell et al., 2013).

9. Oral Etiology of Cardiac Endocarditis

Infective endocarditis (IE) is a rare bacterial infection of endocardial endothelium. The endocarditis is often combined with so called valvulitis in cardiac valves. Endocarditis may be a severe infection with high mortality rate and long intensive care periods (Zoellner, 2011). For some reason men have a double risk for endocarditis compared to women. Especially patients with artificial cardiac valves, less than a year after surgery, have increased risk for endocarditis and valvular problems, their amount in this group being even 1000-fold compared to normal population (Owen and Huang, 2012). Most common site for endocardial infection is the aortic valve (Heiro et al., 2007). The bacterial spectrum, that cause endocarditis is wide: *S. aureus* and *Streptococcus* sp. (particularly *S. epidermidis*) are the two main microbial types; enterococci and pneumococci follow next (Piper et al., 2001). In about 20 % of the IE cases the blood sampling gives negative results (Nonaka et al., 2013). Most common procedures that may cause IE are treatments of teeth (particularly extractions), urologic operations, gastrological procedures and cutaneous cuts or incisions (Heiro, 2006).

10. Oral Biofilms and Endoprotheses

The amount of endoprotheses is growing all the time with the ageing populations. Especially the number of protheses in knee and hip joints is manifold in numbers compared with the situation 30 years ago.

On the surface of endoprotheses, the defence mechanisms of the body system are functioning with much lower level of efficacy than in normal joints. That is the reason for even harmless kinds and small numbers of microbes in blood circulation potentially causing severe joint infections. The fundamental cause for infection in endoprotheses is, in more than 90 % of the cases, some apatogenic microbe of the existing biofilms of the body. In many cases the origin of such microbial invasion is located to the mouth or to urinary mucosa or skin. Oral biofilm is usually situated in periapical lesion or in periodontal pockets of teeth. Therefore, if a patient has endoprosthetic operation planned in near future, it is important to extract bad teeth with high risk of inflammation and contamination of new prostheses via blood circulation.

If endo-operation is already made, it is recommended for a prophylactic reason that an antibiotic would be used for 6 months after operation. After that period of time, it is not necessary to maintain this prophylactic protection.

Conclusion

Oral moist and incessantly warm mucosal environment is a suitable environment for microbial colonization. Therefore biofilms appear almost immediately after birth in the mouth of a newborn baby, and consequently on his or her esophagus and gut. Epithelial microbial balance is based on multifactorial chains of events. Oral fluids, especially saliva, contain many bactericidal functions, exhibit salivary buffer capacity and regulate pH in an environment where microbes are well maintained but under permanent control by the host defenses. Biting and grinding of food boluses causes mechanical stress to mucosa and its biofilm composition.

Healthy gingiva and other oral surfaces with oral enzymes protect the whole body from getting sick and from many spreading infections. Therefore it is important to avoid any unnecessary mechanical traumas especially if patient is under weakened capacity for wound healing, e.g., in case of immunodeficient or elderly people with weakened general health. It is important to understand the mechanisms, how microbes can spread through mucosal barriers and why even basically harmless bacteria can cause severe infections in deeper tissues of oral and neck region. For some patients, green tea and nutrients rich in omega-3 have improved the condition of marginal gingiva. Also other nutritional factors and treatments protecting the oral epithelia and other tissues could be beneficial for the oral health. Mechanisms behind many of these influences are not well-known to this date. More studies are warranted for elucidating the background of the mechanisms, by which the microbial load and invasion of microbes can hinder or even totally prevent infections. At same time, knowledge on many pathogenic microbes is everincreasing and pathogenic mechanisms are known more and more precisely. Eventually, all accumulated research data could lead into increasingly holistic views on microbiological balances in the mouth. This increase in oral microbiology studies has a positive contribution to our general health.

References

Aas, J. A., Paster, B. J., Stokes, L. N., Olsen, I., Dewhirst, F. E. Defining the normal bacterial flora of the oral cavity. *J. Clin. Microbiol.,* 2005; 43(11), 5721-5732.

Aiello, E., Sleigh, M. Ciliary function of the frog oro-pharyngeal epithelium. *Cell. Tissue. Res.,* 1977; 9, 178(2), 267-278.

Beck-Broichsitter, B. E., Dau, H., Moest, T., Jochens, A., Stockmann, P., Wiltfang, J., Becker, S. T. Immunohistological expression of human ß-defensin-1 and human ß-defensin-2 in exacerbation of acute and secondary chronic osteomyelitis of the mandible. *J. Oral Pathol. Med.,* 2014; 16. [Epub ahead of print].

Bisno, A. L., Dismukes, W. E., Durack, D. T., Kaplan, E. L., Karchmer, A. W., Kaye, D., Rahimtoola, S. H., Sande, M. A., Sanford, J. P., Watanakunakorn, C., Wilson, W. R. Antimicrobial Treatment of Infective Endocarditis due to Viridans Streptococci, Enterococci, and Staphylococci. *JAMA,* 1989; 261(10), 1471-1477.

Bollinger, R. R., Everett, M. L., Palestrant, D., Love, S. D., Lin, S. S., Parker, W. Human secretory immunoglobulin A may contribute to biofilm formation in the gut. *Immunology,* 2003; 109, 580-587.

Boronat-Catalá, M., Catalá-Pizarro, M., Bagan, S. Salivary and crevicular fluid interleukins in gingivitis. *J. Clin. Exp. Dent.,* 2014; 1, 6(2):e175-e179.

Braun, A. P. Cigarette smoke and calcium conspire to impair CFTR function in airway epithelia. Channels (Austin). 2014; 22, 8(3). [Epub ahead of print].

Crăiţoiu, M. M., Păuna, M., Crăiţoiu, S., Mercuţ, V. Clinical and histoenzymatic interrelations of the edentulous ridge's mucosa. *Rom. J. Morphol. Embryol.* 2011; 52(1), 99-104.

Dahlen, G., Frandsen, E. Yleistä suuinfektioista. *Suomen Hammaslääkärilehti,* 2002; vol 4, 144-148.

Diaz, *P.,* Xie, Z., Sobue, T., Thompson, A., Biyikoglu, B., Ricker, A., Ikonomou, L., Dongari-Bagtzoglou, A. Synergistic interaction between Candida albicans and commensal oral streptococci in a novel in vitro mucosal model. *Infect. Immun.* 2012; vol. 80, 2620-2632.

Ertugrul, A. S., Sahin, H., Dikilitas, A., Alpaslan, N., Bozoglan, A. Comparison of CCL28, interleukin-8, interleukin-1β and tumor necrosis factor-alpha in subjects with gingivitis, chronic periodontitis and generalized aggressive periodontitis. *J. Periodontal Res.* 2013; 48(1), 44-51.

Fagarasan, S., Honjo, T. Regulation of IgA synthesis at mucosal surfaces. *Curr. Opin. Immunol.,* 2004; 16, 277-283.

Fagundes, J. A., Monoo, L. D., Euzébio Alves, V. T., Pannuti, C. M., Cortelli, S. C., Cortelli, J. R., Holzhausen, M. Porphyromonas gingivalis is associated with protease-activated receptor-2 upregulation in chronic periodontitis. *J. Periodontol.* 2011; 82(11), 1596-1601.

Feller, L., Altini, M., Khammissa, R. A., Chandran, R., Bouckaert, M., Lemmer, J. Oral mucosal immunity. *Oral Surg. Oral Med. Oral Pathol. Oral Radiol.* 2013; 116(5), 576-583.

Giannopoulou, C., Kamma, J. J., Mombelli, A. Effect of inflammation, smoking and stress on gingival crevicular fluid cytokine level. *J. Clin. Periodontol.* 2003; 30(2), 145-153.

Hakalehto, E. Semmelweis' present day follow-up: Updating bacterial sampling and enrichment in clinical hygiene. *Pathophysiology,* 2006; 13, 257-267.

Hakalehto, E. Hygiene monitoring with the Portable Microbe Enrichment Unit (PMEU). *41st R3 -Nordic Symposium. Cleanroom technology, contamination control and cleaning. VTT Publications 266.* Espoo, Finland: VTT (State Research Centre of Finland). 2010. pp. 164-176.

Hakalehto, E. (Ed.). Alimentary microbiome – a PMEU approach. New York, NY, USA: Nova Science Publishers, Inc. 2012; 263 pp.

Hakalehto, E., Kuronen, I. A method for producing jelly sweets, which contain antibodies. WIPO Patent Application WO/1998/043610.

Hakalehto, E., Humppi, T., Paakkanen, H. Dualistic acidic and neutral glucose fermentation balance in small intestine: Simulation *in vitro*. 2008: *Pathophysiology,* 15, 211-220.

Hardie, J. M. The microbiology of dental caries. *Dent. Update, 1982;* 9 (4): 199–200, 202–204, 206–208.

Hattarki, S. A., Pushpa, S. P., Bhat, K. Evaluation of the efficacy of green tea catechins as an adjunct to scaling and root planing in the management of chronic periodontitis using PCR analysis: A clinical and microbiological study. *J. Indian Soc. Periodontol.* 2013; 17(2), 204-209.

Heiro, M., Helenius, H., Mäkilä, S., Hohenthal U., Savunen, T., Engblom, E., Nikoskelainen, J., Kotilainen, P. Infective endocarditis in a Finnish teaching hospital: a study on 326 episodes treated during 1980–2004. *Heart* 2006; 92, 1457-1462.

Heiro, M., Helenius, H., Hurme, S., Savunen, T., Engblom, E., Nikoskelainen, J., Kotilainen, P. Short-term and one-year outcome of infective endocarditis in adult patients treated in a Finnish teaching hospital during 1980-2004. *BMC Infect. Dis.* 2007; 17, 7, 78.

Hell, M., Bernhofer, C., Stalzer, P., Kern, J. M., Claassen, E. Probiotics in Clostridium difficile infection: reviewing the need for a multistrain probiotic. *Benef. Microbes.* 2013; 1;4(1), 39-51.

Holloway, P.J., Moore, W.J. The role of sugar in the etiology of dental caries. *J. Dent.* 1983; 11 (3), 189–213.

Holzhausen, M., Cortelli, J. R., da Silva, V. A., Franco, G. C., Cortelli, S. C., Vergnolle, N. Protease-activated receptor-2 (PAR(2)) in human periodontitis. *J. Dent. Res.* 2010; 89(9), 948-953.

Hupp, J. R. Changing methods of preventing infective endocarditis following dental procedures: 1943 to 1993. *J. Oral. Maxillofac. Surg.* 1993; 51(6), 616-623.

Leishman, S. J., Seymour, G. J., Ford, P. J. Local and systemic inflammatory responses to experimentally induced gingivitis. *Dis. Markers.* 2013; 35(5), 543-549.

Li K. Molecular comparison of the sampling efficiency of four types of airborne bacterial samplers. *Sci. Total Environ.* 2011; 15, 409(24), 5493-5498.

Lockhart, P. B., Brennan, M. T., Sasser, H. C., Fox, P. C., Paster, B. J., Bahrani-Mougeot, F. K. Bacteremia associated with toothbrushing and dental extraction. *Circulation,* 2008; 117, 3118-3125.

Morris, A. M., Webb, G. D. Antibiotics before dental procedures for endocarditis prophylaxis: back to the future. *Heart.* 2001; 86(1), 3-4.

Nance, W. C., Dowd, S. E., Samarian, D., Chludzinski, J., Delli, J., Battista, J., Rickard, A. H. A high-throughput microfluidic dental plaque biofilm system to visualize and quantify the effect of antimicrobials. *J. Antimicrob. Chemother.* 2013; 68(11), 2550-2560.

Nonaka, M., Kusuhara, T., An, K., Nakatsuka, D., Sekine, Y., Iwakura, A., Yamanaka, K. Comparison between early and late prosthetic valve endocarditis: clinical characteristics and outcomes. *J. Heart Valve Dis.* 2013; 22(4), 567-574.

Owen, C. P., Huang, W. H. Antibiotic prophylaxis for dental procedures: is it necessary? *SADJ.* 2012; 67(7), 413-419.

Piper, C., Körfer, R., Horstkotte, D. Prosthetic valve endocarditis. *Heart.* 2001; 85(5), 590-593.

Rabb, D. C., Lesher, J. L Jr. Antibiotic prophylaxis in cutaneous surgery. *Dermatol. Surg.* 1995; 21(6), 550-554.

Reynolds, H. Y. Defense mechanisms against infections. *Curr. Opin. Pulm. Med,* 1999; 5, 136-142.

Rogers, A. H (editor). *Molecular Oral Microbiology.* 2008; Caister Academic Press.

Shale, M., Ghosh, S. How intestinal epithelial cells tolerise dendritic cells and its relevance to inflammatory bowel disease. *Gut.* 2009; 58(9), 1291-1299.

Souto, G. R., Queiroz-Junior, C. M., de Abreu, M. H., Costa, F. O; Mesquita, R. A.Pro-inflammatory, Th1, Th2, Th17 cytokines and dendritic cells: a cross-sectional study in chronic periodontitis. *PLoS. One*. 2014; 26, 9(3):e91636.

Tenovuo, J., Aaltonen, A. S. Antibody responses to mutans streptococci in children. *Proc. Finn. Dent. Soc.,* 1991; 87, 449-461.

Trindade, F., Oppenheim, F. G., Helmerhorst, E. J., Amado, F., Gomes, P. S., Vitorino, R. Uncovering the molecular networks in periodontitis. *Proteomics Clin. Appl.* 2014; 14. (Epub ahead of print).

Wilson, W., Taubert, K. A., Gewitz, M., Lockhart, P. B., Baddour, L. M., Levison, M., Bolger, A., Cabell, C. H., Takahashi, M., Baltimore, R. S., Newburger, J. W., Strom, B. L., Tani, L. Y., Gerber, M., Bonow, R. O., Pallasch, T., Shulman, S. T., Rowley, A. H., Burns, J. C., Ferrieri, P., Gardner, T., Goff, D., Durack, D. T. American Heart Association. Prevention of infective endocarditis: guidelines from the American Heart Association: a guideline from the American Heart Association Rheumatic Fever, Endocarditis and Kawasaki Disease Committee, Council on Cardiovascular Disease in the Young, and the Council on Clinical Cardiology, Council on Cardiovascular Surgery and Anesthesia, and the Quality of Care and Outcomes Research Interdisciplinary Working Group. *J. Am. Dent. Assoc.* 2008; 139, Suppl:3S-24S.

Zoellner, H. Dental infection and vascular disease. *Semin. Thromb. Hemost,* 2011; 37, 181-192.

In: Microbiological Clinical Hygiene
Editor: Eino Elias Hakalehto

ISBN: 978-1-63463-428-1

Chapter 12

Drug Development Regarding the Digestive Microbiota

***Eva M. del Amo*[1] *and Elias Hakalehto*[2]**
[1] School of Pharmacy, University of Eastern Finland, Kuopio, Finland
[2] Department of Environmental Sciences,
University of Eastern Finland, Kuopio, Finland

Abstract

Emerging concern on the potential of colonic microbiota on the disposition of the oral drugs is existing among the scientific circles. The role of the gut microbiota is underestimated in the actual process of drug development of new drug entities. New *in vitro* approaches will improve the understanding on the effects of bacterial metabolism on the oral drug and constitute the input to build promising *in silico* models that could be used in early stages of the drug development process.

In the design of drug delivery systems, the metabolic action of the gut microbiota could be used to deliver anticancer drug into the colon for the treatment of colorectal cancers. This promising approach could be further applied for local treatment of inflammatory bowel diseases or for improving drug absorption into systemic circulation to treat various illnesses.

The potential metabolic function of various microorganisms can as well benefit the pharmaceutical industry in the production of mannitol, an up-and-coming excipient for oral and other drug dosage forms. This production method is cheap, environmentally friendly and efficient. Mannitol has excellent physicochemical properties to accompany the active pharmaceutical ingredient in the dosage form improving the stability, taste and drug release, among others.

1. Gut Microbiota Metabolism in Oral Pharmacokinetics: Predictive Tools

Drug development is a very laborious and expensive process. One of the major reasons for failures during the clinical phases of drug development is the poor pharmacokinetic (PK) properties of the drug candidate. Oral administration is the most common route for drug administration. Absorption, distribution, metabolism and excretion of drugs (abbreviated as ADME) are the PK processes that determine the disposition of the drug within the body and the concentration in the target site. A schematic overview of the gastrointestinal transit of the oral drug is given in Figure 1, paying a special attention to the role of the intestinal microbiota. Within the gastrointestinal tract (GIT), the contents of enzymes in epithelial cells change containing almost no enzymes in the large intestine (Guyton, 2011). In turn, the intestinal microbial colonization increases towards the colon region, reaching the number of 10^{11} microorganisms per gram of gut content. In the upper intestines the microbial cells are functioning in the moving chyme. The microbiota produces a vast number of reductive and hydrolytic enzymes such as azoreductases, glycosidases, and glucuronidases. Both, host and bacterial enzymes distribution are symbolized by red shapes in Figure 1. The host metabolic enzymes primary in liver and also in the GI epithelium produce high molecular weight metabolites via oxidation and conjugation (Phase I and II metabolism). While the bacterial enzymes generate non-polar low molecular weight metabolites by reductive and hydrolytic reactions.

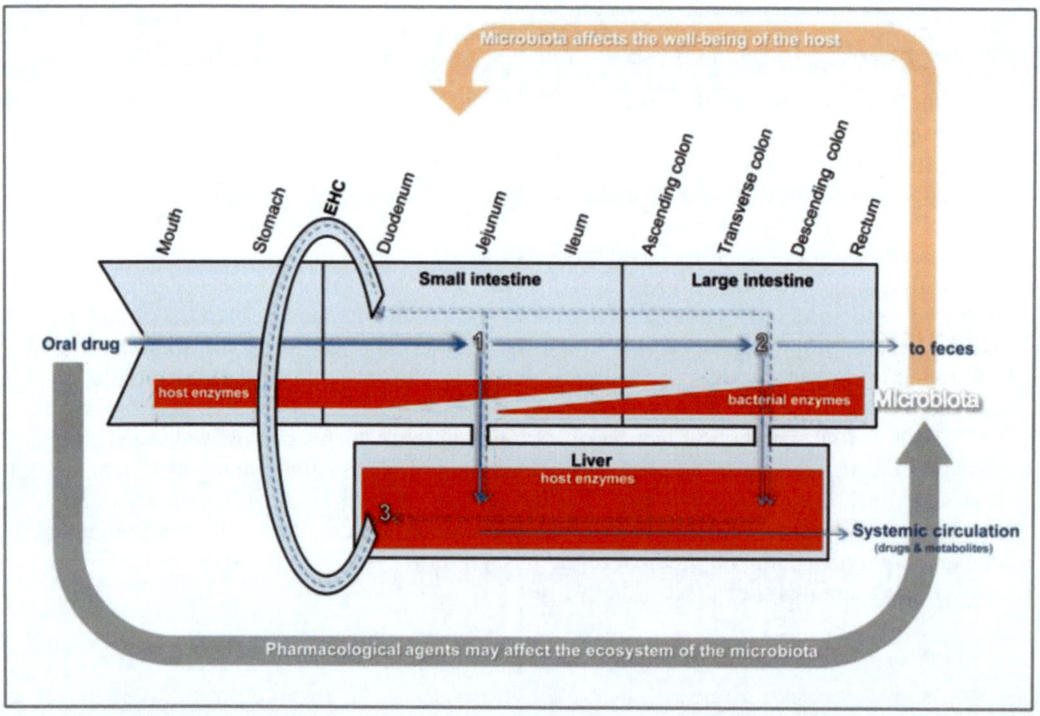

Figure 1. The oral drug fates in the body. The blue arrows show the direction of the drug or metabolites transport in the body and the dashed ones correspond to the enterohepatic circulation (ECH). The distribution of enzymes from the host and gut microbiota is in red.

The absorption of drugs from the intestinal lumen is a very complex process influenced by both physicochemical properties of the drug (drug ionization, solubility, lipophilicity, particle size, endurance of enzymatic actions) and physiological factors of the GIT (such as GIT pH, GIT blood flow, transit time though the different segments, presence of food and various groups of organic and inorganic compounds). After oral administration, drugs are primarily absorbed in the small intestine. This is the region of GIT that has the largest surface area (in Figure 1 marked by number 1). Drug transport across intestinal epithelial surface is mediated basically by one or several of the following processes: passive diffusion and carrier-mediated influx (in the absorptive direction) or efflux transport (in the direction back to the gut lumen). Moreover, the drug is susceptible to intestinal metabolism by cytochrome P-450 enzymes abundant in the intestinal mucosa. This is called intestinal first pass metabolism.

Though the small intestine is considered the dominant site for absorption, some hydrophilic drugs subjected to minimal metabolism in the upper region can reach the colon and be hydrolysed by the enzymatic action of the microbiota. The products of bacterial metabolism can be absorbed in the colon if they are lipophilic enough (in Figure 1 shown by number 2) or eliminated via feces.

The absorbed drug fraction enters the mesenteric blood circulation and reaches the liver via the portal vein. The molecule may experience different fates: be metabolized by hepatic enzymes, be transported from the hepatocyte into the bile or continue to the systemic circulation by the hepatic vein distributing in the organism. In general, more hydrophilic drugs, passes through the liver unchanged, because they cannot permeate the hepatocyte membrane to undergo hepatic metabolism. More lipophilic drugs permeate into the hepatocyte and are metabolized into hydrophilic metabolites. Only a portion of the absorbed drug enters the systemic circulation in unchanged form. The fraction metabolized in the liver undergoes Phase I and/or Phase II reactions, or vice-versa. In Phase I reactions, enzymes introduce reactive, polar groups into the substrates while Phase II consists in conjugation reactions that yield highly polar compounds, e.g., glucuronides. Phase I and Phase II metabolites can be transported into the blood or actively secreted into bile (glucuronides with a molecular weight < 300 preferentially pass into the blood and are eliminated in the urine, while those with molecular weight > 300 enter the bile) (Lüllmann et al., 2000).

The unchanged drug (as well as the resulting metabolites) excreted into the bile (number 3, in Figure 1) are secreted into the duodenum and are accessible for intestinal absorption. Their reabsorption closes in the so-called enterohepatic cycle .

The conjugates are highly polar compounds and so are poorly absorbed from the small intestine. In the colon they can be cleaved by bacterial β-glucuronidases enabling the liberated drug molecule to be reabsorbed. If they remain unhydrolysed they are rapidly eliminated from the body in the feces.

In drug design special attention is given to the first pass elimination where the mammalian enzymes are involved, focusing especially in the hepatic processes. Often the metabolism of gut microbiota is underestimated. For example, the term of "drug first pass elimination" is widely used as the sum of intestinal first pass metabolism and hepatic first pass elimination (hepatic metabolism and biliar excretion), excluding a third factor: the first pass metabolism by the microbiota. Moreover, it is important to notice that microbiota can be also present in the moving chyme in upper regions and there are microbes resistant to the antibacterial properties of bile. Bile acids have been shown to influence intestinal bacteria *in vitro* (Hakalehto et al., 2010). However, it was found out that the bile salt hydrolase (BSH) activity was not related to the resistance to toxicity of bile substance in lactobacilli (Moser and Savage, 2001). In any case, individual bile secretion is an important factor influencing the drug adsorption, also through microbiota. The alteration of its distribution and qualities in various parts of small intestines has been studied (Mallony et al., 1973a). It was also stated that the most normal subjects yielded from their proximal and mid-small bowel small numbers of Gram-positive aerobic bacteria (Mallony et al., 1973b). The anaerobes outnumbered the aerobes 100- or 1000-fold. In some samples, levels of up to 10 000 cells of both coliforms and *Bacteroides* sp. were detected per ml. The presence of antibodies in the bile fluid seemed to be more dependent to local microbiological conditions than on any systematic effect (Hansen and Jackson, 1990). Bile tracts of diseased individuals seemed to contain approximately 1/3 of enterobacterial strains, and 1/3 of enterococci, besides miscellaneous isolates (Hakalehto et al., 2010). Lactobacilli and clostridia were less abundant in this case.

The microbiota may as well affect drug absorption in colon indirectly by altering the physical conditions within the intestinal lumen e.g., the pH that will modify the degree of ionization of ionizable molecules and therefore decreasing the permeability of the compound through the intestinal membrane (Williams et al., 1971). The gut microbiota affects the integrity of the GI epithelial cells, bacteria may promote cell renewal and wound healing and regulation of the mucus layer (Natividad and Verdu, 2013). The gut microbiota is involved in the stimulation of the gut immune system and the regulation of cell proliferation (Kau et al., 2011), in the synthesis of essential vitamins K and B_{12} (Hill, 1997), and providing resistance to colonization by pathogens. Dysregulation of the microbiota community has been linked to diseases ranging from allergies to bowel inflammation and obesity (Natividad and Verdu, 2013). Overall, the maintenance of intestinal barrier homeostasis requires complex interactions between the microbiota, host genes, and other environmental factors such as diet. The alteration of this delicate equilibrium between the host and the microbiota will affect the physiology of the intestine and the intestinal permeability of different compounds, including drugs (Figure 1). In addition, the drug treatments can also affect the intestinal microbiota, the most typical and evident example being the antibiotic administration. Poorly absorbed antibiotic drugs such as ciprofloxacin can reach the colon in active form and suppress quantitatively and qualitatively the intestinal microbiota in an acute manner (Edlund et al., 2000)

In summary, the intestinal microbiome can be involved in different levels of the ADME characteristics of active compounds affecting:

1) the absorption (A): by modifying the physiological conditions within the intestinal lumen or directly when the active drug is a product of the bacterial metabolism in colon (i.e., colonic-targeted drug delivery systems).
2) the distribution (D): when the bacterial metabolism allows the EHC to continue prolonging the distribution of the drugs in the body.
3) the metabolism (M): by degrading the drug in colon by the bacterial enzymatic action

Therefore, potential substrates of the gut microbiota include the numerous drugs that are eliminated via the bile and undergo in some extent EHC (Gao et al., 2013) and those drugs that reach the colon. The latter ones are as well increasing in number due to the emerging design of colon specific drug delivery systems for example, for new drug candidates with poor solubility/permeability (Sousa et al., 2008). The specific bacterial transformations may give products with increased biological properties compared to the parent compounds or lead to extensive degradation of the drug decreasing the bioavailability. However, the bacterial metabolite may as well be toxic. One example is the drug sorivudine that came to the Japanese market as a promising antiviral drug. The drug was metabolized by the gut microbiota and though the bacterial metabolite was not toxic itself, it inhibited the metabolism of the anticancer drug 5-fluorouracil (5-FU) in co-administrated patients leading to toxic levels of 5-FU (Okuda et al., 1998, Sousa et al., 2008). In short, the extensive metabolic potential of the intestinal microbiota could lead to unpredictable diversity of metabolic reactions.

Therefore, in the course of drug development, the metabolism of microbiota should be addressed, whether microbial metabolites are formed and if so, which type: pharmacologically inactive or active or even toxic. Inclusion of microbial metabolic processes in drug bioavailability screening should become a standard practice. Sousa and colleagues reviewed in detail the different available models to elucidate GI bacterial metabolism such as human *in vivo* studies, animal *in vivo* studies and *in vitro* studies (Sousa et al., 2008). In addition, *in silico* studies based on computational models could be used with the advantage that they can be applied in early stages of drug development, reducing the number of the previously mentioned studies, and hence reducing costs and development time. Pieper and Bertau (2010) presented in their review an *in silico* model (Pharmbiosim model) based on a yeast (*Saccharomyces cerevisiae*)for predicting the drug metabolism induced by the GI microbiota (). The *in silico* model is built based on the experimental data on drug metabolism in the yeast, and further experiments can be tested in the living system in order to verify the predictions of the model. Such model is proposed to predict the microbial metabolism in the GIT providing indications of which metabolites may be formed.

For *in vitro* studies, the two most accurate systems of dynamic GIT simulators are the Simulator of the Human Intestinal Microbial Ecosystem *SHIME* (Molly et al.,, 1993) and the GIT model *TIM* by the Dutch research institute TNO (Minekus et al.,, 1999). These bioreactor systems aim to simulate the human intestinal ecosystem of the GIT and have increased understanding of the role of intestinal microbiome on the biotransformations of active compounds. However, a systematic validation is one of their limitations as well as the time required for setting up the systems. Recently, a review that evaluates the *in vitro* models in drug development for oral dosages forms has been published (Kostewick et al., 2014). New *in vitro* tools for the prediction of *in vivo* performance of oral dosage forms are proposed. Among them, the *TIM* system is suggested for simulations of whole GIT including the elucidation of the role of large intestinal microbiota. However, no comments were addressed with respect to the role of microbiota on the new drug entities or advisable *in vitro* studies for its prediction.

More attention should be paid to the microbial potential on ADME together with the improvement of the actual predictive tools. One option is to isolate strains from predeterminated species, and to study their interactions in the PMEU (Portable Microbe Enrichment Unit) (Hakalehto et al., 2008, Hakalehto et al., 2010, Hakalehto and Hänninen, 2012). By the use of combination of *in silico* and *in vitro* methods less *in vivo* studies may be needed to elucidate the role of the GI microbiota on the drug fate.

2. Gut Microbiota Metabolism: Development of Drug Delivery Systems

Drug delivery systems are investigated with the aim to develop more effective therapeutic treatments. These systems are loaded with the therapeutic drug which is released at the specific target site ensuring an effective concentration of the drug and reducing the systemic side effects. For such systems, researchers need move up to adaptive materials for drug delivery (so called smart polymers). These are defined as polymers that undergo reversible large, physical or chemical changes in response to small external changes in the environmental conditions for example temperature, pH, light, etc. In the cancer therapy, one commercial example is ThermoDox® (made by Celsion Corporation) that consist in thermo-sensitive liposomes that encapsulate the antitumor drug doxorubicin. ThermoDox® is administrated by IV infusion and an external hyperthermic (heat-based) treatment is applied on the tumor area. The heat-sensitive liposome rapidly changes structure when heated to a specific temperature, creating openings in the liposome which release doxorubicin directly into the targeted tumor. Currently the drug delivery system has entered Phase III trials for the treatment of primary liver cell carcinoma and is in Phase II clinical trials for the treatment of breast cancer and colorectal liver metastasis. Additionally, in cancer therapy, for example, various combined treatments can be applied for the benefit of a patient. One such application is the study on oxidative stress and free radical biology in the initiation and therapies of malignant tumors (Spiz et al., 2012).

Drug delivery systems are also investigated for colonic targeting after oral administration. They are aiming to treat illnesses such as colonic cancers and inflammatory intestinal diseases (e.g., Crohn's disease, ulcerative colitis). Based on the pH variation along the GIT between 2 (stomach) and 10 (colon), pH-sensitive polymers has been used for colon specific drug delivery. However, pH in GIT varies depending on diet, pathological conditions and between subjects making the release of the drug less predictable. Hence, a suitable alternative to direct drugs to colon is the use of the enzymatic action of the colonic microbiota as a "trigger". Colon-targeting biodegradable polymer systems contain polymers that protect the drug from the environments of stomach and small intestine. Moreover, the polymers are sensible to the microbial degradation in the colon where the drug is delivered and can permeate through the colon epithelium. Some examples are azo-polymeric coating (polymers that are bound to the drug moiety by azo-linkage), polysaccharide based delivery systems (polysaccharides substrates such as amylose, chitosan, and dextran can carry the drug) or combination of polysaccharides (namely lactulose) and materials such as methacrylic acid copolymers in tablet system (Sinha and Kumaria, 2003; Philip and Philip, 2010). The most recently drug delivery technologies for colon specific delivery systems have been reviewed by Kotla and co-workers (Kotla et al., 2014) where COLAL, CODES™,PHLORAL™ tableting technologies are presented as bacteria triggered systems. The first one uses amylose as the coating material, which shows the characteristics of resistance to pancreatic α-amylase but degraded by colonic bacterial enzymes. The CODES™ technology is based on lactulose polymer whose fermentation by the microbiota will indirectly release the drug from the system, first acidifying the microenvironment and then inducing the dissolution of the enteric coating of Eudragit® E. PHLORAL™ technology utilizes a resistant starch that resist the action from the host digestive enzymes but not from the colonic bacterial enzymes. The

Eudragit® S coating prevents the disintegration of the film in the upper GIT and controls swelling of starch. Another example of a colon-specific delivery system currently under research is the one designed by Ma and Coombes (2013) to deliver anticancer drug for colorectal cancer. It consists of alginate microcapsules containing Eudragit®. Alginate is a hydrophilic polysaccharide that forms a compact alginic acid gel at low gastric pH which impedes drug release. Progressively the hydrogel swells giving gradual release of the drug loaded. Additionally, alginate may be degraded by the metabolism of colonic bacteria with the local delivery of the anticancer drug in colon. The alginate microcapsules are coated with Eudragit® S100, which dissolves at pH 7.0, to prevent drug release in the upper GI tract. This system provides a combination of pH, time-delayed and microbiome responsive release of the drug.

Another strategy in the development of colonic-targeted drug delivery systems is the design of prodrugs. A prodrug is a pharmacologically inactive derivative of parent drug molecule that requires spontaneous or enzymatic transformation *in vivo* to release the active drug. For colonic delivery, the hydrophilic prodrug is designed to undergo minimal hydrolysis in the upper tracts of GIT and be susceptible to cleavage by the bacterial enzymes, (so azo-, glucuronide-, glycoside- bond derivatives or cyclodextrin-derivatives) releasing the active drug moiety (more lipophilic than the prodrug) that will be absorbed in the colon (Stella et al., 2007). One example of prodrug is sulfasalazine that was the first bacteria-sensitive system developed for colonic delivery to treat inflammatory bowel disease. The active ingredient is mesalazine (or 5-aminosalicylic acid, an anti-inflammatory drug) linked by azo bond to a carrier molecule, sulfapyridine (Peppercorn and Goldman, 1972). Besides aiming at therapeutic local action, colon specific drug delivery systems may be used as well for biopharmaceutical reasons such as improvement of the oral bioavailability of drugs (avoiding degradation and/or lack of absorption in the upper GIT); prevention of the gastric irritation induce by some drugs such as non-steroidal anti-inflammatory drugs (NSDA); or delay in drug absorption e.g., in case of nocturnal asthma or angina (Sinha and Kumaria, 2003; Philip and Philip, 2010). In connection with NSDA or antibiotic medications, their effects could be supported by the use of pre- and probiotic products for balancing the gut microbiota (Hakalehto and Jaakkola, 2013). See also chapters 18 and 20 of this book.

3. Gut Microbiota Metabolism: Production of Mannitol Excipient

Mannitol is formed from fructose. The theoretical maximum is 67% of the available fructose. Some species, such as *Propionibacterium shermani* and *Lactobacillus xylosus*, can convert lactate to propionate. In 2009 more than half of the propionic acid commercially produced in the US was used as feed or grain preservatives, but the nutritional and pharmaceutical uses are strongly increasing.

Microorganisms can be used as a "factories" for production of compounds. The most typical example is the production of antibiotics. In the present section we will describe an innovative production of mannitol by microorganism fermentation.

Mannitol is a sugar alcohol, $C_6H_8(OH)_6$, with a MW of 182.17 Da. It is a white, crystalline and sweetish powder, water-soluble and not hygroscopic. Mannitol is present in the nature, produce by many organisms such as bacteria, yeast, fungi, algae, lichens, and many plants (Song and Vieille, 2009). It is also a non-toxic substance.

Mannitol is a versatile compound with many applications in the pharmaceutical industry. The most exploited one is as an excipient. An excipient is an inactive substance formulated alongside the drug substance (active pharmaceutical ingredient or API). It should be inert to the API, improve API's stability, enable bioavailability and be inert towards the treated patient. Mannitol is catching more and more attention for its use as an excipient due its excellent physicochemical properties. It can be used in a wide array of dosage forms. In oral dosage forms it can be used as diluent (also called bulking agent or filler), binder (holding the ingredients in a tablet together), plasticizing agent in pills and to enhance material flow. In other dosage forms, it can be utilized as tonicity agent, carrier and lyophilization aid being a popular freeze drying excipient (Rowe et al., 2012). Mannitol is already used also in many sweets and chewing gums.

Mannitol is not hygroscopic and thus reduces the potential for pH-based degradations. It can be used with moisture-sensitive APIs to protect them from hydrolysis or with amorphous materials to protect them from crystallization. Moreover, mannitol does not undergo the Maillard reaction that happens between reducing sugars and amino groups e.g., with lactose and other carbohydrate diluents and the free amines of APIs such as protein drugs leading to APIs' degradation. The mannitol inertness to API together with the conferring protection against degradation makes mannitol the excipient of election for the new drug candidates of biological origin e.g., oligonucleotides or protein drugs which are highly susceptible of hydrolysis and Maillard reactions. Mannitol ensures good stability and storage conditions of the dosage form.

The water solubility of mannitol makes it a good diluent/binder for a fast dissolution or disintegration of the solid dosage form upon contact with the saliva. Moreover, orally given mannitol is not absorbed significantly from the GIT, showing a strong inertness towards the patient. Therefore, mannitol does not increase the levels of blood glucose to such an extent as fructose or lactose are rising it up (Debord et al.,1987). This makes mannitol especially suitable for drug products which are given to diabetics. Further, it is a good alternative to the lactose excipient for drug therapy in case of lactose intolerant patients. The recommended warning labels in USA for oral pharmaceutical formulations containing mannitol indicate that doses over 20 g may cause a mild laxative effect thus showing a safer profile than other polyol excipients (Zumbe et al., 2001).

Mannitol can be used in oral dosage forms as a sweetener that imparts a cooling sensation in the mouth being adequate sweetener as well for diabetic patients. This "mouth feel" property makes it very appealing for the patient, improving the compliance of the treatment.

Recently, Ohrem and co-workers have published a review on mannitol as an excellent excipient for solid oral dosage forms (Ohrem et al., 2014). They described its beneficial physicochemical features as mentioned above. Mannitol can also facilitate a direct compression process in tabletting exhibiting excellent mechanical properties, rapid dissolution and good mouth feel. It is ideal for mouth disintegrating solid doses such as chewable, sublingual, orally disintegrating tablets, and lozenges.

In addition, mannitol has been proposed as an ideal carrier for dry-powder inhaler formulation (Nokhodchi and Larhrib, 2013). Dry-power inhalers have become a popular mean of drug delivery via the lungs, however, they suffer for low drug delivery efficiency. The main reason for that is the insufficient release of the API from the carrier due to strong interparticulate forces. Lactose has been used extensively as a carrier, but present serious drawbacks. It is unsuitable for diabetic and lactose intolerant patients, Maillard reactions (e.g., with budesonide) or interaction with moisture-sensitive APIs. However, mannitol is a potential promising carrier not exhibiting the previous pitfalls. Moreover, mannitol gives an obvious sweet taste sensation that is a useful indicator that the dose has been taken. Nokhodchi and co-workers claim that a particulate engineering is required to tailor the mannitol particles as suitable carriers for specific dry-power inhaler systems. The authors present the modifications required to facilitate API´s detachment from the carrier in their paper (Nokhodchi and Larhrib, 2013). Mannitol is also excellent excipient for freeze-dried formulations for pulmonary drug delivery. The authors suggest that such delivery systems can be applied not only for local treatment of pulmonary diseases but also for systemic release to treat cancer, diabetes and neurological diseases.

Further, mannitol has been considered as an exceptional ternary component e.g., improving the efficiency of lactose based dry-powder inhaler (Kaialy and Nokhodchi, 2013) or upgrade the maintenance of the tablet harness formulated with microcrystalline cellulose during the storage (Ohrem et al., 2014).

However, Ohrem and co-authors remark in their paper that mannitol requires some more effort to be produced than other excipient e.g., lactose (Ohrem et al., 2014). Therefore, the economical point has not been in favor to mannitol so far. The method of its industrial manufacturing is usually by the catalytic or electrolytic reduction of monosaccharides such as mannose or fructose. This process requires higher efforts and brings out lower yield comparing to other polyol excipients. However, the fermentation by microorganisms is an alternative process to the traditional industrial mannitol production. A novel, fast and effective process for mannitol bioconversion has been recently developed in the Finnoflag Oy's laboratory in Finland (Figure 2). This is a promising method with better yields and being more economical. Lactic acid bacteria in a natural mixture obtained from the rumen content could be used in the production of mannitol from fructose-containing biomass (Hakalehto, 2013). In Figure 3, the NMR (Nucleic Magnetic Resonance) graphs of mannitol illustrate the fact that in 20-22 hour process time around 50% of the substrate had been converted into the product. There were still high amounts of sugars remaining in the solution giving a reason to expect still higher yields. The sugar alcohol product, mannitol is then recovered and purified. Novel methods for mannitol downstream processing are under development. They are economically lucrative in comparison with the relative high prices of purified mannitol obtained from other industrial processes. Moreover, the demand for mannitol as excipient in the pharmaceutical formulation development is increasing.

On the other hand, mannitol can be used as an API as well. In osmotherapy, intravenously injected mannitol is excreted rapidly by the kidneys. Not being reabsorbed from the renal tubule, mannitol increases water and Na^+ excretion via its osmotic effect and decrease indirectly the pressure in the brain and eyes. The use of mannitol in intracerebral hemorrhage is well characterized based on decreasing the amount of water in the brain parenchyma to reduce the intracranial pressure. Mannitol has been shown to improve markers of parenchymal metabolic function in patients with intracerebral hemorrhage though investigations on its merits as a clinical treatment is still under way (Corrigan et al., 2013). Mannitol has been used in the short-term management of glaucoma and especially to reduce intra-ocular pressure before ophthalmic surgery. It does not cause the several side-effects associated with traditional glaucoma medications (Levy, 2011). Moreover, mannitol has been injected to increase urine flow in patients with acute renal failure and to promote the excretion of toxic substances by forced diuresis. The adequate rehydration of the patient should be followed-up (Sweetman, 2011). Additionally, its therapeutic role in the treatment of Parkinson disease has been suggested (Shaltiel-Karyo et al., 2013). The authors showed that mannitol presented a general neuroprotective effect in a Parkinson *Drosophila* as well as in the Parkinson mice model.

Mannitol has been investigated in the area of drug delivery to the brain (Passeleu-le Bourdonecc et al., 2013). After intra-carotid injection to the patient, mannitol acts as transient blood-brain barrier disrupter with the aim to deliver drugs into the brain. Their mechanism of action is based on osmotic induction of blood-brain barrier (BBB), the hyperosmolar conditions created on the systemic circulation side of the BBB causes a reversible shrinkage of the endothelial cells, leading to a paracellular opening between endothelial cells. This strategy is primarily used for the treatment of brain tumor when less invasive treatment has not been effective.

Besides, mannitol has been used as a diagnostic agent for kidney function. In pharmaceutical research, mannitol has been used to characterize the paracellular permeation between epithelial cells in *in vitro* studies.

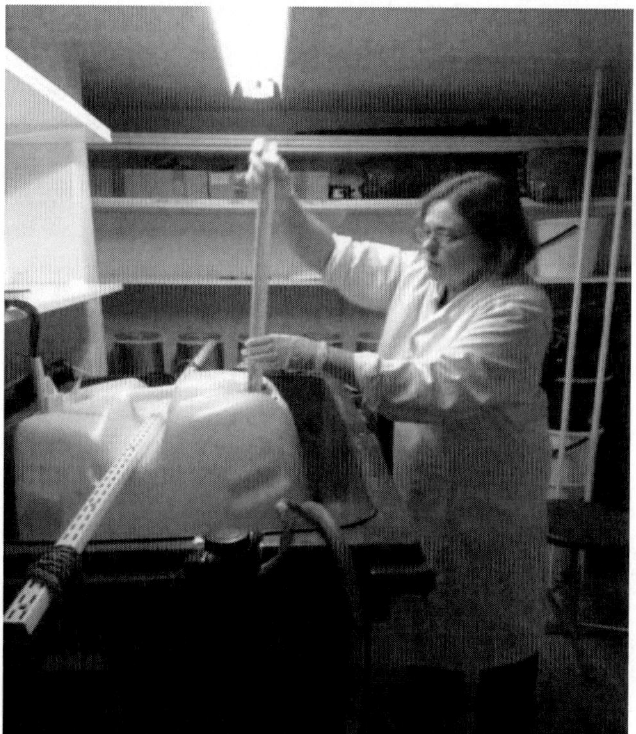

a

Figure 2 a-c. (Continued).

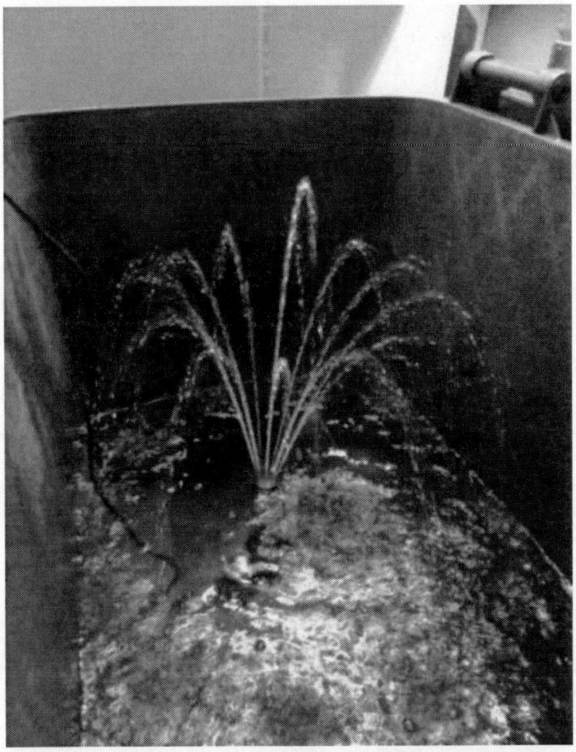

b

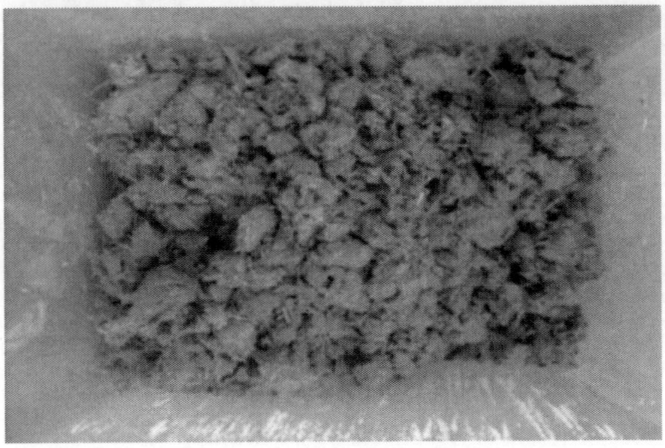

c

Figure 2 a-c. Photographs from pilot experiments for the production of mannitol. a. manual adjustment of the process, b. filling in the water bath, c. fermentation end product, where mannitol and other dissolved organic compounds have been removed. Mannitol concentration reached 20-30% in the experiments at the laboratory of Finnoflag Oy. Mannitol is formed from fructose. The theoretical maximum is 67% of the available fructose. Some species, such as *Propionibacterium shermani* and *Lactobacillus xylosus*, can convert lactate to propionate. In 2009 more than half of the propionic acid produced in the US was used as feed or grain preservatives, but the nutritional and pharmaceutical uses are strongly increasing. Photos: Kevin King.

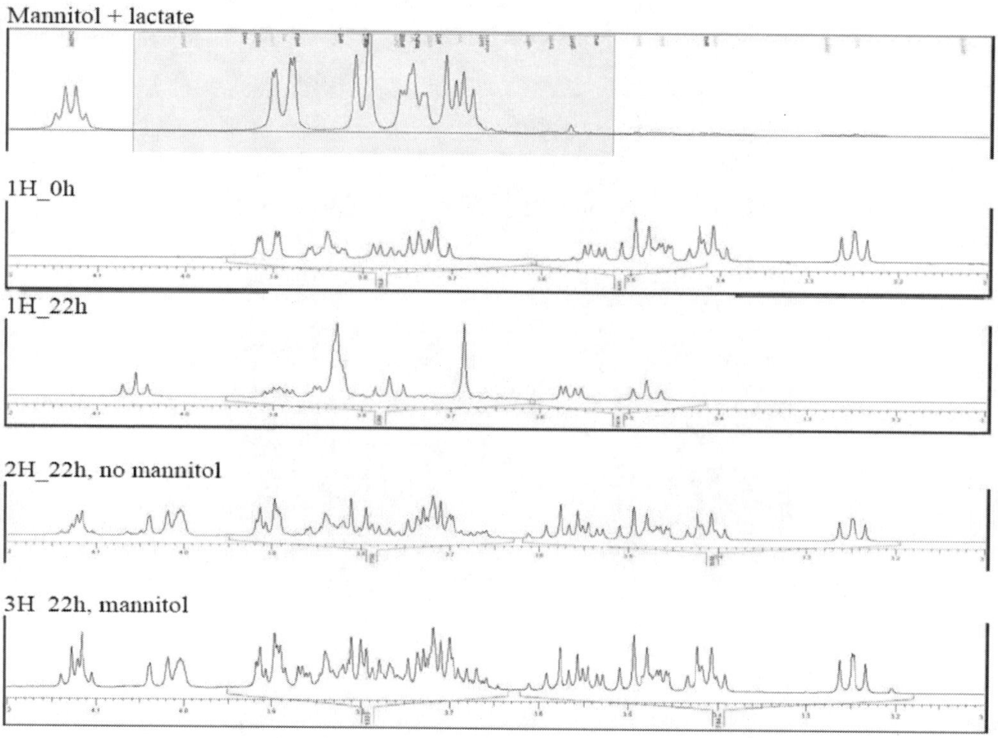

Figure 3. Different NMR graphs on various process phases during fermentative mannitol production. The runs were carried out at the University of Eastern Finland, and results analyzed by Prof. Reino Laatikainen at the Department of Pharmacy.

The wide and versatile applications of mannitol have increased the interest for developing the production processes, especially when larger amounts are required for its use as an excipient. The current methods for its industrial manufacturing seem demanding and with low efficacy. However, the Finnoflag process in mannitol production is exploiting the principles of joint action of mixed bacterial cultures. It is a natural way to arrange the manufacturing of this useful product exploiting the holistic approach where microbial communities are effectively used, and the yield and productivity get significantly increased.

Conclusion

Though challenging, improvement of the actual *in vivo*, *in vitro* and *in silico* models of gut microorganism metabolism and their rational combination are needed. Their implementation in the drug development process will improve the prediction of gut microbiome action on new drug candidates. However, this is not the only relevant aspect of the role of digestive microbiota in drug development. The intestinal microbiome metabolism can be utilized to design drug delivery systems for drug colon targeting for various therapeutic and biopharmaceutical approaches. On the other hand, the potential of microbial metabolism can be applied to produce mannitol, an excellent excipient that may improve the formulation of drugs during the drug development.

References

Corrigan, M. L., Escuro, A. A., Kirby, D. F. *Handbook of Clinical Nutrition and Stroke.* New York: Springer Science + Business Media; 2013

Debord, B., Lefebvre, C., Guyot-Hermann, A. M., Hubert, J., Bouché, R., Cuyot, J. C. Study of different crystalline forms of mannitol: Comparative behaviour under compression. *Drug Development and Industrial Pharmacy*, 1987; 13 , 1533-1546

Edlund, C., Nord, C. E.. Effect on the human normal microflora of oral antibiotics for treatment of urinary tract infections. *Journal of Antimicrobial Chemotherapy*, 2000; 46, 41-48.

Gao, Y., Shao, J., Jiang, Z., Chen, J., Gu, S., Yu, S., Zheng, K., Jia, L. Drug enterohepatic circulation and disposition: Constituents of systems pharmacokinetics. *Drug Discovery Today*, 2013; 19, 326-340.

Guyton, A. C. *Text book of medical physiology.* 7th edition. Saunders College Publishing/Harcourt Brace; 2011

Hill, M. J. Intestinal flora and endogenous vitamin synthesis. *European Journal of Cancer Prevention*, 1977; 6 , 43-45.

Hakalehto, E. Mahalannan biotekninen hyödyntäminen. Finnish Patent Application FI20130286 (in Finnish); 2013.

Hakalehto, E., Hänninen, O. Gaseous CO_2 signal initiate growth of butyric acid producing *Clostridium butyricum* both in pure culture and in mixed cultures with *Lactobacillus brevis*. *Can J Microbiol.*, 2012; 58, 928-931.

Hakalehto, E., Jaakkola, K. Synergistic effect of probiotics and prebiotic flax product on intestinal bacterial balance. *Clinical Nutrition,* 2013; 32 , 200.

Hakalehto, E., Humppi, T., Paakkanen, H. Dualistic acidic and neutral glucose fermentation balance in small intestine: Simulation *in vitro*. *Pathophysiology,* 2008; 15, 211-220.

Hakalehto, E., Hell, M., Bernhofer, C., Heitto, A., Pesola, J., Humppi, T., Paakkanen, H. Growth and gaseous emissions of pure and mixed small intestinal bacterial cultures: Effects of bile and vancomycin. *Pathophysiology*, 2010; 17, 45-53.

Hansen, P. G., Jackson, G. D. The occurance and sources of natural antibody in human bile and serum against the O antigens of two *Escherichia coli* serotypes. *Scan J. Immunol.,*1990; 32, 537-544.

Kaialy, W., Nokhodchi, A. Engineered ternary additives improve dispersion of lactose-salbutamol sulphate dry powder inhalations. *The AAPS Journal*, 2013; 15, 728-743.

Kau, A. L., Ahern, P. P., Griffin, N. W., Goodman, A. L., Gordon, J. I. Human nutrition, the gut microbiome and the immune system. *Nature*, 2011; 474, 327-336.

Kostewicz, E. S., Abrahamsson, B., Brewster, M., Brouwers, J., Butler, J., Carlert, S., Dickinson, P. A., Dressman, J., Holm, R., Klein, S., Mann, J., McAllister, M., Minekus, M., Muenster, U., Müllertz, A., Verwei, M., Vertzoni, M., Weitschies, W., Augustijns, P. In vitro models for the prediction of in vivo performance of oral dosage forms. *European Journal of Pharmaceutical Sciences*, 2014; 57, 342-366.

Kotla, N. G., Shivapooja, A., Yashwant. Recent developments in colon specific drug delivery systems: Approaches promising in targeting colon. *International Journal of Pharmaceutical and Clinical Research*, 2014; 6, 101-106.

Levy, J. Primary congenital glaucoma – A rewiev. In Randbone JM, editor. *Encyclopedia of Infection Research 2/3.* New York, USA:Nova Science Publishers Inc.; 2012

Lüllmann H., Mohr K., Ziegler L., Bieger D. *Color Atlas of Pharmacology*, 2000; 32- 43

Ma, Y., Coombes, A. G. A. Designing colon-specific delivery systems for anticancer drug-loaded nanoparticles: An evaluation of alginate carriers. *Journal of Biomedical Materials Research - Part A*, 2013; 102, 3167-3176.

Mallony, A., Keen Jr F., Smith, J., Savage, D. Patterns of bile acids and microflora in the human small intestine. I. Bile acids. *Gastroenterology*, 1973a; 64, 26-33.

Mallony, A., Savage, D., Keen Jr F., Smith, J. Patterns of bile acids and microflora in the human small intestine. II. Microflora. *Gastroenterology*, 1973b; 64, 34-42.

Minekus, M., Smeets-Peeters, M., Havenaar, R., Bernalier, A., Fonty, G., Marol-Bonnin, S., Alric, M., Marteau, P., Huis In't Veld, J. H. J. A computer-controlled system to simulate conditions of the large intestine with peristaltic mixing, water absorption and absorption of fermentation products. *Applied Microbiology and Biotechnology*, 1999; 53 , 108-114.

Molly, K., VandeWoestyne, M., Verstraete,W. Development of a 5-step multichamber reactor as a simulation of the human intestinal microbial ecosystem. *Appl. Microbiol. Biotechnol.* 1993; 39, 254–258.

Moser, S. A., Savage, D. Bile salt hydrolase activity and resistance to toxicity of conjugated bile salts are unrelated properties in lactobacilli. *Appl. Environ. Microbiol.*, 2001; 67, 3476-3480.

Natividad, J. M. M., Verdu, EF. Modulation of intestinal barrier by intestinal microbiota: Pathological and therapeutic implications. *Pharmacological Research*, 2013; 69 , 42-51.

Nokhodchi, A., Larhrib, H. Overcoming the undesirable properties of dry-powder inhalers with novel engineered mannitol particles. *Therapeutic Delivery*, 2013; 4 , 879-882.

Ohrem, H. L., Schornick, E., Kalivoda, A., Ognibene, R. Why is mannitol becoming more and more popular as a pharmaceutical excipient in solid dosage forms? *Pharmaceutical Development and Technology*, 2014; 19, 257-262.

Okuda, H., Ogura, K., Kato, A., Takubo, H., Watabe, T. A possible mechanism of eighteen patient deaths caused by interactions of sorivudine, a new antiviral drug, with oral 5-fluorouracil prodrugs. *Journal of Pharmacology and Experimental Therapeutics*, 1998; 287, 791-799.

Passeleu-Le Bourdonnec, C., Carrupt, P.-A., Scherrmann, J. M., Martel, S. Methodologies to assess drug permeation through the blood-brain barrier for pharmaceutical research. *Pharmaceutical Research*, 2013; 30, 2729-2756.

Peppercorn, M. A., Goldman, P. The role of intestinal bacteria in the metabolism of salicylazosulfapyridine. *Journal of Pharmacology and Experimental Therapeutics*, 1972; 181, 555-562.

Philip, A. K., Philip, B. Colon targeted drug delivery systems: A review on primary and novel approaches. *Oman Medical Journal*, 2010; 25, 70-78

Pieper, I. A, Bertau, M. Predictive tools for the evaluation of microbial effects on drugs during gastrointestinal passage. *Expert Opinion on Drug Metabolism and Toxicology*, 2010; 6, 747-760.

Rowe, R. C., Sheskey, P. J., Cook, W. G., Fenton, M. E. *Handbook of Pharmaceutical Excipients* 7th edition. London: Pharmaceutical Press; 2012.

Shaltiel-Karyo, R., Frenkel-Pinter, M., Rockenstein, E., Patrick, C., Levy-Sakin, M., Schiller, A., Egoz-Matia, N., Masliah, E., Segal, D., Gazit, E. A Blood-Brain Barrier (BBB) disrupter is also a potent α-synuclein (α-syn) aggregation inhibitor: A novel dual mechanism of mannitol for the treatment of Parkinson Disease (PD). *Journal of Biological Chemistry*, 2013; 288, 17579-17588.

Sinha V. R., Kumaria, R. Microbially triggered drug delivery to the colon. *European Journal of Pharmaceutical Sciences*, 2003; 18, 3–18

Spiz, D. R., Dornfeld, K. J., Krishnan, K., Guis, D. Oxidative stress in cancer biology and therapy. New York, USA: Springer, 2012.

Song, S. H., Vieille, C. Recent advances in the biological production of Mannitol. *Applied Microbiology and Biotechnology,* 2009; 84, 55–62

Sousa, T., Paterson, R., Moore, V., Carlsson, A., Abrahamsson, B., Basit, A. W.. The gastrointestinal microbiota as a site for the biotransformation of drugs. *International Journal of Pharmaceutics*, 2008; 363, 1-25.

Stella, J. V., Borchardt, R. T., Hageman, M. J., Oliyai, R., Maag, H., Tilley, J. W. *Prodrugs: challenges and rewards. Part 1.* New York: Springer Science + Business Media; 2007.

Sweetman, S. C. *Martindale: The complete drug reference.* 37th edition. London: Pharmaceutical Press; 2011.

Williams, R. E. O. Hill, V., Drasar B. S. The influence of intestinal bacteria on the absorption and metabolism of foreign compounds. *Journal of Clinical Pathology. Supplement (Royal College of Pathologists)*, 1971; 5,125

Zumbe, A., Lee, A., Storey, D. Polyols in confectionery: the route to sugar-free, reduced sugar and reduced calorie confectionery. *British Journal of Nutrition*, 2001; 85, 31-45.

In: Microbiological Clinical Hygiene
Editor: Eino Elias Hakalehto

ISBN: 978-1-63463-428-1

Chapter 13

Protection of Immunodeficient Patients from Microbiological Risks

Jouni Pesola[1,*] ***and Elias Hakalehto***[2,†]
[1]Department of Pediatrics, Kuopio University Hospital, Kuopio, Finland
[2]Department of Environmental Sciences,
University of Eastern Finland, Kuopio, Finland

Abstract

The relationship between the human body and intestinal microbiota is essential for good health. Development of intestinal microbiota takes place during the first years of life. On the other hand, the protection against serious infections, if they are to come, is often based on heavy medications. This treatment policy is often necessarily combined with an elevated level of urgency. In these cases the body`s immunological defenses are often weakened and compromised.

In a healthy situation, a symbiotic balance exists between the host and the intestinal microbiota. Malfunctioning of the immune system makes the balance more vulnerable in the early childhood. Different situations and diagnoses related to the immunosuppression of children are prematurity, neonatal period, prolonged infections, malnutrition, specific immunodeficiency syndromes, malignancies and different treatments of cancer.

In lowered health status, microbial penetration into undesired tissues is more readily facilitated.

Immunosuppression makes it easier for harmful microbes to overcome the defense mechanisms of the body. This increases the risk of severe morbidity and mortality related to infections. Certain characteristics unique for different clinical situations are reviewed. In the clinical verification of infections, any sign of inflammation is to be taken seriously in the case of severely vulnerable patients.

* Jouni Pesola: Department of Pediatrics, Kuopio University Hospital, P.O.B. 100, FI-70029 KYS, Kuopio, Finland.
† Elias Hakalehto: Department of Environmental Sciences, University of Eastern Finland, P.O.B. 1627, FI-70211 Kuopio, Finland.

1. Methods for Monitoring the Intestinal Microbiota

The microbiota of the esophagus, ventricle and duodenum can be studied when esophago-gastro-duodenoscopy is performed. In clinical practice only samples for the detection of *Helicobacter pylori* are taken frequently. Although no other microbiological sample is routinely taken during the endoscopies of the alimentary tract, it is possible to get samples from different parts by this method. More active sampling and microbiological surveying of the upper GI tract of healthy and diseased individuals could give an improved view on the pathogenesis of many various diseases of the tract (Coelho et al., 1987; Drumm et al., 1987; Fischer, 1992; Gagliardi et al., 1998).

Microbiological balances have been shown to form between various members of the microflora in the PMEU (Portable Microbe Enrichment Unit) (Hakalehto et al., 2008; Hakalehto et al., 2010). This method gives space for more strains of *Enterobacteriaceae*, for instance (Pesola et al., 2009). Utilizing the PMEU method, the development of the health condition of an individual child was followed for more than two years, starting from birth, indicated the importance of close microbiological examinations for recording the advancement of diseases and the phase of the recovery (Pesola and Hakalehto, 2011). The numbers of isolated enterobacterial species at different ages is shown in Figure 1.

The use of PMEU enrichment was very important in the monitoring of enterobacterial microbiota because 72% of the isolates were detected only after enrichment and some species, like *Klebsiella pneumoniae* and *Proteus mirabilis*, were not at all detectable without the PMEU enrichment (Figure 2).

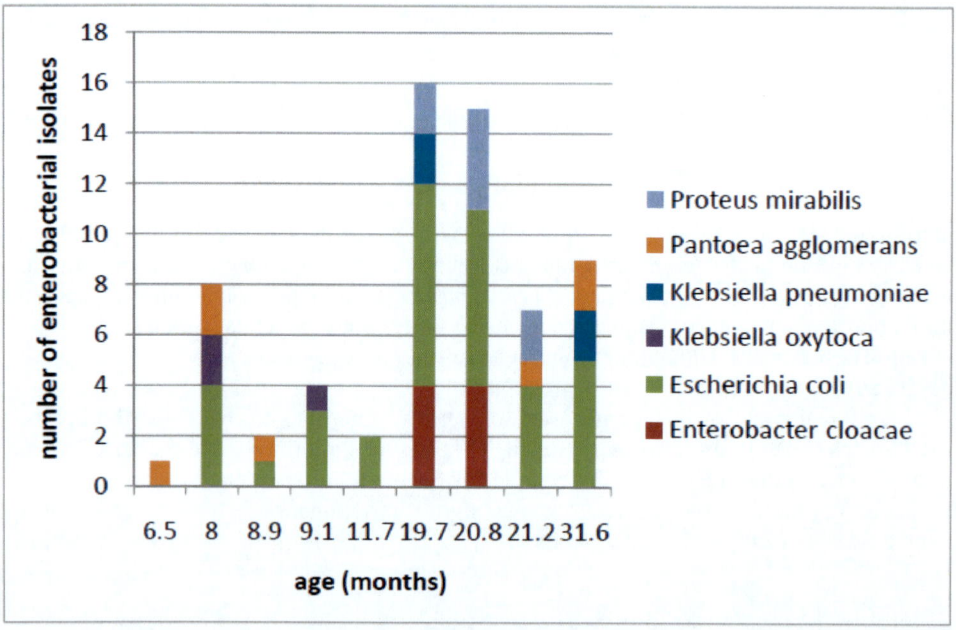

Figure 1. Enterobacterial strains isolated from fecal samples of a child treated by broad-spectrum antibiotics right after birth because of a neonatal septic infection. No enterobacterial strain was detected before the age of 6,5 months.

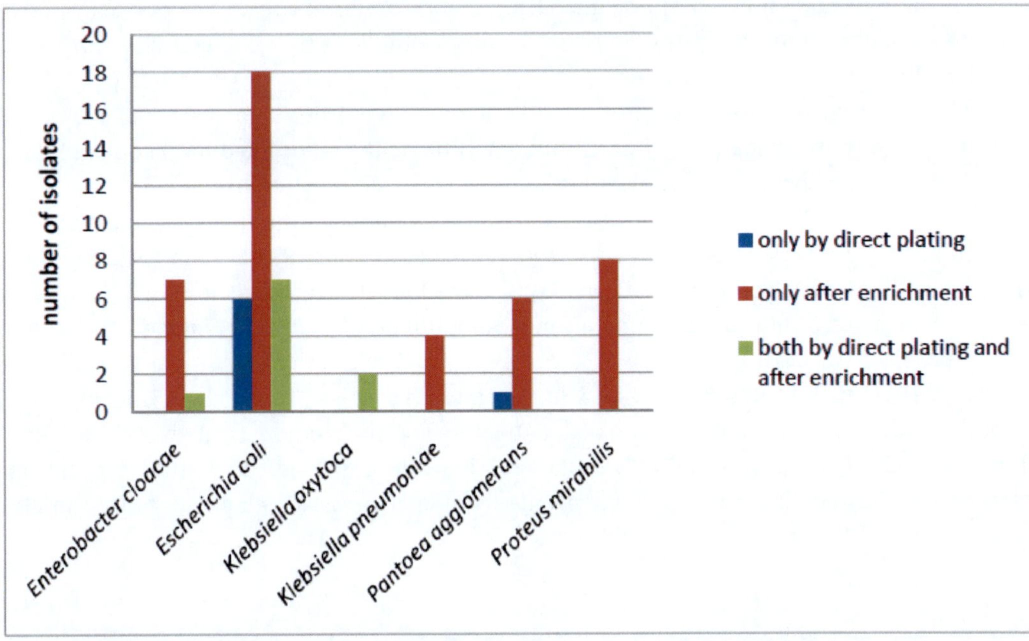

Figure 2. Importance of the PMEU enrichment in the isolation of different enterobacterial species from fecal samples of an infant.

In the pediatric clinical practice the most often performed microbiological examinations from feces are immunological and PCR testing of viruses that are taken when the etiology of viral gastroenteritis is studied. When travel related gastroenteritis is suspected, bacteria from *Campylobacter, Salmonella, Serratia* and *Yersinia* species are studied from the fecal samples (Bottieau et al., 2011), but also toxin-producing *E. coli* strains (Okamoto et al., 1993) and other pathogens are occasionally detected (Serichantalergs et al., 2007; Woo et al., 2005). Other bacteriological tests performed from clinical fecal samples are the detection of *Clostridium difficile* and its toxins and the examination of so-called "dominating flora of the feces" (Kühn et al., 1991; Simojoki, 2011). Surveillance stool cultures have proven especially useful during periods of severe neutropenia in bone marrow transplant patients (Wells et al., 1987). In the research of neonatal blood samples, the septicemia causing bacteria were isolated from the patients' blood after enhanced detection by the gas analysis in the PMEU Scentrion® (Hakalehto et al., 2009). This approach has been validated in the Kuopio University Hospital at the Pediatric Hematology and Oncology Ward and the Neonatal Intensive Care Unit (Pesola et al., 2011). The examination of the dominating flora is occasionally applied during treatment of severely immunocompromised patients, like with patients treated because of an allogenous bone marrow transplant (Simojoki, 2011). Even in this group of patients it is challenging to interpret the results. The clinician would like to have some knowledge about the microbes the patient carries in their intestines and about their antibiotic resistance profile. However, the clinical microbiology laboratory personnel do not know what they should look for and how they should answer the clinicians in a proper way. Also enough suitable methods for monitoring the microbiota have not been available yet.

From the clinician's point of view it has been difficult to determine what to do with the results of the fecal microbiota analysis because the results show only a few strains in a rather random fashion in normal hospital practice. The authors would advocate a wider search with respect to the pathogenic organisms, and also for the interactions between the members of the microbial communities in the body.

The correlation of the examination of dominating flora from samples taken from oral cavity and feces on one hand and blood culture analysis on the other hand has been studied in patients being treated because of allogenous hematological stem cell transplantation.

With present methods in 31% of blood culture positive cases the microbe detected from blood culture were earlier isolated also from dominating microflora samples (Simojoki, 2011). This percentage could have been more than doubled by using a PMEU (Portable Microbe Enrichment Unit; Finnoflag Oy and Samplion Oy, Kuopio, Finland) cultivation method (Pesola et al., 2009).

The PMEU method has been useful in the microbiological mapping of the intestinal microbiota. More strains have been isolated by the PMEU method than by conventional culture methods (Pesola et al., 2009; Pesola and Hakalehto, 2011). The PMEU method has also been used in the study of microbial strains from esofago-gastro-duodenoscopy samples (Hakalehto et al., 2011).

2. Colonization of the Intestines After Birth and Development of the Intestinal Microbiota during the Growth

Intestinal colonization begins immediately after the fetal membranes are pierced (Brook et al., 1979) when the baby is exposed to vaginal and perianal microbes of the mother.

In a couple of days after vaginal delivery, intestinal bacteria similar to those belonging to the mother's vaginal and fecal microbiota can be found in the fecal samples of the baby (Long and Swenson, 1977; Rotimi and Duerden, 1981).

The environment is an important source of colonizing microbes when the infant is born by Caesarean section or nursed apart from the mother, for example in a neonatal intensive care unit.

In this kind of a setting also the cross-spreading of strains between babies by nurses' hands has been documented (Lennox-King et al., 1976). When infants were nursed in a neonatal intensive care unit in Sweden, vertical transmission of Gram-negative bacteria from mother to infant occurred in 12% of vaginally delivered infants and in 0% of 18 infants delivered by Caesarean section (Fryklund et al., 1992). Also here the principal source of the colonizing strains was the fecal flora of other infants.

Delayed acquisition of the intestinal flora is seen, if the baby is born by Caesarean section (Bennet and Nord, 1987; Long and Swenson, 1977) and the formation of the primary gut microbiota may be disturbed. Particularly the acquisition of *Bacteroides fragilis* may be delayed for up to 6 months after the birth (Grönlund et al., 1999).

In the case of enteric coliforms, the antibiotic treatments were documented to delay the colonization for about 6 months (Pesola and Hakalehto, 2011).

There is also evidence that some genetic regulation of the composition of the intestinal microbiota could exist and influence on the joint development of a child and his or her microbiome (Toivanen et al., 2001; van de Merwe et al., 1983; Zoetendal et al., 2002).

De Palma et al. have also shown that some interplay exists between human leukocyte antigen genes and the microbial colonization of the newborn intestine (De Palma et al., 2010). The immunological factors are most likely involved in the determination of the microflora.

3. Microbiota in Different Parts of the Gastrointestinal Tract

The fecal bacterial counts of normal individuals average 10^{10} - 10^{12} CFU / gram representing 400-500 different species (Nord and Kager, 1984). Biochemical and physiological factors have influence on the composition of the microbiota in different parts of the gastrointestinal tract. Diet, gastric acid, exocrine enzymes secreted from salivary glands, pancreas and biliary tract and the velocity of the passage of the digesta play important roles in this process.

The numbers of bacteria cultured from different parts of gastrointestinal tract and the relative proportion of anaerobic and aerobic bacteria investigated by traditional culture methods (Hill, 1995) are presented in Tables 1 and 2.

Oro-pharyngeal area: Different parts of the mouth (tooth surfaces, gingival crevices, the surfaces of the tongue, palatinum, cheek surface and pharynx) have their own characteristic microbiota (Gibbons and Houte, 1975; Könönen, 2000).

The oral microbiota is dominated by Gram-positive rods and cocci (Hill, 1995). The microbiota of the oro-pharyngeal area is discussed in Chapter 11.

Table 1. Numbers of bacteria in different parts of the human gut studied by traditional culture methods (Hill, 1995)

Part of the gastrointestinal tract	cfu / g of luminal content
mouth	$10^7 – 10^8$
stomach	$< 10^3$
jejunum	$< 10^3$
terminal ileum	10^5
colon	10^{11}

cfu, colony forming unit.

Table 2. Relative proportions of anaerobic and aerobic bacteria at various parts of the human gut studied by traditional culture methods (Hill, 1995)

Part of the gastrointestinal tract	counts of anaerobic : aerobic bacteria
mouth	10-100 : 1
stomach	<1 : 1
jejunum	1-10: 1
terminal ileum	1-100 : 1
cecum	100-10000 : 1
colon	100-1000 : 1
colonic mucosa	1-10 : 1

Esophagus and ventricle: The normal resting pH of the gastric juice is below 3 resisting microbial growth, but a hypochlorhydric stomach supports the bacterial growth (Hill, 1995; Väkeväinen et al., 2000). *Helicobacter pylori* is frequently isolated from samples taken from gastric or duodenal ulcerations and it is regarded as a co-carcinogen in the pathogenesis of gastric carcinoma by damaging the mucosa (Misra et al., 2007).

Duodenum and jejunum: Lactobacilli and streptococci are the principal bacterial genera isolated from the upper small intestine (Berg, 1996). On the other hand, in a wide survey of bile tract isolates in an Austrian hospital, a domination of coliformic bacteria and enterococci in the samples was detected (Hakalehto et al., 2010). This could indicate that these genera or groups include the permanent strains of the microbiota their selection being caused by the bile substances which would eventually select the most bile resistant strains in the duodenum. The bacterial colonization of these mucosal areas is reduced, not only by bactericidal biliary and pancreatic secretions, but also by extensive fluid secretion from the mucosa and by the short small bowel transit time (Holzapfel et al., 1998).

On the other hand, the secretions intensely modulate the microbiota of the duodenum and jejunum leading to the selection of bile and pancreatic fluid resistant bacteria.

Ileum: Ileum is colonized both by the microbes transiting from the small bowel and as a result of reflux from the colon through the ileo-cecal junction (Nord and Kager, 1984). The microbiota of the ileum is assumed to be similar to that of the cecum (Hill, 1995). However, it is very difficult to get reliable samples from the terminal ileum.

On the other hand, this region gets inocula also from the upper GI tract, originating from the ventricle and duodenum, which could influence the microbiota composition. These bacteria participate in the bile circulation (Garbutt et al., 1970). For a neonate, the bile secretion is induced as soon as the umbilical supply is interrupted (Beath, 2003).

Duodenal and ileal microbial interactions have been simulated with the PMEU, and these studies are introduced elsewhere in this book (e.g., in Chapter 14).

Large intestines: The largest number of bacteria is found in the large intestines where bacteria comprise approximately 55% of the fecal mass (Stephen and Cummings, 1980). Especially the cecum is densely occupied by mostly anaerobic strains (Hill, 1995). Additionally, there are microbial organisms attached to the intestinal epithelial tissue and within the crypts of the intestinal mucosa (Onderdonk, 1999). These cells may play a role in initiating the microbial growth in the duodenum, associated with the food consumption of the host together with the microbiota (Hakalehto et al., 2008).

The anaerobic bacteria outnumber the aerobic ones within the large bowel (Table 2). The most dominant bacterial genus in this area is *Bacteroides* that accounts for up to 30% of all isolates (Nord and Kager, 1984).

Other culturally dominant anaerobic genera of the colon are *Peptostreptococcus*, *Eubacterium*, *Bifidobacterium*, *Clostridium* and *Fusobacterium*. The proportion of facultatively anaerobic enterobacterial species, such as *Escherichia coli*, is less than 0.1% of the total culturable population of the colon (Onderdonk, 1999). However, they form the most widely used indication of fecal contamination due to their presence in almost all cases of such contamination together with another duodenal group, namely enterococci.

Also other indicator species are studied in order to find more tools for hygiene analysis. For example, the bacteriophages of *Bacteroides* sp. have proven to be a promising means for biological source-tracking and water microbiology (Gomez-Donate et al., 2011; Wicki et al., 2011).

Mucosal-associated flora (MAF): The nutrient-rich mucus covering the mucosa of the intestines provides an excellent niche for bacteria forming an MAF (Savage, 1970; Midtvedt, 1986). Within the MAF the aerobe : anaerobe ratio is approximately 1:1 (Peach et al., 1978; Marks et al., 1979; Hill, 1995) (Table 2). Here the *Enterobacteriaceae* family is well represented (Peach et al., 1978; Marks et al., 1979).

Most of the anaerobes belong to the genus *Bacteroides* (Poxton et al., 1997). The higher proportion of aerobes within the MAF has been explained by the diffusion of oxygen from the capillary vessels through the mucosal membrane (Hill, 1995).

4. Nutrition and Microbiota

The early diet of an infant has a great impact on the development of the intestinal microbiota. In breast milk -fed infants the fecal microbiota consists mostly of *Bifidobacterium* species (Benno et al., 1984; Kleessen et al., 1995; Harmsen et al., 2000; Favier et al., 2002). Formula-fed infants have clearly more enterococci and clostridia than their counterparts fed by breast milk (Kleessen et al., 1995).

After weaning and starting with other foods, the species belonging to the family *Enterobacteriaceae* appear and the microbiota becomes more complex (Pesola et al., 2009; Pesola and Hakalehto, 2011).

Later, after the first years of life when intestinal microbiota has stabilized, the dietary intake does not cause any significant changes in the microbiota (Rautio, 2002). If some changes happen, they are usually reversible.

Different gases, like hydrogen, methane and carbon dioxide, are produced by the microbes of the large intestines. The amounts and proportions of the gases are affected by the diet. The consumption of beans or peas rich in non-absorbable carbohydrates leads to excessive production of gases in the large intestines. This happens also in the case of lactose intolerance when excessive lactose is consumed by the colonic bacteria. The strong odor of the intestinal gas is mainly caused by sulphurhydrogen. The excessive intestinal gases may lead to colic-like abdominal pains resulting from the stretching of the gut wall.

5. Bile and Intestinal Microbiota

Bile secreted through the biliary tract to the duodenum has antibacterial properties. Only some bile resistant bacteria can survive within its presence.

Hence the bile is an important agent causing the selection of microbial species of the intestinal microbiota (Midtvedt and Norman, 1967). From the duodenum, bile-resistant microbes migrate to the lower parts of the intestines (Hakalehto et al., 2010).

Hygiene-indicator bacteria that are used as a sign of fecal contamination in water safety monitoring, are typically bile-resistant bacteria originating from the duodenal area (Midtvedt and Norman, 1967; Edberg et al., 2000; Heitto et al., 2009).

6. Antibiotic Treatments and the Intestinal Microbiota

Neonatal sepsis is a relatively common reason for admission to the neonatal intensive care unit. When the disease is suspected, an empiric broad-scale antibiotic treatment is started right after the collection of diagnostic samples. The duration of the antibiotic treatment depends on the overall condition of the baby and on the results of the microbiological tests, e.g., blood cultures.

Even though the antibiotic treatment of a neonate may last only a few days, it may have a severe impact on the development of intestinal microbiota. It has been shown that the appearance of Gram-negative rods, for example, may be delayed for six months because of a neonatal antibiotic treatment (Pesola and Hakalehto, 2011).

In a murine model the neonatal antibiotic treatment also altered the developmental gene expression of the gastrointestinal tract and the development of gut barrier function (Schumann et al., 2005).

7. The Mutual Relationship between Man and His Microbiota

The microbes of the colon produce several vitamin B group vitamins and vitamin K. They also form some toxic compounds that are normally detoxified by the intestinal mucosa and liver. Also intestinal gases originate partly from bacterial metabolic activity.

There is a certain symbiotic relationship between a man and his intestinal microbiota. The normal flora prevents pathogenic microbes from intruding through the intestinal wall into the body.

If the normal microbiota is disturbed, some symptoms and disorders may appear. Disturbance of the flora may be seen during traveling to different kinds of microbial environments or after antibiotic treatment. This may lead to vomiting, diarrhea, constipation, stomach ache, fatigue or swallowed belly, for example, depending on the situation.

8. Microbiological Factors Related to Immunocompromised Children

There are several factors causing immunosuppression and increasing the proneness to infections in children (Table 3).

a. Immunosuppression and Infections – How to Keep the Weakest Alive?

Immunosuppression makes it easier for the harmful microbes to overcome the defense mechanisms of the body. It increases the risk of severe morbidity and mortality related to different infections. This is common for all the immunocompromised patients. However, there are certain characteristics that are unique in different clinical situations.

Table 3. Factors causing or related to immunosuppression

prematurity neonatal period infections
prolonged infections parvovirus AIDS
specific immunodeficiency syndromes
chronic neutropenia SCID
malnutrition
unusual diets maldigestion starvation anorexia
leukemia and other malignancies chemotherapy

b. Prematurity and Neonatal Period

The basis of the intestinal microbiota is founded during the birth. During their first days, children are vulnerable because of the immaturity of both the immunological system and microbiota.

The pH of the ventricle of babies is higher keeping the colonization window open for the first bacteria that are ready to settle down into the native intestines of the baby. Unfortunately, during this process, also pathogenic microbes can enter the intestines more easily.

Babies treated at the neonatal intensive care units are also prone to nosocomial infections and foreign body related infections. The longer they stay at the hospital the longer is the risk of developing infections caused by some antibiotic resistant bacteria.

c. Infections in Immunocompromised Individuals

Prolonged infection periods lead to a consumption of the compounds of the immune system making the patient even more prone to get new infections. The treatment of infections by antibiotics may unfortunately increase the risk of certain infections because of the changes in the normal microbiota. Viral infections like parvovirus may cause temporary aplasia of the bone marrow leading to cytopenias lasting from weeks to months. In respect to bacterial infections, the most important cytopenia is neutropenia (the low number of neutrophils).

Pulmonary infections may quickly proceed to severe respiratory dysfunction especially in patients receiving chemotherapy. Viral, bacterial and fungal pathogens are frequently detected. Viral infections may not be harmful for healthy relatives or friends, but for a neutropenic patient they may cause admission to an intensive care unit (ICU) because of life-threatening pneumonia.

Pseudomonas is causing remarkable morbidity and mortality among this patient group. That is why neutropenic sepsis should always be treated preferably with two *Pseudomonas* active antibiotics.

Case 1

5-year-old medulloblastoma patient had just got autologous stem cell transplant (ASCT) according to standard protocol. However, two days after the ASCT his condition quickly deteriorated and he started to bleed from his airways. The bleeding stopped, but the patient developed irreversible adult respiratory distress syndrome (ARDS) and multi-organ-failure (MOF). Finally it was shown that *Pseudomonas* was behind the fulminant infection.

The longer the neutropenia lasts - the greater the risk of fungal infection. For example, the treatment of acute lymphatic leukemia (ALL) and acute myeloid leukemia (AML) has intensified. During the treatment of AML or high-intensity chemotherapy used for high-risk ALL neutrophil counts may be at level of severe neutropenia for 3-5 weeks. This is why increasing numbers of pulmonary fungal infections can be seen in clinics. They may be extremely difficult to prove because the radiological imaging is not clear always and because the fungi are very difficult to identify from broncho-alveolar liquid (BAL) or from biopsies. Despite of antifungal prophylaxis the protection from fungal infections is only partial. The microbial diagnostics of fungal infections should be developed in order to get definitive identification results and start the right treatment early enough.

During chronic conditions associated with immunosuppression the risk of mycobacterial diseases increases remarkably. They have to be taken into consideration if respiratory dysfunction is detected or in case of new focal infectious findings in images of the thorax.

AIDS (acquired immune deficiency syndrome) caused by HIV (human immunodeficiency virus) leads to severe vulnerability to infections because the virus attacks specifically the body's defensive mechanisms.

d. Nutritional Abnormalities

Unusual diets, maldigestion, starvation and anorexia may lead to the deterioration of the general condition because of the depletion of the body's nutrition. On the other hand, in certain kidney diseases, like nephrotic syndrome and nephrosis, the permeability of the glomerular capillaries is increased leading to the loss of anti-infective proteins. These conditions make the patients especially prone to infections.

e. Leukemia and Other Malignancies

The most common leukemia in childhood is acute lymphatic leukemia with an incidence of 4% in Nordic population, while acute myeloid leukemia is more rarely seen (incidence 0,7-0,8%) (Heyman et al., 2011). The rapidly growing leukemic blasts take over the bone marrow leaving no space for healthy hematopoietic cells. In addition to the bone marrow at the time of the diagnosis leukemic blasts are also frequently seen in circulating blood. Other organs where infiltration of leukemic blasts may be seen are liver, spleen, kidneys, lymph nodes, intestinal wall, testicles and the central nervous system. Leukemia itself causes a severe risk for life-threatening infections because of the leucopenia resulting from the bone marrow infiltration of the blasts. Furthermore, oncologic treatments cause damage to all dividing cells of the body. That is why the bone marrow is especially sensitive to the chemotherapy. Cytopenias – anemia, thrombocytopenia and leucopenia – are frequently seen. Also mucous membranes are often affected as a side effect of cytostatic drugs.

In the treatment of pediatric malignant diseases roughly half of the work is diagnostics of the malignancy itself but the other half goes for the treatment of infections. Neutropenia means the depletion of specific leucocytes mainly responsible for the protection against bacterial infections, namely neutrophilic granulocytes. Neutropenia may be related to acute leukemia or chemotherapy of the malignancies. During neutropenia, the risk for severe infections is very high.

In the case of Brad Miller a septic shock, however, was not causing fatal consequences (Groopman, 2008). In this particular patient case, the food for the meals was selected to contain low levels of microbes, visitors wore protective clothing, and all other precautions were taken. However, the bacterial infection took over starting from an unnoticed abscess, regardless of the special notion, which the patient received. This example is encouraging when thinking about future diagnostics, in which the microbial parameters would be monitored on a continuous or semi-continuous basis. Also in rapidly developing conditions, such as sepsis or pyelonephritis, the fast tracking of the infection would be an essential improvement (Hakalehto et al., 2009; Pesola et al., 2012; Laitiomäki et al., 2014).

When the first signs of neutropenic septichemia appear, blood culture samples should be taken and empiric antibiotic treatment is started. Blood culture samples are also taken repeatedly during prolonged infections. Blood culture analysis is essential because no clinical or laboratory parameters have been found to differentiate bacterial infections from non-bacterial ones (Riikonen et al., 1993). The speed of the analysis of the blood cultures is of great importance because of the rapid course of neutropenic sepsis. After the detection of fever, remarkable mortality is seen within hours if the onset of wide-spectrum antibiotics is delayed (Castagnola and Faraci, 2009).

In the treatment of neutropenic sepsis it is of great importance to detect the causative agents as quickly as possible (Hakalehto, 2006). Because the bacterial concentration in the circulating blood is low, the samples should be enriched in an incubator before plate culture. There are a few automated incubators of different manufacturers equipped with a built-in monitoring of the microbial growth in the blood culture bottles. 16S rDNA PCR method has also been used in the monitoring of pathogens from blood samples. The specificity of the method can be increased by preanalytical removal of human DNA from the sample (Handschur et al., 2009). Matrix-assisted laser desorption/ionization time-of-flight mass spectrometry (MALDI-TOF MS) offers rapid detection of bacteria from growing colonies but prior enrichment is recommended in order to get more reliable results (Kroumova et al., 2011). Lately, also the PMEU (Portable Microbe Enrichment Unit, Finnoflag Oy and Samplion Oy, Finland) has been used in the examination of blood culture samples offering optimal growth conditions and an ultrasensitive detection method for the microbial growth (Hakalehto et al., 2008; Hakalehto et al., 2009; Hakalehto et al., 2010).

In case of pulmonary fungal infections it is an important issue to understand the interrelationships between space and function in the lung alveoli. In the narrow tubes the fungus can achieve a growth platform if the immune defense is not competent enough to eradicate the inhaled spores and the fungal growth thereof. Proper ventilation in the lungs is naturally important for keeping the airwaves clear.

Especially in the case of fungal pulmonary diseases it is evident that any obstruction of the tubings in the lung airways will cause an elevated risk for the mold strains rooting into the lungs. To some extent this is the case also with respect to the bacterial infections of the lower respiratory tract. For example, *Legionella pneumophila* and *Mycobacterium tuberculosis* are causing the disease, which is spreading step by step in the lungs (Guy et al., 2011).

There are different types of mycobacterial lung diseases that may be difficult to differentiate (Hongfei et al., 2012):

1. pulmonary tuberculosis
2. *Mycobacterium* abscessus lung disease.

In *Mycobacterium* abscessus lung disease micronodules adjacent to the pleura can be seen. Bilateral bronchiectasias without lobar predominance are important features for distinguishing *Mycobacterium* abscessus lung disease from other mycobacterial lung diseases.

Invasive fungal infections are a leading course of morbidity and mortality among hematologic patients. Therefore the general quality of indoor air in the hospital wards is of essential importance. This is even more crucial for the treatment of immunocompromised patients. In the presentation by Fracchiolla et al. (2014) fifteen fungal infections were listed and, eight of them were caused by molds and seven by some candida yeast strains. Most of the molds belonged to the genus *Aspergillus* and one of them was *Fusarium.* All of these molds are generally related to plant origin. These strains are found everywhere globally and because theirs spores are resistant to ultraviolet radiation, they have been isolated at high altitudes (Hakalehto, 2014).

The microbial concentrations in the atmosphere are equally high all over and also it is possible to recognize the sources of emission, which practically means that in the open areas, molds are different from the ones found in the less inhabited reasons. All hospital premises are in need of fresh air, but this fresh air has to be purified from the spores and other agents coming from outside. Many molds and other microfungi can be isolated from soil and therefore it is generally advisable to avoid decorating plants in the wards of extremely sick people.

Because of the high risk of invasive bacterial and fungal infections, wide spectrum antibiotics are used very frequently within this patient group posing a potential risk for the development of the resistance towards the antimicrobial agents (Hakalehto, 2011).

The infectious complications are most difficult when the duration of neutropenia is prolonged. This is the case during the chemotherapy block treatments of high-risk acute lymphatic leukemia (ALL), AML treatment and especially after transplantations of the hematopoietic stem cells. Also the risk for deep fungal infections is markedly increased. The treatment of patients after allogenous is by far the most challenging because of the graft versus host disease resulting from the mismatch between the donor and the recipient. The severity of the graft vs. host disease of the gut may also be related to intestinal microbiota.

Other factors related to an increased risk of infections during oncological treatments are foreign bodies like peripheral and central venous catheters. A biofilm is formed on the surfaces of the foreign bodies.

Because of a remarkable risk of rapidly progressing invasive infections, the patients are taught to bring their child to the hematology/oncology ward at latest within six hours after the appearance of the fever. After blood culture samples, intravenous wide-spectrum antibiotics are introduced at the ward.

Nosocomial infections are complications faced frequently in hematological and oncological patients who have several long-lasting treatments in the hospital. Every means to minimize the infections risk should be done. Laminar chambers or clean room facilities are used by the pharmacological industry but they are also needed in hospitals in preparing medicines for use. The microbiological monitoring is an important part of the work in the clean room facilities (Hakalehto, 2010).

e. Antibiotic Resistance – A Growing Concern

The antibiotic susceptibility monitoring of pathogens is of growing importance because of increasing tendency towards bacterial resistance development (Siu et al., 1999; Ariffin et al., 2000; Ayalew et al., 2003). The antibiotic resistance pressure is highest at hospital wards using long courses of broad-spectrum antibiotics. This goes especially for neonatological, hematological and oncological wards and also for plastic surgery wards. For example, the incidence of extended-spectrum beta-lactamase (ESBL) producing *Klebsiella pneumoniae*, that is an important pathogen causing morbidity and mortality, has increased when oxyimino-cephalosporins, like cefotaxime or ceftazidime, have been used (Abdel-Hady et al., 2008). On the other hand the multi-resistance should be taken into consideration when the response to antibiotic treatment is suboptimal. Among neutropenic cancer patients we have seen carbapenemase producing *Klebsiella pneumonia* in two patients. The first patient was admitted to ICU because of deterioration of general condition and lack of response to empiric antibiotics. Only after initiation of two non-carbapenem antibiotics effective to this particular strain, the patient started to recover. The relatively high incidence of this kind of multi-resistant pathogens has been presented by Martino et al. (2014).

For example, the increasing intensity of the chemotherapy of malignant diseases is inevitably related to more prolonged neutropenias and more difficult infections (Crokaert, 2000). The time for antibiotic susceptibility monitoring should be reduced to minimum. Otherwise the proper treatment would be delayed and the outcome of the patients endangered.

f. Pathogenesis of Infections in Immunocompromised Children

The immune system of neonates and especially preterm babies is still premature. This is why quite high numbers of sepsis, meningitis and necrotizing enterocolitis are seen in these patient groups. Because the mucous membranes are immature as well, the invasion of microbes can easily happen. More protection for neonates is provided by antibodies delivered through the placenta during pregnancy and by breast-feeding containing both antibodies and antibiotic agents.

In case of severe neutropenia, patients are in immediate risk for life-threatening infection. When they get fever it has to be taken as a sign of neutropenic sepsis and treated accordingly. Neutropenia is most commonly related to chemotherapy given against malignant disease. Other important, although rare, causes for neutropenia are aplastic anemia or congenital neutropenia. It is characteristic for these groups of diseases that neutropenia is long-lasting.

Especially patients with congenital neutropenia, e.g., with Kostmann's disease, have extremely low numbers of neutrophils making these patients very prone to infections.

Most infections of neutropenic patients are caused by the strains originating from their own microbiota through mucous membranes of the oral cavity or other parts of the alimentary tract. Also foreign bodies, like indwelling catheters, are important sources of infections.

The spleen has to be removed in some situations, for example after traumatic rupture or in case of difficult, otherwise untreatable autoimmune thrombocytopenia or autoimmune hemolytic anemia. The spleen is important in the defense especially against encapsulated bacteria, like *Haemophilus influenzae, Neisseria meningitidis* and *Streptococcus pneumoniae*. That is why splenectomized patients have to be vaccinated against these bacteria and their infections have to be treated carefully.

9. Invasion of Microbial Agents into Blood Stream from the Digestive Tract

The invasion of microbial agents through the intestinal mucosa is an acute problem especially in the case of immunocompromised or otherwise defensively less competent patients. The interaction between host and microbiota is crucial for the normal development of immunity (Gutzeit et al., 2014). In immunocompromised patients the microbial strains belonging to microbiota may, however, cause severe infections when the mucosal integrity is broken and the balance between microbiota and immunological system disturbed. For example, in neutropenic hematological patients the majority of microbes causing sepsis originate from the host alimentary or skin microbiota (Ali et al., 2014; Rolston et al., 2014). Therefore, it would be important to characterize the microbiota of these patients and investigate also the antimicrobial resistance patterns of the members of the microbiota, in order to get information for choosing right antibiotic treatments during following sepsis episodes. Intestinal mucosa, the microbiota and the immune system normally form a barrier that protects from the invasion or intrusion of pathogenic microbes.

However, bacteria like *Salmonella* and *Yersinia* have also intracellular phases during their invasion. They can live and multiply inside macrophages that have engulfed them by phagocytosis. After phagocytosis macrophages normally degrade the engulfed microbes, cells and tissue debris by enzymes released from their endosomes.

When some part of the preventive measures is declined or totally lacking, the invasive pathogens may find their way into the blood stream. The pathogenic microbes have specific structures for the movement towards the intestinal wall and adhesion to it (Hakalehto et al., 2000; Hakalehto et al., 2007).

10. Association of Microbes and Microflora with Some Common Host Conditions Causing Immunodeficiency

The disturbance of the development of the intestinal microbiota during infancy may result e.g., from antibiotic treatment (Schumann et al., 2005), enteral infections, dietary problems or intestinal food allergy.

Imbalanced intestinal microbiota increases the proneness to infections, but it might also be associated with the risk of developing autoimmune diseases (Lodes et al., 2004).

The links of microbial diseases with allergies or metabolic disorders have been discussed for a long time. The deviation of immunological development of T lymphocytes to T-helper 1 (Th1) type or Th2 type immunity is probably related to the microbiological environment and infections of a developing child. Th1 type immunity is important in the protection from bacterial infections, whereas Th2 seems to be related to higher incidence of atopy and allergic conditions. In earlier publications a clear difference in the immunological deviation was seen between former East and West Germany and between Estonia and Sweden, for example. In the eastern part of Europe Th1 dominated, whereas in western parts of Europe the dominance of Th2 immunity was seen. The differences were at least partly explained by a higher incidence of bacterial infections in Eastern Europe and a higher hygienic level in Western Europe (Kemp and Björkstén, 2003; von Mutius, 2007).

Some factors associated with the deviation of immunity were heating methods used in homes of the children (Howden-Chapman et al., 2008; Pierse et al., 2013) and the number of older siblings (Westergaard et al., 2005). Th1 dominance was associated with heating with charcoil and higher number of older siblings.

Both allergic and autoimmune disorders make the patients more prone to infections. Inflammation caused by any reason causes disturbance of the protective immunity. Also, like in case of diabetes, the increased glucose levels of the body offer the microbes beneficial conditions for survival and multiplication. This goes for both type 1 and type 2 diabetes.

Chronic metabolic disorders, like metabolic syndrome, are also associated with higher incidence of infections. This is possibly due to chronic inflammation related to the metabolic disturbances like obesity (Brandacher et al., 2007).

The etiology of autoimmune diseases is still open. There are different hypotheses how the environmental factors may affect development of autoimmunity. One is the Hygiene Hypothesis suggesting that in modern society, the lack of exposure to pathogens during early childhood prevents the immune system from protecting itself from autoimmune process, like that seen in type 1 diabetes, in genetically predisposed individuals (Wherrett and Daneman, 2009). The connection between autoimmunity and microbiota has been proposed also for many other autoimmune disorders, like Crohn's disease, colitis ulcerosa, reactive arthritis, spondyloarthritis.

The role of bacterial and viral agents has been suspected. Both the lack of contacts to microbes and certain infections may play a role. Enteroviral infections, for example, have been positively associated with the appearance of autoimmune diabetic antibodies (Kondrashova and Hyöty, 2014). Cross-reactions between viral agents and human antigens might be causing autoimmune inflammation (Dagna et al., 2013; Broccolo et al., 2013). Also microbiota of gastro-intestinal tract and skin most probably play some role in the development of autoimmunity. Preceding the diagnosis of autoimmune disease quite often some antibiotic treatment has been used causing major alterations in the microbiota of body. For example, colitis ulcerosa is often diagnosed after some antibiotic treatment.

Therefore, there is a growing interest on the development of microbiota during the first months and years of life when also the development of immunity takes place. The method for characterization of enterobacterial strains from fecal samples of infants has been developed for this purpose (Pesola et al., 2009; Pesola and Hakalehto, 2011).

The molecular communication between host body and the alimentary microbiota has been discussed earlier (Hakalehto, 2012). In the present book this issue is outlined in Chapter 14.

The PMEU method has proven useful in the microbiological mapping of the intestinal microbiota. It has also been developed for the blood culture analysis. It offers also the possibility to compare microbial strains isolated from blood culture samples and intestinal cultures. This approach would be extremely important in order to react fast enough to new infectious challenges by careful monitoring of the symptoms and the antibiotic resistance situation in individual patients. The earlier the antibiotic resistance data is available, the better the antibiotic treatment can be adjusted to a patient's present situation – antibiotic coverage should be wide enough, but excessive use of antibiotics should be avoided. *Clostridium difficile*, a spore-forming Gram-positive rod, is a common member of intestinal microbiota being usually harmless to a healthy host. As a result of broad-spectrum antibiotic treatment or chemotherapy toxin producing strains may, however, cause severe diarrhea and even life-threatening pseudomembraneous colitis. The bacterium cannot normally be eradicated by antibiotics although the symptoms can be cured by e.g., metronidazole or vancomycin. Because the spores of the bacterium are very resistant to the environmental stress and also to ethanol-based disinfectants, they are easily transmitted via hands. Both mechanical washing of hands and the use of disinfectants is recommended after contact with a patient with *C. difficile.* Also the sterilization of the equipment used in the diagnostic examinations, like colonoscopes need to be handled with special attention (Hell et al., 2010).

11. Hospital Validation of the PMEU Scentrion® in the Pediatric Wards

Quite often, despite of clinical signs of sepsis, no infectious agent is found in bacterial cultures of blood samples. From a clinician's point of view it is probable that in reality there are more positive microbial blood stream infections than what can be detected by present methods. In order to improve the blood culture methods, a hospital validation project has been launched. In the project blood samples from septic children treated at the Neonatal Intensive Care Unit and Pediatric Hematology and Oncology Ward in Kuopio University Hospital, Kuopio, Finland are cultivated both by standard method and by PMEU Scentrion® (Finnoflag Oy and Samplion Oy, Kuopio, Finland). The two methods have given similar kind of results complementing each other (Laitiomäki et al., 2014). The PMEU method has also been used in multiple other areas of medical microbiology (Table 4).

12. Prevention of the Infectious Diseases in Immunocompromised Individuals

The risk of infections of other people, can be lowered by isolating the patient during his/her secreting phase of respiratory or gastro-intestinal infection. Contrary during severe neutropenia isolation could be used in order to protect the patient from microbes coming from other persons. Also e.g., during long-lasting neutropenia prophylactic antibacterial, antifungal and antiviral medications can be used (Diorio et al., 2012).

During recent years probiotics and prebiotics have been extensively studied. These products can be used to modify the intestinal flora temporarily, but normally no permanent changes can be achieved.

Table 4. PMEU in medical practice and research

Infection diagnostics
Respiratory infections Gastrointestinal infections
Gastroenteritis Clostridium difficile
Urinary infections CNS infections Blood cultures
Antibiotic resistance testing Enhanced detection of multiresistant bacteria (e.g., MRSA, ESBL, VRE) Monitoring microbiota Interaction between host and microbes Interactions between different microbial strains Hospital hygiene monitoring
Isolation areas Monitoring of clean room facilities (e.g., pharmacological units) Monitoring of sterilization procedures of e.g., endoscopes
Environmental health

Diet has a major impact on the composition of the microbiota. If severe imbalance of the microbiota is seen, e.g., microbial overgrowth syndrome, also antibiotics can be used for the treatment (Ford et al., 2009; Pimentel, 2009).

There is growing interest that focuses on the intestinal microbiota. This seems to be involved in the development of the intestinal immunity, production of some vitamins, immunological defence of the intestines and several pathogenic processes.

The careful investigation of the composition of the microbiota would be important in order to find out indicator microbes that might be related to certain pathogenic processes. But it is still hard to know the best ways to make conclusions on the microbiota.

The intestinal bacteria interact with each other but also with the host. It is a demanding task to investigate these interactions. Especially the study of the flora of the small intestines is rather complicated.

However, the interactions of intestinal microbes can be ideally simulated in the PMEU (Hakalehto, 2011). New interesting interactions have been found using this approach. For example, in mixed culture *E. coli* and *Klebsiella* have been shown to have a dualistic balance being beneficial for both of them and also for the host (Hakalehto et al., 2008). In the PMEU, this kind of symbiosis has been shown to form the basis for building up balanced microbial communities (Hakalehto et al., 2010).

Intensive research has focused on the intestinal microbiota and its impact on human welfare. There are still many open questions: Which are the most important representatives of the intestinal microbiota and how to find them? How could the intestinal microbiota be safely modulated? Further studies are warranted in order to answer these questions.

13. Links between Medication of Cancer and Autoimmune Diseases with Antimicrobial Treatments

The drugs used during chemotherapy are cytostatic or cytotoxic drugs inducing apoptosis of dividing cells. Most of the cells of the host are in a resting state and remain intact. However, there are many tissues that suffer from the chemotherapy because of naturally rapidly dividing cells, such as bone marrow, mucous membranes and hair follicles. As acute side-effects of chemotherapy, cytopenias, pain and ulceration of mucous membranes and loss of hairs are frequently seen, respectively. There are also side-effects that can be seen only after a longer follow-up time. For example, anthracyclins may cause cardiomyopathia that may by diagnosed even decades after the treatment. Vincristin is known for the neuropathy that fortunately is mostly reversible. Cisplatin and ifosfamide may cause renal dysfunction. All these drugs also challenge the body as a whole causing intense stress for the patient.

Some of the drugs used in chemotherapy are closely resembling antibiotics, like anthracyclins (doxorubicin, epirubicin, etc.). Hence some of their action could be a result of the antibacterial characteristics.

Needs for elevated readiness for antibiotic usage have to be considered in context with practical preparedness and well-timed decision-making in the therapy. This has to be followed by careful surveillance of the effects of the chosen treatment. In this "cure validation", rapid diagnostics of the microflora and individual pathogens by the PMEU are valuable tools (Iredell et al., 2006; Pesola and Hakalehto, 2011). The early warning has proven essential in life saving efforts of severely ill infected patients (Grau et al., 2014; Andrijevic et al., 2014). The optimal situation for the patient and cure monitoring during the course of an infection has to be established as a protocol with individually defined indications and timetables for the sampling and analysis. In the case of a rapidly developing bacterial disease such as severe urinary tract infection, early acquisition of relevant information on the agent and its specific features cannot to be too much underlined.

These features include:

- infectivity
- joint effect with the other microflora
- response to the medications and other treatments (including antibiotic susceptibility profiles)
- spread into the host tissues
- emission into secretions or air, or in human-to-human contacts
- environmental preservation, prevalence, distribution and metabolic as well as infective status of the pathogen

This kind of approach extending from the basic microbiology into the host influences and the environmental relevance of various strains will give us a holistic view on the hospital hygiene management. This is particularly important in case of safeguarding the defensively deficient patients. Also, this type of attention is required for protective measures of health care personnel during epidemics and in connection with the treatment of highly infecting diseases. Ultimate examples are the deadly viral diseases such as Ebola or MERS which are reviewed in Chapter 3. Currently in Summer 2014 both of these diseases have been in the headlines, occurring mainly in Central Africa and in the Arabian peninsula, respectively.

It is self-evident that the immunocompromised patients are extremely vulnerable to any kind of epidemics (Whimbey et al., 1997). An elevated risk is associated also with drug misuse (Pol et al., 1998). These patient groups form a risk for the entire hospital system and in extraordinary situations cohort care is easily justified (Weymann et al., 2014).

More common risks relate to the spread of world-widely distributed epidemics such as tuberculosis (see also Chapter 9) and any antibiotic resistant infections (Chapter 21). Moreover, internal risks at hospitals include *Clostridium difficile* (Chapter 15) and legionellosis (Chapter 7). All these risks should be manageable by careful planning of the disease control and facilities and environment for pursuing the treatments. This point of view is reviewed in Chapter 5.

Conclusion

The severely threatened first days of life necessitate special care. No risks can be taken, whatsoever, with respect to microbial infections. At the same time the normal flora should be developing in balanced fashion. Nutrition and the developing immune system set the framework for the growth and recovery. However, in case of seriously diseased child patients, any alarming signs, for example in the blood test results, deserve extreme measures. At this stage it is not always possible to get any idea on the causative reasons, or on the pathogenic agent. The results from the chosen treatment have to be continuously monitored and recorded. The PMEU system has proven to be a valuable tool for fast and efficient follow up in the hospital wards. Also hiding anaerobic agents could be detected from patient samples by this method, thus giving the doctor a possibility to direct effective treatments on these microbes. Also in monitoring blood and blood products this technology could be useful.

References

Abdel-Hady, H., Hawas, S., El-Daker, M., El-Kady, R. Extended-spectrum β-lactamase producing *Klebsiella pneumoniae* in neonatal intensive care unit. *J.Perinatol.,* 2008; 28, 685-690.

Ali, N., Baqir, M., Hamid, A., Khurshid, M. Febrile neutropenia: Median door-to-needle time - Results of an initial audit. *Hematology.* 2014 Apr. 12. [Epub. ahead of print].

Andrijevic, I., Matijasevic, J., Andrijevic, L., Kovacevic, T., Zaric, B. Interleukin-6 and procalcitonin as biomarkers in mortality prediction of hospitalized patients with community acquired pneumonia. *Ann. Thorac. Med.*, 2014; 9, 162-167.

Ariffin, H., Navaratnam, P., Mohamed, M., Arasu, A., Abdullah, W. A., Lee, C. L., Peng, L. H. Ceftazidime-resistant *Klebsiella pneumoniae* bloodstream infection in children with febrile neutropenia. *Int. J. Infect. Dis.,* 2000; 4, 21-25.

Ayalew, K., Nambiar, S., Yasinskaya, Y., Jantausch, B. A. Carbapenems in pediatrics. *Ther. Drug Monit.,* 2003; 25, 593-599.

Beath, S. V. Hepatic function and physiology in the newborn. *Semin. Neonatol.,* 2003; 8, 337-346.

Bennet, R., Nord, C. E. Development of the faecal anaerobic microflora after caesarean section and treatment with antibiotics in newborn infants. *Infection,* 1987; 15, 332-336.

Benno, Y., Sawada, K., Mitsuoka, T. The intestinal microflora of infants: composition of fecal flora in breast-fed and bottle-fed infants. *Microbiol. Immunol.,* 1984; 28, 975-986.

Berg, R. D. The indigenous gastrointestinal microflora. *Trends Microbiol.,* 1996; 4, 430-435.

Bottieau, E., Clerinx, J., Vlieghe, E., Van Esbroeck, M., Jacobs, J., Van Gompel, A., Van Den Ende, J. Epidemiology and outcome of *Shigella, Salmonella* and *Campylobacter* infections in travellers returning from the tropics with fever and diarrhoea. *Acta Clin. Belg.,* 2011; 66, 191-195.

Brandacher, G., Hoeller, E., Fuchs, D., Weiss, H. G. Chronic immune activation underlies morbid obesity: is IDO a key player? *Curr. Drug Metab.*, 2007; 8, 289-295.

Broccolo, F., Fusetti, L., Ceccherini-Nelli, L. Possible role of human herpesvirus 6 as a trigger of autoimmune disease. *Scientific World Journal,* 2013; 2013: 867389.

Brook, I., Barrett, C. T., Brinkman, C. R. 3rd., Martin, W. J., Finegold, S. M. Aerobic and anaerobic bacterial flora of the maternal cervix and newborn gastric fluid and conjunctiva: a prospective study. *Pediatrics,* 1979; 63, 451-455.

Castagnola, E., Faraci, M. Management of bacteremia in patients undergoing hematopoietic stem cell transplantation. *Expert Rev. Anti Infect. Ther.,* 2009; 7, 607-621.

Coelho, L. G., Das, S. S., Karim, Q. N., Walker, M. M., Queiroz, D. M., Mendes, E. N., Lima Junior, G. F., de Oliveira, C. A., Baron, J. H., Castro Lde, P. *Campylobacter pyloridis* in the upper gastrointestinal tract: a Brazilian study. *Arq. Gastroenterol.,* 1987; 24, 5-9.

Crokaert, F. Febrile neutropenia in children. *Int. J. Antimicrob. Agents,* 2000; 16, 173-176.

Dagna, L., Pritchett, J. C., Lusso, P. Immunomodulation and immunosuppression by human herpesvirus 6A and 6B. *Future Virol.*, 2013; 8, 273-287.

De Palma, G., Capilla, A., Nadal, I., Nova, E., Pozo, T., Varea, V., Polanco, I., Castillejo, G., Lopez, A., Garrote, J. A., Calvo, C., Garcia-Novo, M. D., Cilleruelo, M. L., Ribes-Koninckx, C., Palau, F., Sanz, Y. Interplay between human leukocyte antigen genes and the microbial colonization process of the newborn intestine. *Curr. Issues Mol. Biol.,* 2010; 12, 1-10.

Diorio, C., Tomlinson, D., Boydell, K. M., Regier, D. A., Ethier, M.-C., Alli, A., Alexander, S., Gassas, A., Taylor, J., Kellow, C., Mills, D., Sung, L. Attitudes toward infection prophylaxis in pediatric oncology: A qualitative approach. *PLoS ONE*, 2012; 7: e47815. doi:10.1371/journal.pone.0047815.

Drumm, B., O'Brien, A., Cutz, E., Sherman, P. *Campylobacter pyloridis*-associated primary gastritis in children. *Pediatrics,* 1987; 80, 192-195.

Edberg, S. C., Rice, E. W., Karlin, R. J., Allen, M. J. Escherichia coli: the best biological drinking water indicator for public health protection. *Symp. Ser. Soc. Appl. Microbiol.,* 2000; 29, 106S-116S.

Favier, C. F., Vaughan, E. E., De Vos, W. M., Akkermans, A. D. Molecular monitoring of succession of bacterial communities in human neonates. *Appl. Environ. Microbiol.,* 2002; 68, 219-226.

Fischer, R. '*Gastrospirillum hominis*', another gastric spiral bacterium. *Dig. Dis.,* 1992; 10, 144-152.

Ford, A. C., Spiegel, B. M., Talley, N. J., Moayyedi, P. Small intestinal bacterial overgrowth in irritable bowel syndrome: systematic review and meta-analysis. *Clin. Gastroenterol. Hepatol.,* 2009; 7, 1279-1286.

Fracchiolla, N. S., Guidotti, F., Orotino, N., Cortelezzi, A. A single-institution, retrospective analysis of antifungal treatments in onco-hematologic patients (Poster). In: *19th Congress of European Hematology Association*, June 12-15, 2014, Milan, Italy.

Fryklund, B., Tullus, K., Berglund, B., Burman, L. G. Importance of the environment and the faecal flora of infants, nursing staff and parents as sources of gram-negative bacteria colonizing newborns in three neonatal wards. *Infection,* 1992; 20, 253-257.

Gagliardi, D., Makihara, S., Corsi, P. R., Viana Ade, T., Wiczer, M. V., Nakakubo, S., Mimica, L. M. Microbial flora of the normal esophagus. *Dis. Esophagus,* 1998; 11, 248-250.

Garbutt, J. T., Wilkins, R. M., Lack, L., Tyor, M. P. Bacterial modification of taurocholate during enterohepatic recirculation in normal man and patients with small intestinal disease. *Gastroenterology,* 1970; 59, 553-566.

Gibbons, R. J., Houte, J. V. Bacterial adherence in oral microbial ecology. *Annu. Rev. Microbiol.,* 1975; 29, 19-44.

Gomez-Donate, M., Payan, A., Cortes, I., Blanch, A. R., Lucena, F., Jofre, J., Muniesa, M. Isolation of bacteriophage host strains of *Bacteroides* species suitable for tracking sources of animal faecal pollution in water. *Environ. Microbiol.,* 2011; 13, 1622-1631.

Grau, S., Lozano, V., Valladares, A., Cavanillas, R., Xie, Y., Nocea, G. Antibiotic expected effectiveness and cost under real life microbiology: evaluation of ertapenem and ceftriaxone in the treatment of community-acquired pneumonia for elderly patients in Spain. *Clinicoecon. Outcomes Res.*, 2014; 6, 83-92.

Groopman, J. E. *How Doctors Think.* Boston and New York, US. Houghton Mifflin Company. 2008.

Grönlund, M. M., Lehtonen, O. P., Eerola, E., Kero, P. Fecal microflora in healthy infants born by different methods of delivery: permanent changes in intestinal flora after cesarean delivery. *J. Pediatr. Gastroenterol. Nutr.,* 1999; 28, 19-25.

Gutzeit, C., Magri, G., Cerutti, A. Intestinal IgA production and its role in host-microbe interaction. *Immunol. Rev.*, 2014; 260, 76-85.

Guy, S. D., Worth, L. J., Thursky, K. A., Francis, P. A., Slavin, M. A. *Legionella pneumophila* lung abscess associated with immune suppression. *Intern. Med. J.*, 2011; 41, 715-721.

Hakalehto, E. Semmelweis' present day follow-up: Updating bacterial sampling and enrichment in clinical hygiene. *Pathophysiology,* 2006; 13, 257-267.

Hakalehto, E. Hygiene monitoring with the Portable Microbe Enrichment Unit (PMEU). *41st R3 -Nordic Symposium. Cleanroom technology, contamination control and cleaning. VTT Publications 266.* Espoo, Finland: VTT (State Research Centre of Finland); 2010.

Hakalehto, E. Simulation of enhanced growth and metabolism of intestinal *Escherichia coli* in the Portable Microbe Enrichment Unit (PMEU). In: Rogers, M. C., Peterson, N. D., editors. *E. coli infections: causes, treatment and prevention.* New York, US: Nova Publishers; 2011.

Hakalehto, E. (editor). Alimentary microbiome - a PMEU approach. New York, NY, USA: Nova Science Publishers, Inc.; 2012.

Hakalehto, E. Bacteriological indications of human activities in the ecosystems. In: Armon, R., Hänninen, O., editors. *Environmental Bioindicators*. Germany: Springer Verlag; 2014.

Hakalehto, E., Hujakka, H., Airaksinen, S., Ratilainen, J., Närvänen, A. Growth-phase limited expression and rapid detection of *Salmonella* type 1 fimbriae. In: Hakalehto, E., editor. *Characterization of Pectinatus cerevisiiphilus and P. frisingiensis surface components. Use of synthetic peptides in the detection of some Gram-negative bacteria.* Kuopio, Finland: Kuopio University Publications C. Natural and Environmental Sciences 112; 2000.

Hakalehto, E., Pesola, J., Heitto, L., Närvänen, A., Heitto, A. Aerobic and anaerobic growth modes and expression of type 1 fimbriae in *Salmonella*. *Pathophysiology,* 2007; 14, 61-69.

Hakalehto, E., Humppi, T., Paakkanen, H. Dualistic acidic and neutral glucose fermentation balance in small intestine: Simulation in vitro. *Pathophysiology,* 2008; 15, 211-220.

Hakalehto, E., Pesola, J., Heitto, A., Deo, B. B., Rissanen, K., Sankilampi, U., Humppi, T., Paakkanen, H. Fast detection of bacterial growth by using Portable Microbe Enrichment Unit (PMEU) and ChemPro100i® gas sensor. *Pathophysiology,* 2009; 16, 57-62.

Hakalehto, E., Hell, M., Bernhofer, C., Heitto, A., Pesola, J., Humppi, T., Paakkanen, H. Growth and gaseous emissions of pure and mixed small intestinal bacterial cultures: Effects of bile and vancomycin. *Pathophysiology,* 2010; 17, 45-53.

Hakalehto, E., Vilpponen-Salmela, T., Kinnunen, K., von Wright, A. Lactic acid bacteria enriched from human gastric biopsies. *ISRN Gastroenterol.,* 2011; 2011, 109183. doi: 10.5402/2011/109183.

Handschur, M., Karlic, H., Hertel, C., Pfeilstocker, M., Haslberger, A. G. Preanalytic removal of human DNA eliminates false signals in general 16S rDNA PCR monitoring of bacterial pathogens in blood. *Comp. Immunol. Microbiol. Infect. Dis.,* 2009; 32, 207-219.

Harmsen, H. J., Wildeboer-Veloo, A. C., Raangs, G. C., Wagendorp, A. A., Klijn, N., Bindels, J. G., Welling, G. W. Analysis of intestinal flora development in breast-fed and formula-fed infants by using molecular identification and detection methods. *J. Pediatr. Gastroenterol. Nutr.,* 2000; 30, 61-67.

Heitto, L., Heitto, A., Hakalehto, E. Tracing wastewaters with faecal enterococci. (Poster). *Second European Large Lakes Symposium.* Norrtälje, Sweden; 2009.

Hell, M., Bernhofer, C., Huhulescu, S., Indra, A., Allerberger, F., Maass, M., Hakalehto, E. How safe is colonoscope-reprocessing regarding *Clostridium difficile* spores? *Supplement 1: Abstracts, 7th International Congress of the Hospital Infection Society*; 10-13 October 2010; Liverpool, UK; 2010.

Heyman, M., Wesenberg, F., Kock Lie, H., Frandsen, T., Lähteenmäki, P., de Verdier, B. editors. Childhood cancer in the Nordic countries. *Report on epidemiologic and therapeutic results from registries and working groups.* Turku, Finland: Nordic Society of Pediatric Haematology and Oncology; 2011.

Hill, M. J. The normal gut bacterial flora. In: Hill, M. J., editor. *Role of the gut bacteria in human toxicology and pharmacology.* London, United Kingdom: Taylor and Francis Ltd; 1995; 3-17.

Holzapfel, W. H., Haberer, P., Snel, J., Schillinger, U., Huis in't Veld, J. H. Overview of gut flora and probiotics. *Int. J. Food Microbiol.,* 1998; 41, 85-101.

Hongfei, D., Xuerui, H., Jing, W., Naihui, C. *Mycobacterium* abscessus lung disease in a patient with previous pulmonary tuberculosis. *Southeast Asian J. Trop. Med. Public Health,* 2012; 43, 959-963.

Howden-Chapman, P., Pierse, N., Nicholls, S., Gillespie-Bennett, J., Viggers, H., Cunningham, M., Phipps, R., Boulic, M., Fjällström, P., Free, S., Chapman, R., Lloyd, B., Wickens, K., Shields, D., Baker, M., Cunningham, C., Woodward, A., Bullen, C., Crane, J. Effects of improved home heating on asthma in community dwelling children: randomised controlled trial. *BMJ,* 2008; 337, a1411.

Iredell, J., Thomas, L., Espedido, B. Beta-lactam resistance in the gram negatives: increasing complexity of conditional, composite and multiply resistant phenotypes. *Pathology,* 2006; 38, 498-506.

Kemp, A., Björkstén, B. Immune deviation and the hygiene hypothesis: a review of the epidemiological evidence. *Pediatr. Allergy Immunol.*, 2003; 14, 74-80.

Kleessen, B., Bunke, H., Tovar, K., Noack, J., Sawatzki, G. Influence of two infant formulas and human milk on the development of the faecal flora in newborn infants. *Acta Paediatr.,* 1995; 84, 1347-1356.

Kondrashova, A., Hyöty, H. Role of viruses and other microbes in the pathogenesis of type 1 diabetes. *Int. Rev. Immunol.,* 2014; 33, 284-295.

Könönen, E. Development of oral bacterial flora in young children. *Ann. Med.,* 2000; 32, 107-112.

Kroumova, V., Gobbato, E., Basso, E., Mucedola, L., Giani, T., Fortina, G. Direct identification of bacteria in blood culture by matrix-assisted laser desorption/ionization time-of-flight mass spectrometry: a new methodological approach. *Rapid Commun. Mass Spectrom.,* 2011; 25, 2247-2249.

Kühn, I., Allestam, G., Stenstrom, T. A., Mollby, R. Biochemical fingerprinting of water coliform bacteria, a new method for measuring phenotypic diversity and for comparing different bacterial populations. *Appl. Environ. Microbiol.,* 1991; 57, 3171-3177.

Laitiomäki, E., Pesola, J., Hakalehto, E. *Projected improvement in the fast microbiological analysis of neonatal blood samples*. Submitted for publication; 2014.

Lennox-King, S. M., O'Farrell, S. M., Bettelheim, K. A., Shooter, R. A. *Escherichia coli* isolated from babies delivered by caesarean section and their environment. *Infection,* 1976; 4, 139-145.

Lodes, M. J., Cong, Y., Elson, C. O., Mohamath, R., Landers, C. J., Targan, S. R., Fort, M., Hershberg, R. M. Bacterial flagellin is a dominant antigen in Crohn disease. *J. Clin. Invest.,* 2004; 113, 1296-1306.

Long, S. S., Swenson, R. M. Development of anaerobic fecal flora in healthy newborn infants. *J. Pediatr.,* 1977; 91, 298-301.

Marks, C. G., Hawley, P. R., Peach, S. L., Drasar, B. S., Hill, M. J. The effects of phthalylsulphathiazole on the bacteria of the colonic mucosa and intestinal contents as revealed by the examination of surgical samples. *Scand. J. Gastroenterol.,* 1979; 14, 891-896.

Martino, B., Barbaro, A., Ielo, D., Martino, E. A., Alati, C., Rogolino, B. S., Ronco, F., Rotilio, D. Nosocomial multidrug-resistant *Klebsiella pneumoniae* spread as the major cause of severe infections in patients with haematological malignancies (Poster). In: *19th Congress of European Hematology Association*, June 12-15, 2014, Milan, Italy.

Midtvedt, T. Intestinal microflora-associated characteristics. *Microecol. Ther.,* 1986; 16, 121-130.

Midtvedt, T., Norman, A. Bile acid transformations by microbial strains belonging to genera found in intestinal contents. *Acta Pathol. Microbiol. Scand.,* 1967; 71, 629-638.

Misra, V., Misra, S. P., Singh, M. K., Singh, P. A., Dwivedi, M. Prevalence of *H. pylori* in patients with gastric cancer. *Indian J. Pathol. Microbiol.,* 2007; 50, 702-707.

Nord, C. E., Kager, L. The normal flora of the gastrointestinal tract. *Neth. J. Med.,* 1984; 27, 249-252.

Okamoto, K., Fujii, Y., Akashi, N., Hitotsubashi, S., Kurazono, H., Karasawa, T., Takeda, Y. Identification and characterization of heat-stable enterotoxin II-producing *Escherichia coli* from patients with diarrhea. *Microbiol. Immunol.,* 1993; 37, 411-414.

Onderdonk, A. B. The intestinal microflora and intra-abdominal sepsis In: Tannock, G. W., editor. *Medical importance of the normal microflora.* United Kingdom: Kluwer Academic Publishers; 1999; 164-176.

Peach, S., Lock, M. R., Katz, D., Todd, I. P., Tabaqchali, S. Mucosal-associated bacterial flora of the intestine in patients with Crohn's disease and in a control group. *Gut,* 1978; 19, 1034-1042.

Pesola, J., Hakalehto, E. Enterobacterial microflora in infancy - a case study with enhanced enrichment. *Indian J. Pediatr.,* 2011; 78, 562-568.

Pesola, J., Vaarala, O., Heitto, A., Hakalehto, E. Use of portable enrichment unit in rapid characterization of infantile intestinal enterobacterial microbiota. *Microb. Ecol. Health Dis.,* 2009; 21, 203-210.

Pesola, J., Heitto, A., Myöhänen, P., Laitiomäki, E., Sankilampi, U., Paakkanen, H., Riikonen, P., Hakalehto, E. Enhanced bacterial enrichment in the microbial diagnostics of pediatric neutropenic sepsis. (Poster abstract). In: Lähteenmäki, P., Grönroos, M., Salmi, T., editors. *NOPHO 29th Annual Meeting.* Turku, Finland: NOPHO; 2011; 59.

Pesola, J., Paakkanen, H., Hakalehto, E. Enhanced diagnostics of pyelonephritis - A case report. *Int. J. Med. Med. Sci.*, 2012; 2, 273-277.

Pierse, N., Arnold, R., Keall, M., Howden-Chapman, P., Crane, J., Cunningham, M. Heating Housing and Health Study Group. Modelling the effects of low indoor temperatures on the lung function of children with asthma. *J. Epidemiol. Community Health,* 2013; 67, 918-25.

Pimentel, M. Review of rifaximin as treatment for SIBO and IBS. *Expert Opin. Investig. Drugs,* 2009; 18, 349-358.

Pol, S., Fontaine, H., Carnot, F., Zylberberg, H., Berthelot, P., Bréchot, C., Nalpas, B. Predictive factors for development of cirrhosis in parenterally acquired chronic hepatitis C: a comparison between immunocompetent and immunocompromised patients. *J. Hepatol.,* 1998; 29, 12-19.

Poxton, I. R., Brown, R., Sawyerr, A., Ferguson, A. Mucosa-associated bacterial flora of the human colon. *J. Med. Microbiol.,* 1997; 46, 85-91.

Rautio, M. Indigenous intestinal microbiota and disease – different approaches to characterize the composition and products of the human microbiota. Helsinki, Finland: Publications of the National Public Health Institute, A5/2002; 2002.

Riikonen, P., Jalanko, H., Hovi, L., Saarinen, U. M. Fever and neutropenia in children with cancer: diagnostic parameters at presentation. *Acta Paediatr.,* 1993; 82, 271-275.

Rolston, K. V., Besece, D., Lamp, K. C., Yoon, M., McConnell, S. A., White, P. Daptomycin use in neutropenic patients with documented gram-positive infections. *Support. Care Cancer,* 2014; 22, 7-14.

Rotimi, V. O., Duerden, B. I. The development of the bacterial flora in normal neonates. *J. Med. Microbiol.,* 1981; 14, 51-62.

Savage, D. C. Associations of indigenous microorganisms with gastrointestinal mucosal epithelia. *Am. J. Clin. Nutr.,* 1970; 23, 1495-1501.

Schumann, A., Nutten, S., Donnicola, D., Comelli, E. M., Mansourian, R., Cherbut, C., Corthesy-Theulaz, I., Garcia-Rodenas, C. Neonatal antibiotic treatment alters gastrointestinal tract developmental gene expression and intestinal barrier transcriptome. *Physiol. Genomics,* 2005; 23, 235-245.

Serichantalergs, O., Bhuiyan, N. A., Nair, G. B., Chivaratanond, O., Srijan, A., Bodhidatta, L., Anuras, S., Mason, C. J. The dominance of pandemic serovars of *Vibrio parahaemolyticus* in expatriates and sporadic cases of diarrhoea in Thailand, and a new emergent serovar (O3 : K46) with pandemic traits. *J. Med. Microbiol.,* 2007; 56, 608-613.

Simojoki, S.-T. *Kantasolusiirron saaneiden lapsipotilaiden kolonisaatioviljelyt.* (In Finnish.) Helsinki, Finland: University of Helsinki, Faculty of Medicine; 2011.

Siu, L. K., Lu, P. L., Hsueh, P. R., Lin, F. M., Chang, S. C., Luh, K. T., Ho, M., Lee, C. Y. Bacteremia due to extended-spectrum beta-lactamase-producing *Escherichia coli* and *Klebsiella pneumoniae* in a pediatric oncology ward: clinical features and identification of different plasmids carrying both SHV-5 and TEM-1 genes. *J. Clin. Microbiol.,* 1999; 37, 4020-4027.

Stephen, A. M., Cummings, J. H. The microbial contribution to human faecal mass. *J. Med. Microbiol.,* 1980; 13, 45-56.

Toivanen, P., Vaahtovuo, J., Eerola, E. Influence of major histocompatibility complex on bacterial composition of fecal flora. *Infect. Immun.,* 2001; 69, 2372-2377.

Väkeväinen, S., Tillonen, J., Salaspuro, M., Jousimies-Somer, H., Nuutinen, H., Färkkila, M. Hypochlorhydria induced by a proton pump inhibitor leads to intragastric microbial production of acetaldehyde from ethanol. *Aliment. Pharmacol. Ther.,* 2000; 14, 1511-1518.

Van de Merwe, J. P., Stegeman, J. H., Hazenberg, M. P. The resident faecal flora is determined by genetic characteristics of the host. Implications for Crohn's disease? *Antonie Van Leeuwenhoek,* 1983; 49, 119-124.

Von Mutius, E. Allergies, infections and the hygiene hypothesis--the epidemiological evidence. *Immunobiology*, 2007; 212, 433-439.

Wells, C. L., Ferrieri, P., Weisdorf, D. J., Rhame, F. S. The importance of surveillance stool cultures during periods of severe neutropenia. *Infect. Control.,* 1987; 8, 317-319.

Westergaard, T., Rostgaard, K., Wohlfahrt, J., Andersen, P. K., Aaby, P., Melbye, M. Sibship characteristics and risk of allergic rhinitis and asthma. *Am. J. Epidemiol.*, 2005; 162, 125-132.

Weymann, A., Borst, T., Popov, A. F., Sabashnikov, A., Bowles, C., Schmack, B., Veres, G., Chaimow, N., Simon, A. R., Karck, M., Szabo, G. Surgical treatment of infective endocarditis in active intravenous drug users: a justified procedure? *J. Cardiothorac. Surg.*, 2014; 9, 58.

Wherrett, D. K., Daneman, D. Prevention of type 1 diabetes. *Endocrinol. Metab. Clin. North Am.*, 2009; 38, 777-790.

Whimbey, E., Englund, J. A., Couch, R. B. Community respiratory virus infections in immunocompromised patients with cancer. *Am. J. Med.,* 1997; 102, 10-18; discussion 25-26.

Wicki, M., Auckenthaler, A., Felleisen, R., Tanner, M., Baumgartner, A. Novel *Bacteroides* host strains for detection of human- and animal-specific bacteriophages in water. *J. Water Health,* 2011; 9, 159-168.

Woo, P. C., Lau, S. K., Teng, J. L., Yuen, K. Y. Current status and future directions for *Laribacter hongkongensis*, a novel bacterium associated with gastroenteritis and traveller's diarrhoea. *Curr. Opin. Infect. Dis.,* 2005; 18, 413-419.

Zoetendal, E. G., von Wright, A., Vilpponen-Salmela, T., Ben-Amor, K., Akkermans, A. D., de Vos, W. M. Mucosa-associated bacteria in the human gastrointestinal tract are uniformly distributed along the colon and differ from the community recovered from feces. *Appl. Environ. Microbiol.,* 2002; 68, 3401-3407.

In: Microbiological Clinical Hygiene
Editor: Eino Elias Hakalehto

ISBN: 978-1-63463-428-1

Chapter 14

Microbes and Human Digestive System

Elias Hakalehto
Department of Environmental Sciences,
University of Eastern Finland, Kuopio, Finland

Abstract

Digestive system is the powerhouse of our body system. Its proper function is a prerequisite for our good general health. There the food is absorbed into the body, forming sources of chemical energy and building blocks. Microbes have an essential role in these processes. Hygienically, any disturbance in this "locomotive" may and will easily cause problems. Also, our alimentary tract is a port and an opening for many contagious diseases or otherwise harmful microbes or substances to enter the body system.

The natural defenses on the mucosal membranes, as well as the balancing microflora especially on the GI tract surfaces, are protecting us from adverse or deleterious effects of the intruding microbes.

In this sense, it is important to make distinction between those bacterial or other microbial strains, which influence the composition of the chyme or the feces, but do not invade or penetrate the host beneath the gut epithelia, from the microbial agents which directly interfere with the host functions by an intrusion. The latter ones are able to cause pathological consequences within the tissues, whereas harmful microbes in the gut liquid phase (chyme) have more indirect effects on the host. However, they contribute to such syndromes as SIBO (Small Intestinal Bacterial Overgrowth) or IBD (Irritable Bowel Disease), besides interfering with the digestion.

The commensal flora in the intestines can cause problems if it gets distorted. It is also possible, that the hose defenses are somehow compromised which may alter the situation inside the gut. Moreover, many types of medications such as antibiotic therapy, may severely disturb the normal functions of the gut microbiota. Therefore, in order to avoid malfunctions or even dysbiosis, the use of probiotics is often recommended. Some of the functions and misdirected activities of the alimentary microbiome are outlined in this chapter. For the microbiological problems the solution are the microbes!

The digestive process is evaluated with special emphasis on the bacteriological contributions.

1. Introduction

The structures and functions, as well as further characterization of the alimentary microbiome have been previously presented (Midtvedt, 1986; Hill, 1995; Berg, 1996; Kelly, 2010; Hakalehto, 2012a). It can be stated that main "action plan" for an individual intestinal microbial strain could be listed as follows:

- avoid excessive host defenses
- get nutrients and growth factors in an energetically feasible way
- manipulate the environment into favorable direction (if rooted there as a member of larger microbial community)
- establish biofilms as a part of the community (see also Chapter 2)
- dissimilate the biochemical substances inside the host body system

Various gut bacteria interact with each other and with host in order to achieve these goals. In our studies a concept of Bacteriological Intestinal Balance (BIB) has been established as the general goal for metabolic cooperation within the entire microbial communities.

2. Novel Concept of Pathogenicity

In a standard microbiological thinking any particular disease is usually caused by a single pathogen. Such disease is having clear, specific characteristics. Diarrheal diseases often represent such "traditional" type of pathogenic picture (Giannella, 1981; Okamoto et al., 1993). However, nowadays it seems increasingly evident that we need to broaden our view on microbial illnesses. This approach could be called *ecological pathogenesis* or *joint mechanisms of molecular infection*. Often it can even be postulated that the microflora is diseased or imbalanced which cause problems to the host. Typically, these kinds of infectious conditions are progressing inside the body system. Their causative agents may relatively often belong to the normal flora. They have somehow become harmful or disastrous to the host health. Such alteration could be resulting from immunogenic defects caused by some toxication, or pollution effects, for instance. Thus novel pathogens are emerging among microflora with several factors which are able to produce harmful reactions on the molecular level onto the host physiology. For example, various common staphylococci may occupy specific niches in the body, and start secreting their toxins, or superantigens and enzymes, which dramatically influence the host (Smyth et al., 1975; Rossi-George et al., 2005; Bradley and Nizet, 2011). From the medical point of view these pathogens are difficult to get diagnosed and treated with the traditional means. For example, they can make very resistant cell forms in biofilms or microcolonies within the body system. These bacterial intruders can also manipulate the host innate immune system, and often they penetrate into individual host cells (Baxt et al., 2013). Three different mechanisms of intracellular pathogenesis are presented here as examples (according to Wilson et al., 2011):

- *Legionella pneumophila* cells are taken up in a vacuole (phagosome) that does not become acidified or fuse with lysosome. Later on the vacuole becomes surrounded by endoplasmic reticulum. Inside this structure, the legionellas freely replicate, then escape from it and multiply in the cytoplasm of the host cells.
- *Salmonella enterica* serovar Typhimurium is taken up into a phagosome in a macrophage, where it is replicated as the phagosome-lysosome fusion is prevented.
- *Mycobacterium tuberculosis* cells are engulfed also into a phagosome in the macrophage. By the aid of the inhibition of lysosomal enzymes the bacterium is then replicated on the phagolysosome.

As it can be seen from the examples above, the bacteria can sometimes take advantage of the human cell organelles, which are normally used for their eradication.

The above-mentioned novel pathogen types have distanced themselves from the ecological control of the microbiome (Hakalehto, 2012a), or from the control of host defensive mechanisms (Lyte, 2010). They could even establish their own ecological rules of the pathogenesis, where they possibly employ or overtake the same principles that normally restrict and regulate the microbial members of the microbiome. In such case they have only become vectors of malicious activity. However, these effects could often occur during a long period of time. Then observing or documenting of the pathogenic development becomes a real challenging task.

The gut microflora is an important potential source of the slow intrusion of these "hiding pathogens" (Pesola and Hakalehto, 2012). Wounds in the epithelia (or in the skin) can facilitate their dissemination. In the body system they get rooted into favorable locations after breaking through the mucosal barrier. One of these "risky sites" is the heart and its veins, where oxygen-rich blood is creating a niche for energetically favorable colonization for many facultative strains (Hakalehto et al., 2007). Subacute bacterial endocarditis is caused by α-hemolytic streptococci. From mouth opportunistic infections without measurable virulence factors, these harmful organisms could disseminate elsewhere in the body system (Wilson et al., 2011). Although these streptococci are normally highly susceptible to penicillin, sometimes restricted circulation of blood or inadequate diffusion of the medicines is not allowing enough antibiotic molecules to be delivered on site. In a similar fashion, it is possible that intestinal intrusions of opportunistic pathogens may cause troublesome infections elsewhere in the body. For example, such antibiotic resistant strains as vancomycin resistant *Enterococcus* sp. can cause a bloodstream invasion (Ubeda et al., 2010).

Another rather easily contaminated area is the lung tissue, where the oxygen provides many bacteria with beneficial surroundings for a continuing presence and for developing a disease even in a relatively low phase. This is potentially leading to the high prevalence of pneumonia in the ageing populations (Aliberti and Kaye, 2013). (They can originate from the digestive tract.) Resulting from low oxygen levels, also the CO_2 bursts inside the heart and in the lungs could effectively boost the slow pathogenesis (Hakalehto and Hänninen, 2012). The stimulating effect of CO_2 on the onset of bacterial growth has been known for a long time (Walker, 1932).

Also artificial objects in the body may serve as platforms for the bacterial colonization. For example, intravenous catheters may get colonized with staphylococci or other bacteria, as well as the plastic joints or equivalent (see also Chapter 8). These bacteria may also reside in the mineral-rich bone tissue, which possibly gives them extra protection. Some staphylococcal strains could produce hydrophobic capsules of teichoic acids, polysaccharides or lipids (Fox et al., 1998; O'Riordan and Lee, 2004). The polysaccharide capsules promote mucosal colonization and persistence of staphylococci in blood (and lymphatic) circulation. The growth of staphylococcal capsules is enhanced by the presence of whey (Watson, 1989).

In our own studies, *Bacillus cereus* was accumulating milk casein on the bacterial cell surfaces (results not shown here). This implies to the capabilities of the intestinal intruders to acquire protective shields from external compounds, *e.g.,* of food origin. Staphylococcal capsular forms have been found in the intestines as well as in the peritoneal cavity of a severely ill patient (Hakalehto, unpublished results).

Patient condition with somehow weakened defenses is often required for the development of this type "hiding" or "sneaking" infection. For example, *Klebsiella pneumoniae* is a member of normal infantile gut flora (Pesola et al., 2009; Pesola and Hakalehto, 2011; Hakalehto, 2013). However, it can also cause fatal lung infections for individuals with compromised immunodefenses. *Klebsiella pneumonia*e has been shown to possess mechanisms to withstand host inflammatory responses by producing a polysaccharide-rich layer around the cells (Lawlor et al., 2005). Moreover, this bacterium could establish a symbiosis with other strains as it acts as a member of the normal flora (Hakalehto et al., 2008). It is an important contributor to the BIB (Bacterial Intestinal Balance) (Hakalehto, 2013). Since many disturbances in the microbiome are caused by defective nutrition, it is obvious that any inadequancies in our diet will cause an increased risk of pathogenic action also outside the alimentary tract (Jaakkola and Hakalehto, 2012).

In the intestinal milieu gases play an important role in keeping up and regulating the microbial action (Hakalehto, 2011a; Hakalehto and Hänninen, 2012). They have been studied in the PMEU Scentrion® where the liberated gas is used for the ultrasensitive detection of pathogens in various body fluids, such as blood or urine (Hakalehto et al., 2009; Pesola et al., 2012), and in water samples (Pitkänen et al., 2009; Hakalehto et al., 2011a). The host and the symbiotic microflora create a gas phase inside the body. The eukaryotic cells have to acquire the required oxygen into the cell for their respiratory chain in the mitochondrias. Inside the cells the microtubules and microfilaments transport the oxygen supply (Denis, 2014). It is noteworthy, that many intracellular pathogens are facultative anaerobes. *Salmonella* sp. may benefit from the oxygen transported by the blood circulation (Hakalehto et al., 2007).

In fact, it could be supposed that in the body a competition for oxygen is a prevailing condition. If parasitic aerobic organisms wander around in the body, in its fluids or organs, they seek for oxygen supplies. Therefore, it could be assumed that *e.g.,* salmonellas from the intestines attempt to invade the tissues in order to get access to the blood oxygen (Hakalehto et al., 2007). If we continue this line of thinking, it is possible to hypothetize, that the intracellular mode of many bacterial pathogens could be caused by their strive to obtain energy and building bloc molecules by using parasitic means. Besides the actual intracellular pathogens typically represented by *Borrelia burgdorferi* (Tilly et al., 2008), there are several common bacteria occasionally residing inside the host cells (Torcato et al., 2013; Gorgojo et al., 2012).

3. Role of Antioxidants in the Prevention of Infections

Bacterial cells and other microflora in the human body live in "a molecular universe". There they are subjected to the host functions beside their own regulatory system. Biochemically this is an extremely complicated situation, where various interactions play crucial roles. The microbial associations as such are not necessarily competitive but inside the body system it is often possible to see tendencies toward cooperation between different strains (Hakalehto, 2012b). These kinds of "enhanced" or "concentrated" ecosystems force their members into the cooperative approach in the above-mentioned molecular universe. In fact, it has been documented that within the alimentary tract of different individuals, various bacterial strains may fulfill specific roles in the microbial community within the body matrix.

If the microbial existence inside human tissues, or on their surfaces, is causing additional stress, this stress could be further divided into:

- Oxidative stress
- pH stress
- Pseudoregulation of the host
- Provoking the immunosystem

All these activities may enhance also the cleansing action of the body. In long term, the stress caused by the microbial presence is thus consuming various resources of the body. Consequently, this causes increasing oxidative stress and lack of nutritives. Therefore, the storages of the antioxidant molecules need a substitution. It is also noteworthy that besides overwhelming oxidative stress, also the high level of intestinal hydrogen production may cause health threats caused by distorting of the redox balance inside the body tissues.

4. Microbial Ecosystems of the Human Body in Health and Disease

As a whole, the various micro-organisms in our body system take part in ecosystemic functions which are integrated with the host body activities (Lyte, 2010). During early infancy the intestines get colonized by bacteria. The early life diet can modify the colonization process (Benno et al., 1984). This scope of making observations taking the microflora development into account is giving novel views into the healthcare. For example, gaseous substances emitted by the bacteria, or by the host cells, could contribute to the microbiological distribution of strains and their mode of action (Hakalehto and Hänninen, 2012). The lactobacilli (and most other bacteria) produce CO_2 when they actively metabolize. In an arrangement using the PMEU method it was possible to demonstrate the boosting effect of CO_2 produced by lactobacilli on some anaerobic clostridia (butyric acid bacteria). The latter bacteria belonging to genus *Clostridium*, in turn, have been considered as a group as being a potential health hazard amongst the intestinal flora, even though *C. butyricum* is a member of the normal flora. Paradoxically enough, the CO_2 emitted by the "benign" lactic acid bacteria (LAB) is preventing the "malicious" putrefactive anaerobes from rooting into the gut. This effective "bubbling" inside the large intestines is probably mimicked in the PMEU as a boosting effect for growth and metabolism (Hakalehto and Hänninen, 2012; Hakalehto 2013; Hakalehto et al., 2013).

Besides the various phases; solid, gaseous and liquid ones, also other physical phenomena influence both the host cells and the microbes. This has been exploited in treatments for various illnesses. For example, the pulsed electromagnetic fields have been used for curing osteoarthritis (Trock et al., 1994). In fact, it is of high importance to overcome the "hiding infections" in bone tissues, and elsewhere in the body. For this "molecular level victory" on the hideous pathogens, it is of crucial importance that the antioxidant levels of an individual correspond to the ones needed for true recovery (Jaakkola and Hakalehto, 2012). The hiding infections can be monitored by following up the leucosyte level, for instance (Knight et al., 2013).

The intestinal ecosystem forms a continuum, whose starting point is in the duodenum (Kendall et al., 1927). There acidic chyme is neutralized with pancreatic bicarbonates, and also with the enterobacterial balancing action (Hakalehto et al., 2008).

The microbial ecosystem is "enhanced" by nature, as the existing and invasing microbes are integrated into rapidly moving mass of intestinal chyme, which is digested while in motion (Hakalehto, 2012b). There the food is degraded and absorbed with high effectivity, and the bile substances are secreted into the chyme together with many enzymatic components (Hakalehto et al., 2012).

These processes are influenced by complicated host hormonal regulations. In order to understand the microbiology of the small intestines we need to comprehend the functions of these rapidly changing conditions where the microbial strains are taking part in the efficient uptake of nutrients taking place in the host small bowel.

Simulation in the PMEU is providing data on the behavior of individual cells and subcultures, as well as on their interactions. In the digestive tract, various strains in microbial communities can together metabolize many substances which would remain unprocessed by a pure culture (Dalton and Stirling, 1982).

It has been documented that the absence of bile (biliary atresia) in a neonate will lead to a dominance of enterobacteria in the gut (Kobayashi et al., 1988). This is probably due to the fast growth speed of these intestinal bacteria, which are relatively bile-tolerant in general. In case of the bottle-fed infants, bifidobacteria were the bacterial type which lowered the most in proportion, from 75% of total flora in healthy cases in comparison with only 2.4% in case of the biliary atresia.

As the bifidobacteria are considered to be the primary group of bacterial strains in the healthy neonatal intestines, this example illustrates the importance of proper bile functions for the healthy development of the intestinal flora and gut ecosystem. However, one has to keep in mind that the above-mentioned consequences were measured from the fecal flora, not directly in the duodenum. In case of the developing gut microflora, a monotonous microbial community is more vulnerable to imbalances and diseases than a versatile one (Bennet and Nord, 1987; Kühn et al., 1993; Keesing et al., 2010).

The processing of the food within the digestive tract takes place during a few hours. The period required for the chyme to passage through the small bowel is about 6-7 hours. The bile acids are recovered in the terminal ileum to be transported to liver, and back to the duodenum. In the end of the small intestines the intestinal chyme is led into the microbe-rich cecum through the ileocecal valve. At this point the enterobacterial and enterococcal main flora is ultimately losing their majority in cell number to the lactic acid bacteria and obligate anaerobes. The facultative members of *Enterobacteriaceae* maintain the pH balance in the small bowel (Hakalehto et al., 2008; Hakalehto et al., 2010), whereas the lactic acid bacteria keep gaseous flow active during the movement of healthy intestines, especially in the colon (Hakalehto and Hänninen, 2012). If the colonic microflora is transforming into a stagnant phase, this imposes the risk that the anaerobes start producing secondary metabolites, many of them being harmful to our health.

4. Distribution of Pathogenic or Symbiotic Effects, and the Research on Them

What makes a pathogen? – There are certain bacteria and other microbes, which in majority of cases cause a contagious disease. However, even salmonellas could form latent strains (Ahiwale et al., 2013). Which factors are then preventing them from causing an illness? Which provokes them? Immunoprotection is undoubtedly one part of the answer to these questions, as well as the protection offered by other host defense mechanisms. An additional reason for the latent infections could be the interactive regulation between the microbial strains, and between the strains and the host body system. It keeps the opportunistic or other pathogens dormant, with respect to pathogenesis, as long as the host is *e.g.,* in good general health.

Although we tend to consider the pathogenicity often as defined by the Koch's postulates (Segre, 2013) this concept of microbes as causative agents for illnesses is generally still a wider one. Since the microbes extend their influence beyond the direct impact of the intruding cells, we have to take into account the immunogenic molecules, toxins, structures and signal substances, which all have their effects on the host body. Many bacteria, for example, have common antigens, such as ECA (Enterobacterial Common Antigen) (Gozdziewicz et al., 2014). The bacterial fimbriae contain rather universal antigenic structures within some groups (Hakalehto, 1995), and their flagellar proteins also bear close similarities to each other (Hakalehto et al., 1997). All these molecular structures are closely resembling each other also with respect to their function. There detection can be exploited for the early verification of the pathogens.

Since the microbes inhabit niches smaller than our visual perception is able to observe, we need to adjust our reasoning accordingly. For example, on human skin most bacteria are anaerobic ones, prevailing in small niches. Correspondingly, in a brewery, the contaminations of an obligately anaerobic *Pectinatus* bacteria were largely spreading as air-borne "infections" inside liquid droplets in aerosols (Hakalehto, 2000).

In principle the microbiological conditions could be roughly divided into:

- survival conditions
- spreading up conditions
- multiplication conditions
- specific metabolic conditions

It is of crucial importance to make a difference between these various sets of conditions. Any particular "subcondition" (niche) for any member of the microbial community needs to be evaluated with respect to all different factors that constitute the overall "condition" (ecosystem). For example, joint culture of *E. coli* and *K. mobilis* produced different pH conditions in different partial pressures of oxygen, which has a profound effect on the entire microbiome (Hakalehto et al., 2008).

If we are going to measure the presence, growth or metabolism of any particular microbe in any sample, we need to take into account the considerations above. All microbes function in different ways in changing conditions. It is still possible to make an argument that this would be irrelevant if specific genes for indicating or enumerating the presence of various microbes specifically were screened. However, there is a conceptual "trap" where we get easily caught as a result of the tremendous development of molecular biology. However, counting or typing the molecular data alone is *not* an indication of the past, present or future condition *in vivo*. The numerical or on/off data always requires interpretation on the basis of understanding the specific conditions in various categories of existence for any members of microbiota. An excellent example is that by knowing all bacterial species in an intestinal sample, or even their genetic markers for antibiotic resistance at any time point, we cannot deduce the best possible treatment for those strains which we consider as pathogens. For optimal care, the actual behavior of and interactions in the microflora need to be examined during various medications and combined treatments. The PMEU method is offering a tool for this type of investigation.

This cascade of thinking may look out too speculative or philosophical one in the beginning. However, that kind of mental effort is necessary for a successful microbiological evaluation of any microbiological sample, if our goal is the optimal treatment of any microbiological illness. This evaluation of conditions is not or will not be successful by physico-chemical measurements only, however broad or representative they potentially could be. For truthful simulation of the sample situation, data on the *reactions of the microbe* is an essential factor and piece of information most urgently needed for understanding the status of any particular strain. This is relevant line of thinking if we aim for an ultimate understanding, which could give an optimal view on patient condition, disease, contamination characteristics *etc*. In real laboratory world, often just on/off answer is quite adequate. However, if we want to develop our understanding on pathogenesis, and our procedures, it simply is not enough.

In order to captivate by research the most authentic expressions of bacterial or other microbial life we need to be extremely cautious in determining the scope of investigation, and the specific conditions, in different test vials or rounds. This is a necessity if correct information is expected.

5. Conditions of the Duodenal Tract and the Origin of BIB (Bacteriological Intestinal Balance)

It was stated almost one hundred years ago by Kendall and coworkers (1927): "The duodenal tract of normal individual is an important part of the alimentary tract, not only it receives secretions from the neighboring glandular organs, but also because it is the place of the initial development of that vast column of bacteria, numbering some thirty millions, which is excreted daily in the fecal mass." This reflects the importance of the upper small intestinal areas, besides in nutrient uptake, also as the origin of the intestinal microbial ecosystem. This point of view has often been neglected. In any case, duodenal tract seems to harbor enterobacterial strains, which maintain the pH balance, as well as protect the intestinal microflora and its internal balance (Bacteriological Intestinal Balance) from excess osmotic shock when food is arriving into the intestines (Hakalehto et al., 2008; Hakalehto, 2012a). Some lactic acid bacteria, for example, may inoculate the food already in the ventricle (Hakalehto et al., 2011b).

The duodenal microflora has to cope with many environmental stresses. They are encountered by *e.g.,* the gradient of gastric acidity, bile substances and various host defenses. These conditions, which are mostly strenuous for the microbes, largely explain the relatively low numbers of microbes found in the epithelia of the upper intestinal tract when compared to the billions of cells in the colon. Most of these effects are caused by human body defenses, or by the overall conditions in the alimentary tract:

- low pH, acidic stomach
- abrupt pH regulation by *e.g.,* pancreatic bicarbonates
- food arriving in bursts into the duodenum
- toxicity of the bile substances toward many microbes (see also part 5 of this chapter)
- gut movements
- immunodefences
- defensins

Also, some bacterial strains "attenuate" the growth of the others (Hakalehto and Jaakkola, 2013).

On the other hand, the vast surface area of the small intestinal epithelia could provide the bacteria with plenty of space for attachment, and even sites for invasive purposes. However, the above-mentioned mechanisms keep the duodenal epithelial surfaces relatively sparsely covered with bacterial strains. Perhaps most importantly, the absorption of most nutrients by the host deprive the necessary factors from the reach of excessive bacterial population growth. Nevertheless, this growth is occasionally made possible by the arriving new food. The duodenal bacteria inoculate and then flourish in the degrading food particles and molecules, and in the intestinal chyme derived from them (Hakalehto et al., 2012). Some main microbial components and their activities contributing to the Bacteriological Intestinal Balance (BIB) are illustrated in Figure 1 (Hakalehto 2011a, 2012a, 2013).

The flow downwards makes the original bacterial strains of duodenum "the onset of vast column" (Kendall et al., 1927). They multiply on the way in the chyme during its movement in the intestines. From there the bacteria take actively part in the nutrient uptake by the host body. Many of their enzymatic activities benefit the host and *vice versa* (Hakalehto, 2012a). Some cells remain, partially in a resting state, on the epithelial membranes, expecting for new bursts of nutrients. The origins of these populations can possibly be found also from the food but some interactive and immunological factors are probably determining the basic composition of the individual normal flora. When a newborn child had lost his most natural enterobacterial strains as a consequence of antibiotic treatment during his first days of life, he could recover from this deprivation and regain these bacterial types during a period of half a year when getting solid food, instead of hygienically safeguarded milk formulas (Pesola and Hakalehto, 2011). In the intestines microbial strains are not likely to grow against the food flow. In a mature adult alimentary microbiota the relative cell number is increasing when chyme is moving downwards. In different parts of the intestines, different species often form the majority. The bacterial "gradients" are partially associated with the bacterial contribution to circulation of bile substances. This circulation, in turn, is essential for our healthy fat uptake, for example.

6. Human Microbiome Studies

In Science News it was stated that "We humans co-evolved with our microbial communities." (Balter, 2012). This is not necessarily representing any darwinistic views, but merely the rapid fluctuation of microbial composition. Program Director Lita Proctor of the Human Microbiome Project (HMP) (170 M$ in 5 years) US National Institutes of Health (NIH), Bethesda, MA, has said: "It is this co-evolved relationship that has expanded our capabilities beyond what is coded in our genomes to defend against diseases, adapt to new environments, exploit a diverse diet, and thrive as a species." Human Microbiome Project together with the corresponding European program called "Metagenomics of the Human Intestinal Tract" (MetaHIT) run by governmental agencies of *e.g.,* France, Japan and Canada is striving for increasingly accurate definition of the intestinal microflora.

However, this flora is somewhat like a "moveable feast", which makes all definitions to become approximations, at least from the functional point of view.

David Reiman, microbiologist at Stanford University, Palo Alto, California, who has been involved for 15 years in microbiome research in "raising visibility and attracting a much larger number of people to the field", has summed up the following on the development of the microbiological methods: when started (the career), he and others lacked good tools to identify the microbes teeming in the human gut, skin, mouth, nose and reproductive tract. S. Dusko Erlich, a molecular biologist at the French research agency INRA, a coordinator of MetaHIT, has emphasized new methods for the characterization of our microflora: high throughput DNA sequencing: millions of sequences without culturing also using short rRNA (16S) as a taxonomic marker. In this approach, no physiological data is collected. The study of 124 subjects (persons) from Denmark and Spain with average of 160 microbial species located in their gut areas (about 1000 different bacterial species totally) lead to the finding of three "enterotypes" globally (Wu et al., 2011).

Dr. Rob Knight is a biologist of the University of Colorado, Boulder, and is involved in Human Microbiome Project. He has characterized the continuation project: HMP2 to follow thousands of individuals between 0-20 years of age. Kjersti Aagaard, an obstetrician-gynecologist and microbiome researcher from Baylor College of Medicine, Houston, Texas, has stated that "My hope is that this will be one of the most rapid translations from [lab] bench to bedside seen to date", and "Unlike the human genome, the microbiome is changeable, and it is this changeability which holds real promise." In a citation of Costello et al. (2012): "Only a handful of studies have used cultivation independent surveys to examine the consequences of therapeutic doses of antibiotics on gut microbiota." However, there is a fundamental mistake occurring, if the following basic principle is neglected: Ecological study should include enrichment cultivations in various sets of selected conditions in order to understand the microbiological interactions.

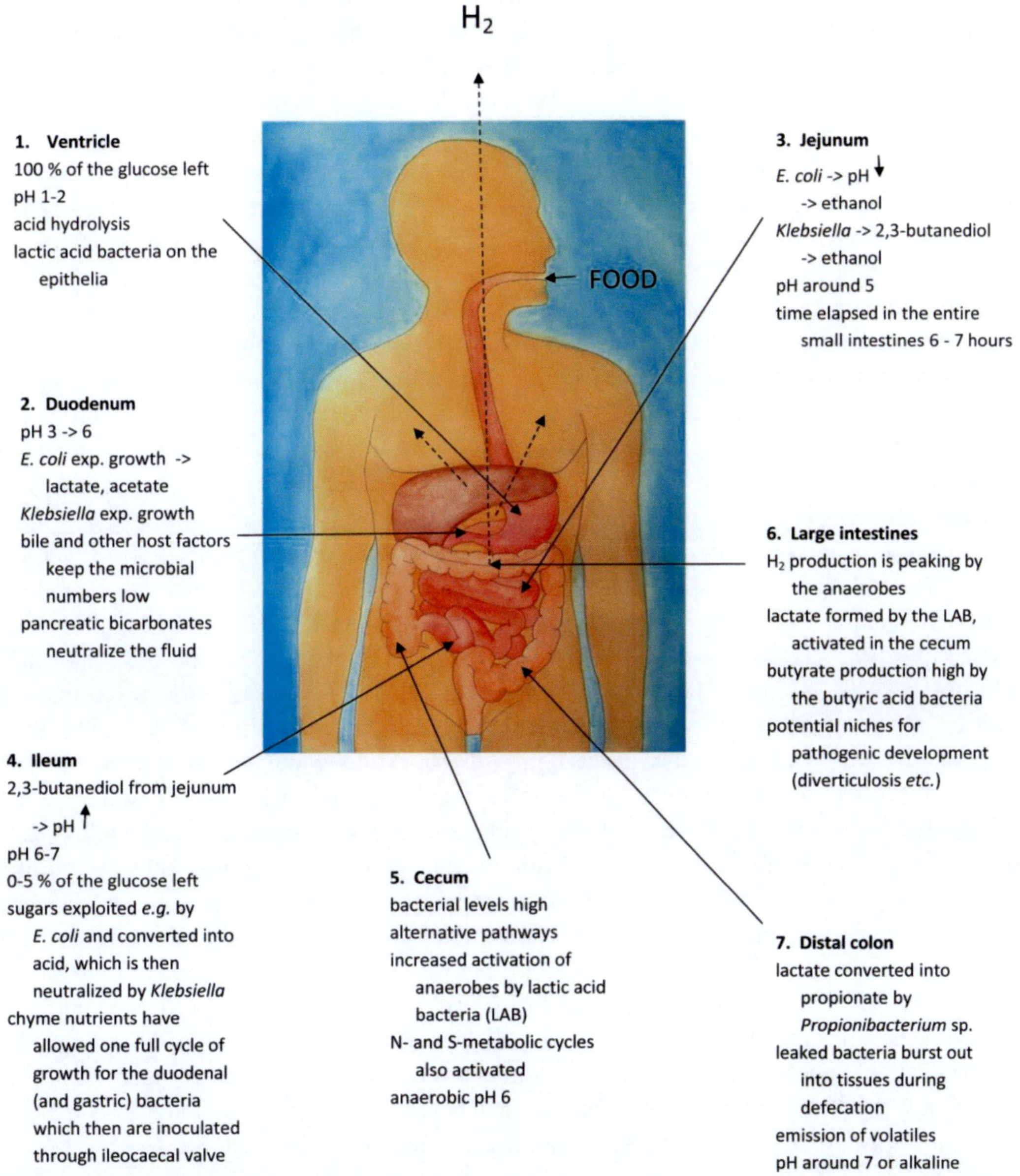

Figure 1. Some basics of the Bacteriological Intestinal Balance (BIB) according to the PMEU studies.

7. Bacteriological Intestinal Balance (BIB)

Growth-phase-associated protein patterns of different *Lactobacillus plantarum* strains have been mapped in the lag-phase, early-exponential, late-exponential and early-stationary phases (Koistinen et al., 2007). The corresponding proteins were mainly associated with the catalytic pathways (glycolysis, phosphoketolase pathway and ribose metabolism). The strain (REB1) isolated from spontaneously fermented cereals had more stable pattern than the other strain (MLBPL1) isolated from white cabbage. The latter one had energy metabolism which was more agitated during active growth phases. This could be a sign of more profound penetration and integration of the strain in question into the soft plant tissue, whereas the REB1 strain was more surface associated on the kernels. This has an implication to the mode of food degradation in the intestines where the lactic acid bacteria (LAB) are directly connected with the enzymatic degradation of plant derived macromolecules. This basic activity of the microbiota in the intestinal chyme is offering them an "upper hand" in formulating the Bacteriological Intestinal Balance (BIB) (Hakalehto, 2011a, 2012a, 2013). This is including the mechanisms of enterobacterial duodenal flora when inoculating the newly forming chyme in the upper intestines. There the pancreatic and bile substances are mixed into the degradable food materials, and the LAB strains produce the seed inoculation from the food sources (especially from the fermented milk and plant materials). Additionally, it could be possible that the gastric surfaces host some microcolonies of these basically beneficial bacterial strains, capable of inoculating the chyme at its origin. Some proof has been collected about the LAB incorporating the gastric epithelia of healthy individuals (Hakalehto et al., 2011b). Inside the chyme different bacterial groups then search for a dynamic balance between each other.

The basic metabolism of lactic acid formation by many intestinal bacteria is, in fact, the second driving force in the BIB, besides the enterobacterial dualistic balance of pH and the osmotic regulation associated with it (Hakalehto et al., 2008; Hakalehto, 2012a). In further elucidation of the digestive role of LAB we have simulated their effects on other intestinal flora in the PMEU system (Hakalehto and Jaakkola, 2013). It has been proven out that the LAB exercise certain "attenuation" on the other members of the microflora. (The term "attenuation" was concluded in a discussion with Dr. Mike Wakeman in Helsinki in Fall 2013.) This effect is not entirely based on lactate formation, but also on other so far unidentified influences. However, together with prebiotic flax substance and antioxidants some probiotics repeatedly produced a 100-fold attenuation of overwhelming other microflora components. Correspondingly, the prebiotic potential of cereal arabinoxylo-oligosaccharides has been documented together with the bifidobacterial probiotic strains (Pastell, 2010). This indicates the existence of a significant basic mechanism which is a key factor in most of the health promoting effects associated with the LAB. Additionally, they also modulate the human intestinal epithelia (O'Hara et al., 2006). This is an example of "molecular communication" phenomena between the human host and his intestinal microbes. It is noteworthy, that this communication maintained between a bacterial culture in a moving state, and not only in conjunction with surface associated microflora or biofilms.

Interestingly, if the reasons for obesity are seeked for from the bacteriological point of view, some specific reactions in the intestines deserve special attention, namely:

2,3-butanediol fermentation in the small intestines	optimal pH around 6.0
lactic acid fermentation during the passage of chyme in the small intestines	optimal pH 5.2
conversion of lactated into propionate in the intestines	optimal pH 6.4
butyric acid fermentation in the colon	optimal pH 5.9

The various sites of microbiological action in the intestines are illustrated in Figure 1. The consequences of the metabolic actions of the microflora in the upper intestines may be the cause for different bacterial compositions in the cecum (Ley et al., 2006; Turnbaugh et al., 2006; Hakalehto, 2012a).

The more neutral substances are formed, the more favorable are the conditions for propionic acid fermentation, and consequently for butyric acid fermentation in colon. A part of these organic acids are further converted into alcohols by anaerobic bacteria. These reactions, in turn, partially replace the acetate and lactate formation. In some cases, acetate and propionate condence into valeric acid. Lactate is also effectively metabolized into propionate by the *Propionibacterium* sp. This reaction has been followed in an industrial waste treatment process on slaughterhouse wastes, in which process almost all lactate was eventually converted into propionate and butyrate. Subsequently, the anaerobic flora is then converting the acids into alcohols. This formation of alcohols instead of short-chain acids is causing increased absorption of the chemical energy into the host body system. This is the case both when the alcoholic fraction is mainly consisting of ethanol (*e.g.,* in ethanol or 2,3-butanediol fermentations) and in case of higher propionate and butyrate concentrations, with subsequent conversions into propanol and butanol. As a result, tendency for host developing obesity is established, whereas in case of individuals with more dominant lactic and acetic acid production by their gut microbes the energy is more effectively transferred out of the reach of the body system. Also, some carbon and hydrogen evaporated into gases. Then the lowering pH is also decelerating the microbial metabolism. All these effects are accumulating during the course of digestion which is casting the foundation for the characteristic metabolic type of any individual microflora, and thus for the entire body system. This links the overall microbial metabolism of the alimentary tract with that of the host, and constitutes a built-in pattern of interdependence. The colonic consequences of all this metabolic action are often screened by investigating the stool composition (Hakalehto et al., 2012).

Human feces are normally alkaline which is a result from *e.g.,* degradation of proteins. However, if the fecal pH lowers below 5.5, this is considered as a sign of a digestive problem, such as lactose intolerance, or contagion with *e.g., E. coli* or rotavirus (Bonheur et al., 2011). This ends up into the considerations of pH in the chain of food-chyme-feces. As a thumb rule it can be stated that at around pH 4.5 the dominant organic acid is the acetic acid, at pH 5.5 it is the butyric acid and at pH 6.5 the propionic acid. Correspondingly, the dualistic balance between acid producing and neutral substances forming enterobacterial strains in the intestines is causing first the lowering of the pH, which is then elevated in the end of the process (Hakalehto et al., 2008). The pH increase is more observable in increasingly oxidative conditions. In the PMEU culture cycle of a symbiotic *Escherichia coli – Klebsiella* population the pH finally sets up around pH 8 in aerobiosis. In microaerobic conditions this value could be around 7, and in anaerobiosis it is approximately 6. The latter is corresponding to the pH of duodenal tract. Microbiologically the numbers of the so called mixed-acid forming coliforms and their neutral substances liberating relatives (*e.g., Klebsiella – Enterobacter* group) tend to constitute a dualistic balance in healthy intestines.

On the basis of their pH optima, the *Propionibacterium* sp. strains and their strictly anaerobic relatives situate mainly in the most distal areas of intestines. There they metabolize also the excessive lactate produced by other microflora during the course of the overall digestive process. This lactate would otherwise increasingly accumulate into the feces (lactate is the slowest absorbing small organic molecule in the gut). This leads to the enrichment of these strains close to the sigmoidic part of colon and the rectum. During defecation the intrarectal pressure extends the gut wall which is causing leakage and intrusion of microbes into the surrounding tissues. Anatomically these areas are in the proximity of the lower lumbar vertebrae and the pelvic joints. This could be a root cause behind the surprising finding of potential association of propionic acid bacteria with the lower back problems (Albert et al., 2013). The researchers have proposed that around 40% of the cases with lower back disorders could be caused by these bacteria. The mechanism for this particular disturbance could be further hypothetized, since lactate is the principle energy source for the neural tissues. Therefore, anaerobes such as the members of the genus *Propionibacterium* can cause deprivation and exhaustion of the adjacent energy sources of the neural cells leading into the development of chronic pain and other related symptoms. In fact, these anaerobes are also a group of harmful bacteria associated with postoperative infections and can cause damage to the axons.

It is also a lucrative possibility to think about the link between oxidative stress and carcinogenesis (Ahmad and Abdalla, 2012; Spitz et al., 2012) in this microbiological contest. The above-mentioned reductive effect on the neural tissues by the anaerobic bacteria could hence lead to a cancerous development. In our studies with lactobacilli and butyric acid bacteria in the PMEU, it was demonstrated that vigorous gas production could prevent the harmful strains from rooting into the intestines (Hakalehto and Hänninen, 2012). Similar phenomenon occurred in silage as a result of low oxygen generation (Borreani and Tabacco, 2008).

8. Hygienic Link and Health Aspects of the Intestinal Flora

Human body is one of the most obvious and richest source of potential contaminants in the clinical setting. Personal hygiene including proper toilet hygiene is therefore a key to prevent transmission, but it cannot guarantee microbiological safety alone. Different body fluids and secretions are continuously contaminating hospital milieu, and they provide niches for various microbes. There these strains survive and propagate within the microscale environments. Numerous bacteria and other microbes are breathed out or otherwise emitted into the air. Besides, there is the environmental responsibility of the clinical practices also existing, since at worst the hospitals are causing a source of infection to the visitors, and to the society around. Also the hospital waste waters need to be paid attention to in order to avoid dissemination of pathogenic strains or antibiotic resistance (Hakalehto, 2011b).

In case of 2,3-butanediol production by *Klebsiella* cultures, we have come to the conclusion that the pathways to this metabolic "platform" product are versatile, including some shunts of overflow metabolism in conditions, where the klebsiellas

- are under osmotic pressure caused by overmetabolism of glucose residues.
- have experienced rich growth conditions preceding this environmental stress phase.

The available carbon sources influence on the surface functions of the microbial cells (Chang et al., 2004). Circulation of immobilized and assimilated CO_2 and the initialization of storage hydrocarbon formation (*e.g.,* 3-β-hydroxybutyrate), as well as the emission of hydrogen contribute to the maintenance of pH, osmotic and redox balances in the intestinal milieu.

In their efforts to control the pH, redox and osmotic conditions in different parts of the intestines, many bacteria have established joint activities, such as the "dualistic balance" between acid-producing (*e.g., E. coli*) and neutral substances producing (*e.g., Klebsiella* sp.) enterobacterial species (Hakalehto et al., 2008) This balance is not easily shaken by the other microflora, and it includes the conversion of acetic acid into other substances, such as 2,3-butanediol (Hakalehto et al., 2010; Hakalehto, 2014), or its condensation with propionate into valeric acid. Ultimately the stream of protons into molecular hydrogen is compensating the pH drop.

Emitted hydrogen penetrates through the tissues, epithelia and skin. In the chyme, or in the stools, it alone is not necessarily forming detectable bubbling, but is mostly being exchanged between the phases by the above mentioned enzymatic reactions, and diffusion. As implied earlier, the effective pH areas of these enzymes is surprisingly low in many cases. It is likely to be reflecting the intracellular milieu, whose pH is lower than in the close proximity of the cells. Then the proton flow is necessary for undisturbed energy production. Lower pH limits of many dehydrogenases make it possible for them to effectively operate both in the intracellular and extracellular pH conditions *in vivo.* Since the hydrogen gas produced in high volumes in specific circumstances on the interfaces is a sign of niche formation by a multitude on bacteria, it is therefore of crucial importance for the microbes to keep this potential existent even though pH or other environmental parameters were unfavorable. Moreover, this postulation is compatible with the idea that in the "enhanced" ecosystem microbes do not compete out each other, but favor the metabolic versatility and cooperation. This is enabling a "metabolic field" to be formed (Hakalehto, 2012b). In this field of numerous simultaneous metabolic activities, different micro-organisms are selecting from various substrates as potential driving forces the ones being energetically feasible sources. Therefore, the direction of the reactions can even turn back, as a joint result of metabolic activities of multiple strains. The direction of the metabolism at any specific point cannot be precisely predicted, but accumulative information makes it possible to deduce and calculate those directions in a community of numerous microbial members. This kind of ecosystem thinking in healthcare could produce new practices for both diagnostics and treatments, as well as for clearing up the wards and maintaining adequate level of microbiological awareness.

Yoghurt is a product where billions of bacterial cells metabolize in the organic molecules in the food product. It is often a monoculture, and such an "ecosystem" is seldom normal in "natural" surroundings. In the intestines, as like in any sediment, or in sewage sludge, or even on hospital surfaces in the accumulating dirt, microbes constitute interactive metabolic networks. In these circumstances the traditional microbiological research on the pure cultures is not giving answers to the questions regarding more versatile reality in the microbial world. Accordingly, only if the laboratory surfaces were contaminated with a single strain, the PMEU curves on the bacterial growth were sigmoid ones (Hakalehto, 2010). However, more fruitful thinking is represented by a "microbiological or metabolic field theory", where the "field" is in constant change, and could be formed within a biofilm structure. The biofilm formation is illustrated in the Chapter 2 of this book.

Intestines are by far the biggest integrated and partially also inherited reservoir of microbes in our body system. The intestinal microflora strives for balance with our immune system. The foundation of this interaction is being laid in the early childhood (Walker, 2013). Therefore, permanent implementation of new strains into the basic flora is hardly possible. For the same reason, such treatments as fecal transplantation (Sha et al., 2014) can be effective in rebuilding the BIB (Bacteriological Intestinal Balance) (Hakalehto, 2011b, 2012a, 2013).

9. 'Hydrogen Economy' in the Body System

The "hydrogen space", or diffusion of the H_2 gas in our body system, is from its part determining such phenomena as tissue build up, removal of metabolic wastes, disease protection, ageing, etc. Anatomically, the abdomen is pressing the lungs as like the bellows when pressed in, and also pressurizing the internal and intestinal organs into their cavities or either side of the abdomen. This pressure, in turn, is straining the lower back, as well as the reproductive organs, which both have a crucial role in human existence. The postulated impacts of propionate formation on the spine were already discussed briefly earlier in this chapter. At the same time the hardening adipose tissues (as a result of the hydrogen flow) are making the joints and cartilages stiffer, which increases the health problems. Correspondingly, in order to protect the internal organs and the genetic material in there, adipose tissue is formed also downwards from the digestive tract. Paradoxically, the more unsaturated lipid molecules have been absorbed, the more the metabolic burden of their dehydrogenation is increasing. In fact, it is the antioxidant protection inside both the intestinal contents and in the body tissues and fluids, which safeguards our health. But essentially it is the saturation of the fatty acids, which is merely indicating metabolic turmoil than being a root cause of it.

In the light of healthy or unhealthy microbial living or microbial presence, it is of crucial importance, how well our body system can protect the adipose and lymphatic tissues from the detrimental microbial colonization. It makes a point to assume that if fat soluble antimicrobial agents could be produced, such substances could also make novel classes of antibiotic medicines capable of penetrating into the hydrophobic tissues in the body.

The hydrogen balance, i.e., the balance between dehydrogenating activities among the microflora and the counteracting hydrogenation and hydration on the other, is influencing the actual concentration of emitted hydrogen. It consequently penetrates the host tissues. The cavities of the body, as well as the lineups for the blood and lymphatic vessels, are leading the hydrogen flow toward topical tissues, and the brains, mainly in the upright position. Therefore, extensive hydrogen formation leads to tiredness, fatigue, depression, and other symptoms of mental malfunction and dysfunction. The active agents producing this hydrogen flow are the microbes in our digestive tract, especially in the colonic microflora.

Consequently, even though the large intestines are a big drainage of solid and liquid substances positioned as wastes by the body, it could well be possible that in adequate stool formation we may have a protective mechanism against excessive biologically produced hydrogen. In case of ruminants, such as cow, the microbial biomass is degraded in the parts of digestive system subsequent to the rumen, where anaerobic microflora is dominating. Further degradation of the feed and the microbes is binding hydrogen into the manure, which protects the animal from its adverse effects. In case of fasting, decreased microbiological activities in the gut eventually lower the hydrogen formation. However, this requires proper movements of the gut, prevention of excess acid formation, and adequate ventilation by such metabolic gases as carbon dioxide. Therefore, a healthy LAB (lactic acid bacteria) flora together with alkaline substances producing bacterial flora, such as klebsiellas, is balancing the intestinal milieu (Hakalehto, 2013; Hakalehto and Jaakkola, 2013).

The circulation and liberation of water in our body system and particularly in the digestive tract is coherent with the "hydrogen economy" of the gut. This integrated balance of hydrogenation and dehydrogenation, on the one hand, and between hydration and dehydration on the other is maintained by the enzymes, which are both of microbial and human origins. Since water is lost from the tissues by sweating and is subjected to regulation of different physiological, anatomical, hormonal or neurological factors, microbes have only a partial but remarkable impact on its circulation.

The large intestines are an active site in the human body system, where microbes take part in the circulation of water, as well as in defining the water balance of their host´s body. Both diarrhea and constipation are not normal conditions for the body system. When the colon is taking up water or relieving it into stools, its regulation system is inevitably linked with the joint metabolism of colonic bacteria *and* the microbes from upper intestines, from where the strains are arriving into the colon in the chyme flow. Hydrogen is bound into organic matter as water, and liberated as a proton flow, and eventually as gaseous hydrogen molecules. The protons are joined to each other, and with a stream of electrons on the border of liquid and gas phases, or even when moving out from microbes harboring food particles are led directly into the gas phase as molecular hydrogen. Many microbial dehydrogenases are active within a pH range which includes conditions both permissive and non-permissive for extensive population growth. This indicates that their role is associated also with the beneficial conditions for microbial cells in a resting state. In general, the proper functioning of the hydrogen flow, or "hydrogen economy" is important for both host and the microbiota. In these conditions carbon metabolism and liberation of carbon dioxide is decreased. This carbon is saved for "better times" by the microbes, whereas hydrogen is emitted for preventing the excessive lowering of the pH. This is essential for the gut microflora to stay active in the GI tract, where many acidic metabolites tend to lower the pH. Without balancing action this would cause metabolic stagnation detrimental also to the host.

10. Intestinal Ecosystem is a Column Contributing to Our Health

In the intestines, especially in the colon, there is the most abundant zone of *concentrated* microbial activity. The colon microflora is a consequence of:

- initial inoculation of the intestines in the childhood
- neurological, hormonal and immunological activity and control of the GI functions by the host

- host defense mechanisms (gastric acid, gut movement, bile substances, mucosal antibodies, defensins etc.)
- duodenal microflora as a “starter” for the food degradation process and microbial nutrient utilization in the chyme
- host neutralizing bicarbonates, and enzymes, acting on the food substances in the gut
- microbial interactions and metabolic activities in the small intestines along the small intestines as the chyme is traversing through this region where 80% our nutrients are absorbed (duration 6-7 hours)
- additional inoculum by the microflora reservoir of the cecal region

All these preceding factors contribute to the individual features of the colonic activities and to the development of the microbiota in it.

It could be hypothetized that in the upper small intestines of obese people there are more bacteria performing the 2,3-butanediol (butylene glycole) fermentation than in the corresponding part of the small bowel of more skinny individuals. Nevertheless, in all human digestive tracts, most 2,3-butanediol is moving into the cecumpartially non-metabolized. The bacterial species forming it are capable of binding acetate into the butanediol and thus neutralize their surroundings (Hakalehto, 2014). These strains also lower the osmotic pressure by converting glucose derived from food into 2,3-butanediol, ethanol and hydrogen. The ethanol is readily taken up as the most readily absorbed small organic molecule. Hydrogen formation is also relieving the metabolic restrictions which the microbes are facing in the form of sinking pH, which in turn is a consequence of the action of *e.g.,* the mixed acid fermenting enterobacteria, such as *E. coli*, butyric acid bacteria, acetic acid bacteria, and many other members of the intestinal flora.

In the course of the small intestines and in the cecum there are several metabolic cycles prevailing, such as the rapidly circulating carbon flow between the acetic acid, 2,3-butanediol, cell storage 3-β-polyhydroxybutyrate, and dissolved butyrate. In the pool of active microbes, and plentiful of metabolites, the butyrate is hypothetically reacting with any glucose molecule liberated from the macromolecules. This accelerated reaction of the bacterial metabolic sideways, via overflow metabolism, is thus resulting in the formation of 2,3-butanediol and ethanol, the latter of which is absorbed into the host body. Carbon dioxide is then emitted from this reaction, and it activates the butyric acid bacteria of the colon (Hakalehto and Hänninen, 2012). The storage polysaccharide, β-polyhydroxybutyrate from within the bacterial cells is triggering and possibly speeding up the 2,3-butanediol formation (Hakalehto et al., 2014).

Excess 2,3-butanediol derived from the upper parts of the digestive system is mostly formed together with acetic acid and ethanol, which then make the carbon circles moving on. The lactic acid formed by the LAB (lactic acid bacteria) is also incorporated into the 2,3-butanediol together with excess acetate in case of them not being absorbed by the host. The gradient of the lactic acid produced by LAB attached onto fibrous materials, such as probiotic flax, can partially explain the control (or attenuation) exercised by the LAB onto the rest of the gut microbiota (Hakalehto and Jaakkola, 2013). This gradient could provoke the metabolic mode of 2,3-butanediol formation to spread into the bacterial population, which accelerates the circles of overflow metabolism by the microbiota and nutrient absorption by the host provided that the glucose is not the limiting factor for bacterial growth.

In the large intestines the main functions of the rich microflora are associated with such activities (from the host point) as balancing the moisture content of the feces (and that of the body system), immunological regulation, production of some vitamins etc. (Ottman et al., 2012). In fact, one neglected major factor contributing to our general health is the production of emissible hydrogen (Hakalehto, 2014). This gas flow is penetrating into all tissues from the large intestines, and influences on the acidity of the whole body. In the upright position it is liberated and flowing towards the head which effects our brain and neural functions. On its way through various tissues and cavities of our body, hydrogen is influencing on the regulation of many important enzymes, such as hydrogenases. Inside the colon, hydrase enzymes contribute to the binding of new water molecules into the fecal biomass, into its organic molecules. These molecules, in turn, are still subjected to the fecal enzymatic activities of many microbes and also of the host.

As a matter of fact, the gaseous hydrogen penetrating the host tissues is also hydrogenating them. In case of fatty acids, for example, this leads to the breakage of double bonds, and to conversion of unsaturated fats into saturated ones. Such development is downgrading the elasticity of the body organs, such as blood and lymphatic vessels, epithelial membranes, neutral tissues etc. In other words: the continuous hydrogen flow originating largely from the colon microbial biomass is supposed to provoke the aging of our body. Therefore, an explanation to the mid-abdominal obesity could be the protection of the inner organs around the intestines from the effects of hydrogenation. Consequently, the more adipose tissue build up is taking place, the more the risk of microbial inversion into it is increasing. As long as the intracellular metabolic proton flow is producing more hydrogen as a result of the bacterial metabolism, the more unsaturated lipids are required for blocking or compensating its adverse health effects.

On the cellular level, water absorption is replacing the liberated hydrogen in fermentations. Consequently, the binding of water into organic compounds of the body and its microflora are essential factors of good health. Otherwise risks of cellular malfunctions, reading-frame mistakes, metabolic defects, and carcinogenesis will increase. This partially hypothetic consideration of the microflora functions could give us a new view into the onset of many chronic diseases, such as cancer, cardiovascular diseases, arthritis, as well as neural defects and pain. This preamble is underlining the importance of balanced gut microflora as a manifestation of good health. In our studies with the PMEU, it has been revealed that the carbon dioxide emitted as a product of metabolism is provoking microbial growth inside the gut (Hakalehto, 2011a, 2013; Hakalehto and Hänninen, 2012). The liberation of hydrogen by the microflora is having a still more direct impact on all human tissues.

11. Formation of Intestinal Microbial Communities and Some of Their Effects on the Host

Leakage of bacterial strains from their major colonic reservoir could be facilitated by some anatomical preconditions. For example, this is the case in diverticulosis that is commonly staged according to Hinchey classification (Hinchey et al., 1978):

- stage 1a phlegmon
- stage 1b diverticulitis with pericolic or mesenteric abscess
- stage 2 - diverticulitis with walled off pelvic abscess
- stage 3 - diverticulitis with generalized purulent peritonitis
- stage 4 - diverticulitis with generalized fecal peritonitis

These stages allow step-by-step worsening infections to develop as a consequence of the original confinement. Bacterial strains develop isolated communities where pathogenic development may occur and spread elsewhere in the body through ruptures in the epithelia. In normally structured parts of the intestines, however, penetration of bacterial strains can be facilitated by the so called leaky gut syndrome (Jaakkola and Hakalehto, 2012). More disruptive consequences are produced by ulcerative diseases as well as by different digestive hemorrhages and ulcersAll these host conditions offer an option for the microbial pathogens to invade into the body system. This causes inflammatory reactions of numerous kinds contributing to chronic inflammations such as seen in Crohn's disease and pseudomembranous colitis. The bacterial origin of these diseases has been anticipated. They could also be provoked by excessive use of *e.g.,* cephalosporins which could be explained by the selection of monotonous, harmful outgrowth of bacteria or even dysbiosis (Jaakkola and Hakalehto, 2012). From the microbiological standpoint we could further postulate on the invasion of mixed cultures into the underlying tissues behind the intestinal walls. Those epithelial walls are often covered by microbial biofilms (Bernstein et al., 2014). These biofilms have been shown to get structured within a relatively short course of time. We have micrographed this type of unspecified bacterial cultures in our laboratory (see Chapter 2). There the regulatory mechanisms determine the fate a single bacterial cell, whether it becomes a swarmer cell or a biofilm cell. They are controlled by overall cell metabolism. In this case, it is important to keep in mind that in such situations, the collective molecular regulation by extracellular signal molecules plays an essential role, *e.g.,* as in quarum sensing phenomena (Amara et al., 2009) or in the disassembly of biofilms (Oppenheimer-Shaanan et al., 2013).

Many intestinal functions relate to the gas pressures inside the GI tract. As indicated above it has been postulated that the growth of *Propionibacterium* sp. could be responsible for many severe lower back problems (Albert et al., 2013). This could be explained by the close proximity of the distal colon, and its increased pressure during defecation. Similar phenomena have been measured in the stomach. In the gastric areas, various blood gas pressures were determined, and charges were observed *e.g.,* during various medications (Parviainen et al., 1995; Parviainen, 1997). In the upper parts of the intestines, gas pressures, pH and redox characteristics of the gases emitted by the microbes are varying with respect to the eating habits, biorhythms etc.

In fact, there have been detected a relatively short-cycled oscillation of 1-2 hours in *Klebsiella aerogenes* cultures (Harrison and Pirt, 1967). We have detected similar kind of cycles in the expression and deprivation of fimbrial structures of *Salmonella* from waste water treatment plants (Hakalehto, unpublished results). Also shorter cycles of 2-5 min (oscillations with higher frequency) have been detected in the NADH fluorescense of a chemostat culture of *K. aerogenes* (Harrison, 1970). Continuing oscillations in well-regulated chemostat cultures are indicative of a more complex system and may occur through feedback interaction between cell metabolism and the environment or by the synchronization of oscillations based on entirely intracellular feedback mechanisms (Harrison, 1973). Similar rhythms occur also in human cells and tissues (Palmer, 1976). It could be postulated that in the intestines these microbial biorhythms are somewhat interrelated with the rhythms of the host body.

12. Bacterial Cell Attachment and Movements During Colonization

There are several interfaces which all have utmost importance the survival and activity of all intestinal micro-organisms. They inhabit the lipid molecule - water interfaces having hydrophobic surfaces in emulsions (Ellwood et al., 1982). These strains are important in the degradation and assimilation of lipids in the gastrointestinal tract (Zhao et al., 2005). For example, there is a sensitive balance between the supply and catabolism of the cholesterol (Dietschy et al., 1993). Excess cholesterol in the body is mainly converted to bile acids in the liver (Russell and Setchell, 1992). After the meals, gallbladder is secreting bile acids to duodenum through the *papilla vateri*. They are conjugated with taurine or glycine. In the duodenum they are converted to secondary and tertiary bile acids by intestinal bacteria. The bile acids emulsify the lipids in the intestines, thus forming the above-mentioned interfaces (Hylemon et al., 2009). They also act as signal molecules for the uptake of fat substances. Also the pathogens have sophisticated methods for facilitating their entry into the body system. For example, the MMTV virus uses lipopolysaccharides (LPS) from gut bacteria to avoid the human immune system (Pennis, 2011).

13. Protective Microbiome and its Manipulation of Environmental Conditions and Energy Metabolism

Besides the above-mentioned conditions, many biological regulators contribute and modulate microbial metabolism and the behavior of the strains. For example, molecules produced by other microbes may stimulate or make pace of the growth of a particular strain.

Alternatively, many microbes produce antibiotic substances which could slow down, hinder or prevent the growth of the other strains. This formation of different organic acids, if excessive, could influence remarkably also on the metabolism of the acid-producing microbes themselves. For example, *E. coli* belongs to the mixed-acid fermenting bacteria. It secretes significant amounts of *e.g.,* formic and acetic acids. Simultaneously, a drop in the pH results from its own activities and can cause self-limitation. In the duodenum there has been revealed to exist an intriguing mechanism regulating the pH levels (Hakalehto et al., 2008). Besides *E. coli* and other mixed-acid fermenters in these areas there occur strains of the *Klebsiella / Enterobacter* group, which perform *e.g.,* 2,3 –butanediol fermentation. In this metabolic pattern, 2,3 –butanediol, ethanol, CO_2 and H_2 are formed besides some acidic compounds (Mitzscherling, 2009). The production of the neutral substances, such as 2,3 –butanediol and ethanol slow down the pH drop. This activity of the biochemical pathways is fast, and is counteracting the acid production of some other species. Meanwhile, the gaseous H_2 "leaks away" the protons, which would otherwise cause the decrease in the pH. In the experiments with *Klebsiella mobilis* we have detected that the CO_2 is in some cases produced less, if the production of the neutral substances is increasing (Hakalehto et al., 2014). This observations implies to the existence of another metabolic route for the production of 2,3 –butanediol besides the sideline reaction of the anabolic production of the amino acid valine (Blomqvist et al., 1993). The idea is supported *e.g.,* by the finding that the 2,3 –butanediol is produced in large amounts without concomitant cell growth, which could be explained by a form of previously unknown overflow metabolism (Hakalehto et al., 2014).

It could be deduced, in anyway, that the H_2 production is keeping up the gradient of protons across the cell membranes, which is crucial for all bacteria for their energy metabolism. The power house of the cells, the proton pump, is functioning in connection with the membranes, and is also most likely the foundation of most electrochemical phenomena within the cells (Smirnov et al., 2011).

In order to preserve this option the klebsiellas and their kind of facultative bacteria are carrying out an important task not only for themselves, but for the entire intestinal microbial community, by preventing the pH from sinking down.

In the particular symbiotic relation between the mixed-acid fermenters, such as *E. coli*, and the 2,3 –butanediol producing species, such as *Klebsiella mobilis* (known earlier as *Enterobacter aerogenes* or *Aerobacter aerogenes*) grow in mixed cultures equally well than in the separate pure cultures (Hakalehto et al., 2008).

This finding has been repeatedly documented, and the symbiotic relationship between these facultative bacteria is:

- promoting the energy metabolism of the entire microbial population
- regulating the duodenal pH (at around 6), and
- keeping the mixed-acid fermenters and the 2,3 –butanediol producers in a dualistic balance, which well could be the foundation of the BIB (Bacterial Intestinal Balance).

In further studies with the PMEU (Portable Microbe Enrichment Unit) we have documented that the newcoming strains of *Staphylococcus aureus* and/or *Bacillus cereus* do not interrupt the balance between *E. coli* and *K. mobilis* (Hakalehto et al., 2010). The facultative bacteria were also relatively indifferent to the effects of oxgall (a bile substance) or vancomycin. Interestingly, these coliformic bacteria, together with enterococci, are the most commonly used bacterial hygienic indicators (Hakalehto et al., 2011a, Heitto et al., 2012, Hakalehto et al. 2013). These species are also the most resistant ones toward the antimicrobial action of the bile substances (Hakalehto et al., 2010). Therefore, they survive the best in the duodenum, being one of the most abundant bacterial group in the fecal samples, and the intestinal areas. The production of the 2,3 –butanediol by the klebsiellas has shown to be activated by the acetic acid (Hakalehto et al., 2008). Therefore, the symbiosis with *E. coli* is strengthened also by this signal effect. The activity of the *Klebsiella* / *Enterobacter* group is likely to take place especially in nutritional situations where excessive sugar or starch is suddenly appearing. In these circumstances, the 2,3-butanediol producers have been shown to increase dramatically their corresponding metabolic activities without simultaneous population growth (Hakalehto et al., 2008; Hakalehto, 2011b; Hakalehto et al. 2014). This function is protecting the bacterial population against the pH drop and from the destructive osmotic pressures. The proposed mechanism of the Gram-negative bacteria in question includes some periplasmic enzymes. The ethanol is instantaneously consumed by the human body, and its rigorous uptake prevents the accumulation inside the gut. Thus the ethanol inhibition, which could otherwise restrict the normal flora is avoided. Shaken microbial balance in the gut may lead to hazardous situations, such as candidiasis, which occasionally could lead to dysbiosis (Xuan et al., 2014).

Also the gaseous compounds may transmit information among bacterial populations. *E. coli* cultures have been shown to get stimulated, and have a shortened lag phase, or earlier onset of growth, by the production of CO_2 by the microbes themselves (Hakalehto, 2011b). This stimulation or signaling effect has been documented also in the case of interspecies association between lactobacilli and butyric acid bacteria (Hakalehto and Hänninen, 2012). This kind of bacterial coculture is found also in the silage, where getting the optimal preserving result requires that the butyric acid levels remain low enough. In the intestines the stimulation and activation of the clostridia could serve as a preventive factor for their spore formation, or attachment, and thus indirectly prevent the colonization of the intestinal walls by these potentially health compromising, putrefacient bacteria. The anaerobic clostridia and especially the butyric acid producing ones, nevertheless, grow extensively in the cecum, the proximal part of the human large intestines. There they have been found more numerous in obese individuals (Vrieze et al., 2010). This could imply to a mechanism which is taking into use the 2,3-butanediol, which otherwise is relatively slowly consumed by the bacterial communities. In soil, for example, the 2,3 –butanediol is degraded into simple organic compounds, such as acetic acid and ethanol (Han et al., 2011). The site for its assimilation in the gut areas could well be the colon, where clostridia are carrying out this task. However, for the benefit of the human body and its entire microbiota, it is more beneficial that the clostridia do not conquer too much space. This kind of undesired situation is occurring in the case of *Clostridium difficile* colonizing the intestinal tract after heavy antibiotic medications (Coakley et al., 2011). Such infections could be life-threatening, and it is of utmost importance to monitor *C. difficile* most carefully (Hell et al., 2010).

The cells energize their membranes by the electron flow across the lipid bilayer. Therefore, the membrane potential plays an important role in bacterial energy metabolism. The electric flow across the cell surface is recharging the phosphorylated energy reserves as the ATP (adenoside triphosphate) (Malakooti et al., 2011).

In broader sense, these electron transport chains through the bacterial cell walls are the powerhouses of the cells. Their functioning is entirely dependent on the gradients formed across the cell membranes. Therefore, the diffusion rates of nutrients and waste substances in close proximity of the cells have enormous impacts on the cell metabolism. It has been generally believed that the anaerobic bacterial metabolism would be much less effective than the aerobic one (Hentges, 1996). This has been explained *e.g.,* by the mobilization of the citric acid cycle (Krebs cycle) enzymes in the latter one. However, in the experiments with the PMEU cultivator and detector unit, it has been documented that the anaerobic metabolic activity of *e.g.,* some facultative bacteria is at the same level as it is in the aerobic growth mode (Hakalehto et al., 2007; Hakalehto, 2011a).

Three different modes of bacterial metabolism can be distinguished:

- Catabolism
- Anabolism
- Overflow metabolism

The overflow metamolism is important for the survival of strains in some extreme conditions. We have documented that without any population growth the facultative klebsiellas can carry out rapid pH shifts (Hakalehto et al., 2008). It is not likely that these extensive reactions where remarkable amount of 2,3-butanediol is produced could occur as a branch of a biosynthetic pathway only as it is generally suggested (Rao et al., 2012).

In the experiments with PMEU we have also documented that these reactions, which rapidly consume the glucose from the medium, did not combine with either population growth or increases in gas production (Hakalehto et al., 2014). In fact, the volatiles emission was diminished regardless of the increased production of 2,3-butanediol. Therefore we suggest that with some Gram-negative facultatively anaerobic bacteria there could exist a previously unknown route for the overflow metabolism. This rapid mechanism would protect the bacterial cells from high osmotic pressures caused by elevated sugar concentrations, and also from the lowering of the pH in their microenvironment.

14. Microbial Coverage of the Epithelial Surfaces and Various Niches Inside the Alimentary Tract

Bacterial surface structures are essential part of their movement and attachment (Hakalehto, 2000). See also the Chapter 2. The eubacterial flagellin and fimbrin molecules are synthesized in ribosomes adjacent to the cell membranes. They are transported out of their site of action by different mechanisms. Bacterial flagellins (the actual structural proteins of the flagellar filaments) are transported within the tubular filament as linear molecules (see also Figure 1 in Chapter 2). The type-1 fimbriae have been shown to act in the formation of bacterial layers onto surfaces. They are not expressed at 20 °C but are readily produced at 37 °C by salmonellas. These pathogens are capable of building up the fimbrial structures during a short period of time for attachment purposes. The N-terminal sequences of all eubacterial flagellins resemble very closely each other, which also is indicating their important roles in cell movements, as well as in relocation and adsorption (Hakalehto et al., 1997). The fimbriae, on the other hand, are shorter filaments which facilitate the attachment onto the mucosal membranes and then can also get deprived from the cells for liberating them from the surfaces. This mechanism is helping the pathogens (and also other bacteria) to colonize the intestines rapidly. What is then the ecological consequence of this phenomenon?

Type 1 fimbriae are used for attachment by many bacterial strains (Baek et al., 2011). It was shown that the cells rapidly loose these protrudements, if these are not needed in the culture (Hakalehto et al., 2000). *Salmonella* species seem to express the structures more readily in the presence of oxygen than in complete anaerobiosis (Hakalehto et al., 2007). This is a sign of the importance of oxidative conditions for the facultative bacteria. These bacteria form a big part of the intestinal flora especially in the upper alimentary regions in some cases.

It could be possible that their functions are somewhat controlled by the blood circulation in the intestinal epithelia. The blood is transporting oxygen into the minor veins in the areas where the nutrients are taken up. Such pathogens as salmonellas search for these niches in order to root into the alimentary tract. In case of the intrusion of fimbriated bacteria, these organelles act as like anchors onto the gut walls, in order to facilitate colony formation in different areas.

Microbes are living things being incredibly fast in their use of the preferred nutrients. According to the PMEU studies and simulations, the intestinal bacteria seem to collaborate with each other for the optimal use of available nutrients (Hakalehto et al., 2008, Hakalehto et al., 2010, Hakalehto et al., 2011b). This balance between different bacterial strains found in the PMEU experiments is somewhat antagonistic piece of evidence to the "nutrient-niche hypothesis", according to which every microbial strain has its own niche in the intestines determined by its abilities to exploit carbon sources, or simple sugars (Freter and Jones, 1983). From the PMEU results we can see that different bacterial strains tend to build up a kind of balance where the metabolic end-products of one strain could be instantaneously consumed by another strain thus fading the boundaries between niches (Hakalehto et al., 2010). For instance, *E. coli* and klebsiellas are able to cooperate when living together in the small bowel. In the PMEU they produce equal concentrations of cells with the concentrations produced by each strain in pure cultures (Hakalehto et al., 2008). They also regulate the duodenal pH for the benefit of the host, and thus maintain the balance of the local microflora and perhaps also that of the microbiota of the rest of the intestines to some extent.

15. Role of Bacterial Surface Structures in Establishment of Ecosystems and in Host-Microbe Interactions

In order to understand the bacterial behavior in the alimentary tract we need to pay further attention to their extracellular organelles and outer surfaces. These structures mediate the contacts between the bacterial cells, and between them and the surfaces. Also the contacts with human cells, tissues and organelles take place with the aid of these molecular matrices or structures of our prokaryotic microflora. Some 5-10% of protein molecules can be of flagellar origin (Macnab and Castle, 1987). The N-terminal sequences of the eubacterial flagellar filament proteins are rather similar from species to species (Hakalehto et al., 1997). This part of the molecule is in dissolved form when produced inside the cells, on the inner side of the membranes. Then the steric structures direct it toward the growing filament from the ribosomes attached to the membrane, and further into the tube-like growing filament. These filaments can be expressed in a few seconds of time. They can also disappear in a short while. This could occur *e.g.,* when the acidic conditions in the stomach remove them from the cell surfaces, or when the bacterial cell has deliberately cut them off. The detachment may also be a result of need for quick detachment due to exhausting resources in the case of fimbriae (Hakalehto et al., 2010), or alternatively due to flagellar or fimbrial phase variation intended for camouflaging the bacterial cells against the host immune system (Rhen et al., 1983). If present, the flagellae are actively moving the bacterial cells toward beneficial niches and conditions. Their contribution to the orientation of the cells, and to their relocation in the GI tract is of utmost importance for the bacterial search of optimal nutritional conditions, for instance. Fimbrial structures, and other molecular tools for attachment such as adhesins, are responsible for the rapid adsorption of many bacteria onto the epithelial surfaces. As like flagellins, also fimbrial structures are synthesized within an extremely short period of time, in a few seconds (Farfan et al., 2011). The fimbriated bacteria are able to detach these fibrils at once. For example, the salmonellas express type 1 fimbriae during the exponential growth phase, and later give them up as the population density on the surface is increasing, and the resources are being exhausted (Hakalehto et al., 2000). This mechanism enables the rapid bacterial colonization of the small intestines together with the enhanced anaerobic metabolism of the facultatives (Hakalehto et al., 2007). If the space or nutrients are deprived from the bacterial cells, they leave the fimbriae behind, and possibly consume them as raw material for their own novel biosynthesis. The cells are then also liberated from their previous location, and free to move into new sites on the gut walls. In order to avoid host immune defences they may carry out flagellar or fimbrial phase variation (Chen et al., 2010; Morowitz et al., 2011). In practice this means that the same strain is expressing an altering flagellin or fimbrin epitopes in order to mislead the immune system. The production of fimbrial subunits could count for 95% of the intracellular protein precursors at the time point of 1.5 hours in *E. coli* cultures (Abraham and Beachey, 1987).

Besides the antibodies against the above-mentioned surface organelles or their subunits, the host body is producing different types of antibodies against capsular polysaccharides (K antigens), or the O-specific side chains of the lipopolysaccharides (O antigens) (Hood et al., 2004). The so called H antigens are the flagellar antigens. Some structures on the cell surfaces are universally present on the surfaces of a certain group of bacteria, such as the enterobacterial common antigen (ECA) (Gilbreath et al., 2011).

When the expression of antigens against type 1 fimbriae was studied in the case of *Salmonella* sp. it was observed that these immunological reactions were stronger and prevailed for a longer period of time in aerobiosis (Hakalehto et al., 2007). This finding could indicate the preferencies among salmonellas toward aerobic conditions also *in vivo*. They could get oxygen rich blood available when penetrating across the one host cell deep surface of the small bowel epithelium. Therefore, the stronger expression of fimbriae in the presence of oxygen in cultures with equal growth rates aerobically and anaerobically, could imply to active search for aerobic conditions by the facultatively anaerobic, pathogenic salmonellas. In turn, this preference is probably making the salmonellas basically unfit to the intestinal microbial community. This very characteristic is possibly also making them causative agents of contagious intestinal diseases.

16. Bacterial Interference Caused by Intrusions from the Alimentary Tract

As a general rule we could assume that the micro-organisms would prefer staying in the alimentary tract as an integral part of this complex ecosystem. They also form symbiotic relationships between different strains and with the host. Any singular bacterial or other microbial strain that breaks this rule could become a true pathogen. Consequently, it is escaping the regulation from both the host body and the other microbial strains, and that of the entire microbial community.

In many cases, due to some neurological, hormonal or nutritional malfunction, some strain or strains make the balance (BIB; Bacterial Intestinal Balance) to collapse (Hakalehto, 2012a).

This situation is both detrimental to the host and offensive against the regular members of the microflora. If the newcoming intruders, or "trouble-makers" within the normal flora contain several members, the situation could develop into a mixed infection. In this case the microflora may seek for a new balance which, however, is less beneficial to the host. This could lead to a "pathological state of balanced flora". The interactions between commencal organisms, opportunistic pathogens, and disease causing microbes could be studied in the PMEU device by simulating the cocultures in the intestines (Hakalehto et al., 2010). Some invasive pathogens, such as salmonellas, start penetrating the intestinal membranes (Hakalehto et al., 2007).

The molecular mechanisms of this attack, as well as the host defense option, are surveyed earlier in this chapter. However, for the balanced and healthy function of a human body, it would be important to maintain or revert the BIB rather than to try to repair the damage only. This means that the body has to struggle against any invading strain which rapidly disturbs the balance, converting it towards less a supportive, or stabilized, situation.

In order to permanently eradicate the pathogens, often strong antibiotic medications are required. In the clinical practices it is of utmost importance to stabilize the body with infusion therapy in order to help the body system to sustain the infection, and to develop improved immunological responses.

Some methods, such as novel probiotics, or passive immunization as well as antioxidant therapy, could be attempted for returning the BIB, which is the best option for getting rid of the pathogenic function. In fact, it is often possible that the once pathogenic strain has "escaped" the control of the human host body as well as the microbial community. Consequently, the re-establishment of the balance could return the opportunistically pathogenic strain into commensal status, For example, the species *Klebsiella pneumoniae* is found in the intestines of many individual where it is a common part of the ecosystem. However, in some undesired circumstances the same bacterium could find its way to the respiratory tract and occur as a pathogen there (Parm et al., 2011).

17. Intracellular Pathogens

One of the most severe forms of pathogenecity is the intracellular pathogenesis. Such pathogenic species as *Chlamydia* sp., *Borrelia burgdorferi*, *Treponema pallidum*, some yersinias and salmonellas could penetrate through human cell membranes and cause serious infections, which could also include latent periods (Guttman et al., 2006). These diseases are difficult to get diagnosed, and their treatments are often very complicated. For example, the *B. burgdorferi* IgAG antibodies could be detected from human serum with such rapid molecular methods as dot blot, MarDx, and VIDAS enzyme immunoassays (Jespersen et al., 2002). The two former methods were found to require a Western Blot confirmation due to their low specificities. One big challenge in researching this type of pathogens which penetrate the cells, is the sampling threshold. When can we be sure of having a reliable amount or type of specimen material, without the risk of the pathogens continuously hiding inside the human cells?

Since many bacteria are able to colonize the host cell intracellularly, there is a need for a mechanism of autophagy for the degradation and removal of these intruding pathogens such as *Staphylococcus aureus*, for example (Amano et al., 2006). Such intestinal microbes as *Escherichia coli* and *Candida albicans* and *Streptococcus pneumoniae* influence the complement cascade depriving its full activity (Zipfel et al., 2007). Regardless of the multitude of mechanisms which are exploited by the host, and by the microbial strains to control each other, the decisive studies on the microbial behavior in the alimentary ecosystem remain to be elucidated. Since it is extremely tedious to monitor the events inside the gut, effective means are required for the simulations of these effects *in vitro*. The PMEU method has been developed in order to facilitate the evaluation of the relations between micro-organisms, as well as to study their reactions to various host parameters (Hakalehto, 2006, 2010, 2011a).

Besides the commonly known intracellular pathogens, it has been suggested that intracellular forms may explain such phenomena as persistence of pathogenic *E.coli* infections against antibiotic treatments (Kerrn et al., 2005). It seems possible that some organisms may penetrate the epithelium and remain in there during antibiotic treatments. In these cases, flushing the pathogens out of the epithelium with some intracellular cAMP (cyclic adenosine monophosphate) increasing drugs could be a useful strategy in the cure of disease (Bishop et al., 2007). The cAMP is an important mediator in the regulation of the intracellular effects of several hormones. It is also evident that for proper functions of gastrointestinal tract or the urinary tract it is of utmost importance to keep the intracellular bacterial strains or viruses out of the cell interior. Therefore, it can be deduced that in the development of microflora it is essential to find microbial ecosystems which would be capable of overgrowing any of these intruding strains. Also, the innate immunity is needed for maintaining such a flora, and for supporting it.

The mechanisms of severe infections often include taking over of the host body, or directing its actions. For example, the borrelias as like some other serious pathogens, such as HIV virus and tuberculosis bacteria (*Mycobacterium tuberculosis*) are blocking the vitamin D receptors (Khoo et al., 2011; Spector, 2011). These, in turn, would be key factors in building up the innate immunity, which is the first line defense against infections. This is due to the central role of vitamin D in this immunity (Gleisner et al., 2011). Moreover, the same receptors function also as receptors for lipocacheic acid which is one of the important bile acids (Steiner et al., 2011). By preventing the binding of the vitamin D and the bile salt the pathogen is regenerating the defenses both immunologically, and by weakening the fatty acid dissimilation, which in turn is damaging the cell membranes.

Many bacteria, such as *Escherichia coli* and *Bacteroides* sp. in the large intestine, can synthesize vitamin K_2 (menaquinone-7), but not vitamin K_1 (phylloquinone) (Vermeer and Braam, 2001). In these bacteria, menaquinone will receive two electrons from small molecules, such as lactate, formate, or NADH, in a process called anaerobic respiration (Jones et al., 2011). The menaquinone, with the help of another enzyme, will in turn in another enzymatic reaction transfer these electrons to an oxidant, such as fumarate or nitrate. Adding two electrons to fumarate or nitrate will convert the molecules to succinate or nitrite + water, respectively. These reactions resemble the generation of cellular energy by eukaryotic cell in aerobic respiration, except that the final electron acceptor is not molecular oxygen, but fumarate or nitrate, for example. Thus the vitamin K2 synthesis offers some intestinal bacteria means for carrying out oxidative respiration in the anaerobiosis. This provides them with more options in their energy metabolism.

In the host body, the lack of vitamin K2 produced by bacteria may cause the blocking of the coronary arteries. Therefore, calcium and vitamin D supplementation needs to be completed with an adequate vitamin K2 supply. Vitamin K2 activates osteocalcin hormone, produced by osteoblasts, which is needed to bind calcium into the bones. If this activation is inadequate, the calcium may end up into the arteries. The vitamin K2 also improves the bone health in our body. This example is an indication of the continuous interdependence between man and the microbiome.

18. We Are Linked with Our Environment via the Microbiome

In microbiological metabolism different end-products are formed. They are in turn regulating their own production and inside the microbial ecosystems there is a complex network of different regulatory events occurring. Very often the microbes are combining their metabolic action into a co-metabolic mode of action (Dalton and Stirling, 1982). The products of the microbial metabolism can be liquid substances, dissolved in solutions, or they can be emitted as volatile compounds, or sometimes they might precipitate. Besides their internal metabolic capabilities, microbes often produce also extracellular enzymes which take part in specific reactions outside the cell compartment. In case of Gram-negative bacteria, some of these enzymes are remaining in the periplasmic space which is situating in between the cell membrane and the Gram-negative outer membrane. This periplasmic space is the site of several metabolic activities, as further described in Chapter 2.

The metabolic products of different micro-organisms could be measured with several sophisticated methods such as mass-spectrometry or NMR (Nucleic Magnetic Resonance). PMEU Scentrion® device has several sensors for detecting the volatile organic compounds on the basis of the changes in the electric resistance on the probes. According to the results or signals from different sensors the origin and qualifications of the microbes in the sample can be deduced (Hakalehto et al., 2008; Hakalehto et al., 2009).

All essential elements in Nature are taking part in the circulation which is activated and performed by the environmental microbes (Hakalehto, 2014). In the biosphere the nitrogen compounds are present in all forms of life. In the plants the symbiotic bacteria of the root nodules, for example, can effectively fix the atmospheric nitrogen which is then utilized also by the plant. This kind of symbiotic association is less studied in case of animals. Also many intestinal bacteria such as *Klebsiella* sp. are known for their ability to fix atmospheric nitrogen. Besides the nitrogen as such, also many other simple inorganic nitrogen compounds are utilized and circulated by various groups of microbes (Moat and Foster, 1988).

In soil and elsewhere in natural ecosystems the nitrites are converted to ammonia which is then the starting point for organic nitrogen compounds. And the denitrification process is making nitric oxide out of nitrites and nitrification produces the nitrates. The nitric oxides are liberated as gased, whereas the nitrites can be reversibly converted back to nitrite (Mortenson,

1962). And there is a continued flow of nitrogen between all these different forms of simple compounds. In the conversion of nitrite into ammonia, six electrons are bound into the nitrogen backbones of organic compounds as reductive (or antioxidant).

Many intestinal bacteria are actively taking part in the nitrogen cycles which is also connected with the human nutrition. In fact, the revolved diet of an individual is determining largely the basic type of the intestinal microbiota. In a recent comprehensive study different intestinal communities were compared worldwide. It was found out that basically three types were occurring (Wu et al., 2011). According to this study three predominant basic types of intestinal microflora could be recognized. It was also found out that even though different individuals can have different composition of the microflora, distribution of metabolic activities between the various microbes can be arranged in similar fashion within every metabolic main type, and in the intestines of each individuals. This means that the microbial communities have to perform a task which is essentially important also for the human body system. It can be also deduced that on this basis our body is also directing the conditions in the intestines into the positive direction for the bacterial community. This is establishing the universal baseline for the existence of human gastrointestinal microbiota. From this point of view the individual bacteriological intestinal balance (BIB) can be estimated (Hakalehto, 2012a).

Oxidative stress is a challenge for our body system, and a damaged immune system makes us vulnerable to microbial attacks. Glucose depletion causes cytotoxicity and oxidative stress in many kinds of cell types. Transformed or malignant cells have appeared to be more susceptible to glucose deprivation-induced cytotoxicity and oxidative stress than normal cells (Ahmad and Abdalla, 2012). When transformed cells seem to exhibit defective oxidative metabolism this phenomenon could possibly be used in the treatment of malignancies. This, in turn, is giving us an option to deliberately “treat” the microbiome into a direction, which could be favorable for the host. This chain of thinking inevitably leads to the applications in the personalized medicine using probiotics in an increasingly focused manner for the protection of the general health.

However, various environmental stresses, and chemical toxication, may alter the relationship between man and his microflora. Impaired functions of human neutrophils has been associated with some types of colitis (Uzel et al., 2001).

It has been also reported that superantigens derived from such lumen-associated intestinal bacteria as enterotoxigenic *Staphylococcus aureus* or nitrogenic *Yersinia pseudotuberculosis* could elicit a local inflammation and aggregate enteric inflammatory disorders (Lu et al., 2003). Thus the above-mentioned superantigenic effects were not the primary cause of the disease, but evoked an inflammatory response and exaggregated the disease of the experimental animals. It has also been documented that enterotoxin-producing staphylococci cause intestinal inflammation, which is a combined result from epithelial cytopathy and superantigen-mediated T-cell activation (Edwards et al., 2012). In our studies we investigated a patient who had, besides severe intestinal and digestive problems, also an intrusion of *Staphylococcus haemolyticus* strains in his peritoneum. This implies to the leakage of the bacterial strains from the intestines. This patient also had a gastritis and dysbiotic bacterial and yeast growth in his duodenum, as verified by endoscopy. The duodenal pH was exceptionally low (between 1 and 2).

Globalization, including changes in human nutrition, increased use of medicines, worldwide trade and tourism, together with pollution and overcrowding in many areas, has contributed to altered patterns of bacterial diseases (Hakalehto, 2014).

Mixed infections with novel symptoms, emerging infections and increasing prevalence of antibiotic resistant strains have caused new problems and challenges to our immune system and other defenses. Here the case of the above-mentioned teenaged patient is briefly described. He had a life-threatening staphylococcal infection caused by *Staphylococcus haemolyticus* and *S. aureus* strains, which made possible the collapse of the nutrient uptake functions and the immunoprotection of the patient's body system. These were probably originally caused by some chemical intoxication. Recovery from the tissues destroying bacterial inflammation and enzymatic activity was achieved by long-lasting doxycycline medication. This prevented the staphylococcal hemolytic, proteolytic and lipolytic enzymes from utilizing the nutrients and from destroying the patient's tissues. In a somewhat similar case another patient, this time a 30 year old young mother with collapsed health after delivery, was having bacterial strains which crossreacted with the antibodies of the teenager patient (results not shown here).

Both of these geographically remote patients obviously suffered from a commensal bacterial outgrowth, which was not under the control of the deteriorated defensive mechanisms of the body system. The first patient also exhibited signs of pancreatitis. This type of symptoms combined abrupt malnutrition with cachexia and immunodeficiency, being curable with tetracyclines or other antibiotics, could possibly be a sign of novel type of modern-age bacterial illnesses?

Conclusion

Our alimentary tract includes a food processing system for digesting and absorbing catabolic chemical energy and organic building blocks for anabolic building up of our body system. These metabolic objectives of the human host are connected with the microbial metabolism in the gut. The outcome of this joint activity is influencing our health to a large extent. We need more studies on the host-microbe interactions, as well as on the interactions between different microbes in order to understand the total picture of the digestive functions. In any case, the GI tract is consisting of several different environments for the microbes. Since the food (or chyme) is in constant movement, the microflora is acting and developing in successions along this movement. Therefore, it is the entire alimentary microflora that deserves and needs to be studied, not only the colonic one.

References

Abraham, S. N., Beachey, E. H. Assembly of a chemically synthesized peptide of *Escherichia coli* type 1 fimbriae into fimbria-like antigenic structures. *J. Bacteriol,,* 1987; 169, 2460-2465.

Ahiwale, S. S., Bankar, A. V., Tagunde, S. N., Zinjarde, S., Ackermann, H. W., Kapadnis, B. P. Isolation and characterization of a rare waterborne lytic phage of *Salmonella enterica* serovar Paratyphi B. *Can. J. Microbiol.*, 2013; 59, 318-323.

Ahmad, I. M., Abdalla, M. Y. Mitochondria-mediated oxidative stress and cancer therapy. In: Spitz, D. R., Dornfeld, K. J., Krishnan, K., Guis, D., editors. *Oxidative Stress in Cancer Biology and Therapy.* New York, USA: Springer Science+Business Media; 2012, pp. 3-20.

Albert, H. B., Lambert, P., Rollason, J., Sorensen, J. S., Worthington, T., Pedersen, M. B., Nørgaard, H. S., Vernallis, A., Busch, F., Manniche, C., Elliott, T. Does nuclear tissue infected with bacteria following disc herniations lead to Modic changes in the adjacent vertebrae? Eur. Spine J., 2013; 22, 690-696.

Aliberti, S., Kaye, K. S. The changing microbiologic epidemiology of community-acquired pneumonia. *Postgrad. Med.,* 2013; 125, 31-42.Amano, A., Nakagawa, I., Yoshimori, T. Autophagy in innate immunity against intracellular bacteria. *J. Biochem.*, 2006; 140, 161-166.

Amara, N., Mashiach, R., Amar, D., Krief, P., Spieser, S. A., Bottomley, M. J., Aharoni, A., Meijler, M. M. Covalent inhibition of bacterial quorum sensing. *J. Am. Chem. Soc.,* 2009; 131, 10610-10619.

Baek, C. H., Kang, H. Y., Roland, K. L., Curtiss, R., 3rd. Lrp acts as both a positive and negative regulator for type 1 fimbriae production in *Salmonella enterica* serovar Typhimurium. *PLoS One,* 2011; 6, e26896.

Balter, M. Taking stock of the human microbiome and disease. *Science*, 2012; 336, 1246-1247.

Baxt, L. A., Garza-Mayers, A. C., Goldberg, M. B. Bacterial subversion of host innate immune pathways. *Science,* 2013; 340, 697-701.

Bennet, R., Nord, C. E. Development of the faecal anaerobic microflora after caesarean section and treatment with antibiotics in newborn infants. *Infection,* 1987; 15, 332-336.

Benno, Y., Sawada, K., Mitsuoka, T. The intestinal microflora of infants: composition of fecal flora in breast-fed and bottle-fed infants. *Microbiol. Immunol.,* 1984; 28, 975-986.

Berg, R. D. The indigenous gastrointestinal microflora. *Trends Microbiol.,* 1996; 4, 430-435.

Bernstein, R., Freger, V., Lee, J. H., Kim, Y. G., Lee, J., Herzberg, M. 'Should I stay or should I go?' Bacterial attachment vs biofilm formation on surface-modified membranes. Biofouling, 2014; 30, 367-376.

Bishop, B. L., Duncan, M. J., Song, J., Li, G., Zaas, D., Abraham, S. N. Cyclic AMP-regulated exocytosis of *Escherichia coli* from infected bladder epithelial cells. *Nat. Med.,* 2007; 13, 625-630.

Blomqvist, K., Nikkola, M., Lehtovaara, P., Suihko, M. L., Airaksinen, U., Stråby, K. B., Knowles, J. K., Penttilä, M. E. Characterization of the genes of the 2,3-butanediol operons from *Klebsiella terrigena* and *Enterobacter aerogenes*. *J. Bacteriol.,* 1993; 175, 1392-1404.

Bonheur, J. L., Arya, M., Tamer, M. A. Bacterial gastroenteritis. *Medscape Reference*, 2014.

Borreani, G., Tabacco, E. Low permeability to oxygen of a new barrier film prevents butyric acid bacteria spore formation in farm corn silage. *J. Dairy Sci.,* 2008; 91, 4272-4281.

Bradley, J. S., Nizet, V. Staphylococcal infections. In: Remington, J. S., Klein, J. O., Wilson, C. O., Nizet, V., Malconado, Y. A., editors. *Infectious Diseases of the Fetus and Newborn Infant*. Philadelphia, PA, USA: Saunders, Elsevier Inc.; 2011.

Chang, D.-E., Smalley, D. J., Tucker, D. L., Leatham, M. P., Norris, W. E., Stevenson, S. J., Anderson, A. B., Grissom, J. E., Laux, D. C., Cohen, P. S., Conway, T. Carbon nutrition of *Escherichia coli* in the mouse intestine. *PNAS*, 2004; 101, 7427-7432.

Chen, Q., Decker, K. B., Boucher, P. E., Hinton, D., Stibitz, S. Novel architectural features of *Bordetella pertussis* fimbrial subunit promoters and their activation by the global virulence regulator BvgA. *Mol. Microbiol.,* 2010; 77, 1326-1340.

Coakley, B. A., Sussman, E. S., Wolfson, T. S., Bhagavath, A. S., Choi, J. J., Ranasinghe, N. E., Lynn, E. T., Divino, C. M. Postoperative antibiotics correlate with worse outcomes after appendectomy for nonperforated appendicitis. *J. Am. Coll. Surg.,* 2011; 213, 778-783.

Costello, E. K., Stagaman, K., Dethlefsen, L., Bohannan, B. J., Relman, D. A. The application of ecological theory toward an understanding of the human microbiome. *Science,* 2012; 336, 1255-1262.

Dalton, H., Stirling, D. I. Co-metabolism. *Philos. Trans. R. Soc. Lond. B. Biol. Sci.,* 1982; 297, 481-496.

Denis, P. A. Heuristic consequences of a load of oxygen in microtubules. *BioSystems*, 2014; 118, 17-30.

Dietschy, J. M., Woollett, L. A., Spady, D. K. The interaction of dietary cholesterol and specific fatty acids in the regulation of LDL receptor activity and plasma LDL-cholesterol concentrations. *Ann. N. Y. Acad. Sci.,* 1993; 676, 11-26.

Edwards, L. A., O'Neill, C., Furman, M. A., Hicks, S., Torrente, F., Pérez-Machado, M., Wellington, E. M., Phillips, A. D., Murch, S. H. Enterotoxin-producing staphylococci cause intestinal inflammation by a combination of direct epithelial cytopathy and superantigen-mediated T-cell activation. *Inflamm. Bowel Dis.*, 2012; 18, 624-640.

Ellwood, D. C., Keevil, C. W., Marsh, P. D., Brown, C. M., Wardell, J. N. Surface-associated growth. *Philos. Trans. R. Soc. Lond. B. Biol. Sci.*, 1982; 297, 517-532.Farfan, M. J., Cantero, L., Vidal, R., Botkin, D. J., Torres, A. G. Long polar fimbriae of enterohemorrhagic *Escherichia coli* O157:H7 bind to extracellular matrix proteins. *Infect. Immun.*, 2011; 79, 3744-3750.

Fox, K. F,. Stewart, G. C., Fox, A. Synthesis of microcapsule is not responsive to environmental phosphate concentrations. *Infect. Immun.,* 1998; 66, 4004-4007.Freter, R., Jones, G. W. Models for studying the role of bacterial attachment in virulence and pathogenesis. *Rev. Infect. Dis.*, 1983; 5 (Suppl 4), S647-658.

Giannella, R. A. Pathogenesis of acute bacterial diarrheal disorders. *Annu. Rev. Med.,* 1981; 32, 341-357. Gilbreath, J. J., Colvocoresses Dodds, J., Rick, P. D., Soloski, M. J., Merrell, D. S., Metcalf, E. S. Enterobacterial common antigen mutants of *Salmonella enterica* serovar Typhimurium establish a persistent infection and provide protection against subsequent lethal challenge. *Infect. Immun.,* 2011; 80, 441-450.

Gleisner, M. A., Rosemblatt, M., Fierro, J. A., Bono, M. R. Delivery of alloantigens via apoptotic cells generates dendritic cells with an immature tolerogenic phenotype. *Transplant. Proc.,* 2011; 43, 2325-2333.

Gorgojo, J., Lamberti, Y., Valdez, H., Harvill, E. T., Rodríguez, M. E. *Bordetella parapertussis* survives the innate interaction with human neutrophils by impairing bactericidal trafficking inside the cell through a lipid raft-dependent mechanism mediated by the lipopolysaccharide O antigen. *Infect. Immun.,* 2012; 80, 4309-4316.

Gozdziewicz, T. K., Lugowski, C., Lukasiewicz, J. First evidence for a covalent linkage between enterobacterial common antigen and lipopolysaccharide in *Shigella sonnei* phase II ECALPS. *J. Biol. Chem.,* 2014; 289, 2745-2754.

Guttman, J. A., Li, Y., Wickham, M. E., Deng, W., Vogl, A. W., Finlay, B. B. Attaching and effacing pathogen-induced tight junction disruption in vivo. *Cell. Microbiol.*, 2006; 8, 634-645.

Hakalehto, E. Patent Application. 1995 950253 Fimbria-antigeeneja, –vasta-aineita, –osoitusmenetelmiä ja –rokotteita; 1995.

Hakalehto, E. Characterization of *Pectinatus cerevisiiphilus* and *P.frisingiensis* surface components. Use of synthetic peptides in the detection of some gram-negative bacteria, PhD Thesis, Kuopio University Publications C, Natural and Environmental Sciences 112, Kuopio, Finland; 2000.

Hakalehto, E. Semmelweis' present day follow-up: Updating bacterial sampling and enrichment in clinical hygiene. *Pathophysiology,* 2006; 13, 257-267.

Hakalehto, E. Hygiene monitoring with the Portable Microbe Enrichment Unit (PMEU). *41st R3 -Nordic Symposium. Cleanroom technology, contamination control and cleaning. VTT Publications 266.* Espoo, Finland: VTT (State Research Centre of Finland); 2010.

Hakalehto, E. Simulation of enhanced growth and metabolism of intestinal *Escherichia coli* in the Portable Microbe Enrichment Unit (PMEU). In: Rogers MC, Peterson ND, editors. *E. coli infections: causes, treatment and prevention.* New York, USA: Nova Publishers; 2011a.

Hakalehto, E. Antibiotic resistant traits of facultative *Enterobacter cloacae* strain studied with the PMEU (Portable Microbe Enrichment Unit). In: Méndez-Vilas, A., editor. *Science against microbial pathogens: communicating current research and technological advances. Microbiology book series Nr. 3.* Badajoz, Spain: Formatex Research Center; 2011b.

Hakalehto, E., editor. Alimentary microbiome - a PMEU approach. New York, NY, USA: Nova Science Publishers, Inc.; 2012a.Hakalehto, E. Development of microbial ecosystems. In: Hakalehto, E., editor. *Alimentary Microbiome - a PMEU Approach.* New York, NY, USA: Nova Science Publishers, Inc.; 2012b, pp. 95-125.

Hakalehto, E. Interactions of *Klebsiella* sp. with other intestinal flora. In: Pereira, L. A., Santos, A., editors. *Klebsiella Infections: Epidemiology, Pathogenesis and Clinical Outcomes.* New York, USA: Nova Science Publishers, Inc.; 2013, pp. 1-33.

Hakalehto, E. Bacteriological indications of human activities in the ecosystems. In: Armon, R., Hänninen, O., editors. *Environmental Bioindicators.* Germany: Springer Verlag; 2014.

Hakalehto, E., Hänninen, O. Gaseous CO_2 signal initiate growth of butyric acid producing *Clostridium butyricum* both in pure culture and in mixed cultures with *Lactobacillus brevis. Can. J. Microbiol.,* 2012; 58, 928-931.

Hakalehto, E., Jaakkola, K. Synergistic effect of probiotics and prebiotic flax product on intestinal bacterial balance. *Clinical Nutrition,* 2013; 32 (Suppl. 1), S200.Hakalehto, E., Santa, H., Vepsäläinen, J., Laatikainen, R., Finne, J. Identification of a common structural motif in the disordered N-terminal region of bacterial flagellins. Evidence for a new class of fibril-forming peptides. *Eur. J. Biochem.,* 1997; 250, 19-29.

Hakalehto, E., Hujakka, H., Airaksinen, S., Ratilainen, J., Närvänen, A. Growth-phase limited expression and rapid detection of *Salmonella* type 1 fimbriae. In: Hakalehto, E., editor.

Characterization of Pectinatus cerevisiiphilus and P. frisingiensis surface components. Use of synthetic peptides in the detection of some Gram-negative bacteria. Kuopio, Finland: Kuopio University Publications C. Natural and Environmental Sciences 112; 2000.

Hakalehto, E., Pesola, J., Heitto, L., Närvänen, A., Heitto, A. Aerobic and anaerobic growth modes and expression of type 1 fimbriae in *Salmonella. Pathophysiology,* 2007; 14, 61-69.

Hakalehto, E., Humppi, T., Paakkanen, H. Dualistic acidic and neutral glucose fermentation balance in small intestine: Simulation in vitro. *Pathophysiology,* 2008; 15, 211-220.

Hakalehto, E., Pesola, J., Heitto, A., Bhanj Deo, B., Rissanen, K., Sankilampi, U., Humppi, T., Paakkanen, H. Fast detection of bacterial growth by using Portable Microbe Enrichment Unit (PMEU) and ChemPro100i® gas sensor. *Pathophysiology,* 2009; 16, 57-62.

Hakalehto, E., Hell, M., Bernhofer, C., Heitto, A., Pesola, J., Humppi, T., Paakkanen, H. Growth and gaseous emissions of pure and mixed small intestinal bacterial cultures: Effects of bile and vancomycin. *Pathophysiology,* 2010; 17, 45-53.

Hakalehto, E., Heitto, A., Heitto, L., Humppi, T., Rissanen, K., Jääskeläinen, A., Hänninen, O. Fast monitoring of water distribution system with portable enrichment unit – Measurement of volatile compounds of coliforms and *Salmonella* sp. in tap water. *Journal of Toxicology and Environmental Health Sciences,* 2011a; 3, 223-233.

Hakalehto, E., Vilpponen-Salmela, T., Kinnunen, K., von Wright, A. Lactic acid bacteria enriched from human gastric biopsies. *ISRN Gastroenterol.,* 2011b; 2011, 109183.

Hakalehto, E., Pesola, J., del Amo, E. M., Hänninen, O. Bacterial interactions in the small intestine and their contribution to host nutrient uptake. In: Hakalehto, E., editor. *Alimentary microbiome - a PMEU approach.* New York, NY, USA: Nova Science Publishers, Inc.; 2012, pp. 61-94.Hakalehto, E., Heitto, A., Heitto, L. Fast coliform detection in portable microbe enrichment unit (PMEU) with Colilert® medium and bubbling. *Pathophysiology*, 2013; 20, 257-262.

Hakalehto, E., Tiainen, M., Laatikainen, R., Paakkanen, H., Humppi, T., Hänninen, O. *Klebsiella* sp. ferments hydrolyzed cellulose by overflow metabolism to 2,3-butanediol and ethanol by overflow metabolism to 2,3-butanediol and ethanol balancing pH and osmotic stress without bacterial growth. 2014. Manuscript in preparation.

Han, W., Wang, Z., Chen, H., Yao, X., Li, Y. Simultaneous biohydrogen and bioethanol production from anaerobic fermentation with immobilized sludge. *J. Biomed. Biotechnol.,* 2011; 2011, 343791. Harrison, D. E. Undamped oscillations of pyridine nucleotide and oxygen tension in chemostat cultures of *Klebsiella aerogenes. J. Cell. Biol.,* 1970; 45, 514-521.

Harrison, D. E. Studies on the affinity of methanol--and methane--utilizing bacteria for their carbon substrates. *J. Appl. Bacteriol.,* 1973; 36, 301-308.

Harrison, D. E., Pirt, S. J. The influence of dissolved oxygen concentration on the respiration and glucose metabolism of *Klebsiella aerogenes* during growth. *J. Gen. Microbiol.*, 1967; 46, 193-211.

Heitto, L., Heitto, A., Hakalehto, E. Environmental monitoring using the enrichment of hygienic indicators. In: Hakalehto, E., editor. *Alimentary microbiome - a PMEU approach.* New York, NY, USA: Nova Science Publishers, Inc.; 2012, pp. 215-231.

Hell, M., Bernhofer, C., Huhulescu, S., Indra, A., Allerberger, F., Maass, M., Hakalehto, E. How safe is colonoscope-reprocessing regarding *Clostridium difficile* spores*? The Journal of Hospital Infection*, 2010; 76 (Suppl. 1), S21-22. Abstracts, 8th International Congress of the Hospital Infection Society, 10-13 October 2010, Liverpool, UK.

Hentges, D. J. Anaerobes: general characteristics. In: Baron, S., editor. *Medical Microbiology*. 4th edition. Galveston (TX): University of Texas Medical Branch at Galveston; 1996. Chapter 17.

Hill, M. J. The normal gut bacterial flora. In: Hill, M. J., editor. *Role of the gut bacteria in human toxicology and pharmacology*. London, United Kingdom: Taylor and Francis Ltd.; 1995, pp. 3-17.

Hinchey, E. J., Schaal, P. G., Richards, G. K. Treatment of perforated diverticular disease of the colon. *Adv. Surg*., 1978; 12, 85-109.

Hood, D. W., Randle, G., Cox, A. D., Makepeace, K., Li, J., Schweda, E. K., Richards, J. C., Moxon, E. R. Biosynthesis of cryptic lipopolysaccharide glycoforms in *Haemophilus influenzae* involves a mechanism similar to that required for O-antigen synthesis. *J. Bacteriol.,* 2004; 186, 7429-7439.

Hylemon, P. B., Zhou, H., Pandak, W. M., Ren, S., Gil, G., Dent, P. Bile acids as regulatory molecules. *J. Lipid Res*., 2009; 50, 1509-1520.

Jaakkola, K., Hakalehto, E. Intestinal imbalances and diseases of the digestive tract. In: Hakalehto, E., editor. Alimentary microbiome - a PMEU approach. New York, NY, USA: Nova Science Publishers, Inc.; 2012, pp. 127-160.

Jespersen, D. J., Smith, T. F., Rosenblatt, J. E., Cockerill, F. R., 3rd. Comparison of the *Borrelia* DotBlot G, MarDx, and VIDAS enzyme immunoassays for detecting immunoglobulin G antibodies to *Borrelia burgdorferi* in human serum. *J. Clin. Microbiol.,* 2002; 40, 4782-4784.Jones, S. A., Gibson, T., Maltby, R. C., Chowdhury, F. Z., Stewart, V., Cohen, P. S., Conway, T. Anaerobic respiration of *Escherichia coli* in the mouse intestine. *Infect. Immun.,* 2011; 79, 4218-4226.

Keesing, F., Belden, L. K., Daszak, P., Dobson, A., Harvell, C. D., Holt, R. D., Hudson, P., Jolles, A., Jones, K. E., Mitchell, C. E., Myers, S. S., Bogich, T., Ostfeld, R. S. Impacts on biodiversity on the emergence and transmission of infectious diseases. *Nature*, 2010; 468, 647-652.Kelly, P. Nutrition, intestinal defence and the microbiome. *Proc. Nutr. Soc.,* 2010; 69, 261-268. Kendall, A. I., Alexander, A. D., Walker, A. W., Haner, B. C. The bacteriology and chemistry of adult duodenal contents. Studies in Bacterial Metabolism LXXXII. *The Journal of Infectious Diseases*, 1927; 40, 677-688.

Kerrn, M. B., Struve, C., Blom, J., Frimodt-Moller, N., Krogfelt, K. A. Intracellular persistence of *Escherichia coli* in urinary bladders from mecillinam-treated mice. *J. Antimicrob. Chemother.,* 2005; 55, 383-386.

Khoo, A. L., Chai, L. Y., Koenen, H. J., Oosting, M., Steinmeyer, A., Zuegel, U., Joosten, I., Netea, M. G., van der Ven, A. J. Vitamin D(3) down-regulates proinflammatory cytokine response to *Mycobacterium tuberculosis* through pattern recognition receptors while inducing protective cathelicidin production. *Cytokine,* 2011; 55, 294-300.

Knight, J., Reeves, J., Wakeman, M. ABEL-Sport Test for assessing overtraining syndrome and detecting infection. Poster in: International Sports Science + Sports Medicine Conference, 2013.

Kobayashi, A., Kawai, S., Ohbe, Y., Benno, Y. Fecal flora of infants with biliary atresia: effects of the absence of bile on fecal flora. *Am. J. Clin. Nutr.,* 1988; 48, 1211-1213.

Koistinen, K. M., Plumed-Ferrer, C., Lehesranta, S. J., Kärenlampi, S. O., von Wright, A. Comparison of growth-phase-dependent cytosolic proteomes of two *Lactobacillus plantarum* strains used in food and feed fermentations. *FEMS Microbiol. Lett.*, 2007; 273, 12-21.

Kühn, I., Ayling-Smith, B., Tullus, K., Burman, L. G. The use of colonization rate and epidemic index as tools to illustrate the epidemiology of faecal *Enterobacteriaceae* strains in Swedish neonatal wards. *J. Hosp. Infect.,* 1993; 23, 287-297.

Ley, R. E., Turnbaugh, P. J., Klein, S., Gordon, J. I. Microbial ecology: human gut microbes associated with obesity. *Nature,* 2006; 444, 1022-1023.

Lu, J., Wang, A., Ansari, S., Hershberg, R. M., McKay, D. M. Colonic bacterial superantigens evoke an inflammatory response and exaggerate disease in mice recovering from colitis. *Gastroenterology*, 2003; 125, 1785-1795.

Lyte, M. The microbial organ in the gut as a driver of homeostasis and disease. *Med. Hypotheses,* 2010; 74, 634-638.

Macnab, R. M., Castle, A. M. A variable stoichiometry model for pH homeostasis in bacteria. *Biophys. J.,* 1987; 52, 637-647.

Malakooti, J., Saksena, S., Gill, R. K., Dudeja, P. K.Transcriptional regulation of the intestinal luminal Na^+ and Cl^- transporters. *Biochem. J.*, 2011; 435, 313-325.

Midtvedt, T. Intestinal microflora-associated characteristics. *Microecol. Ther.,* 1986; 16, 121-130. Mitzscherling. K., Volynets, V., Parlesak, A. Phosphatidylcholine reverses ethanol-induced increase in transepithelial endotoxin permeability and abolishes transepithelial leukocyte activation. *Alcohol Clin. Exp. Res.,* 2009; 33, 557-562.

Moat, A. G., Foster, J. W. Microbial physiology, 2nd edition. New York, USA: John Wiley & Sons; 1988.

Morowitz, M. J., Denef, V. J., Costello, E. K., Thomas, B. C., Poroyko, V., Relman, D. A., Banfield, J. F. Strain-resolved community genomic analysis of gut microbial colonization in a premature infant. *Proc. Natl. Acad. Sci. U S A,* 2011; 108, 1128-1133.

Mortenson, L. E. Inorganic nitrogen? Assimilation an ammonia in corporation. In: Consalus, I. C., Stanier, R., editors. *The Bacteria*, Vol. 3. New York, USA: Academic press; 1962.

O'Hara, A. M., O'Regan, P., Fanning, A., O'Mahony, C., Macsharry, J., Lyons, A., Bienenstock, J., O'Mahony, L., Shanahan, F. Functional modulation of human intestinal epithelial cell responses by *Bifidobacterium infantis* and *Lactobacillus salivarius*. *Immunology*, 2006; 118, 202-215.

Okamoto, K., Fujii, Y., Akashi, N., Hitotsubashi, S., Kurazono, H., Karasawa, T., Takeda, Y. Identification and characterization of heat-stable enterotoxin II-producing *Escherichia coli* from patients with diarrhea. *Microbiol. Immunol.,* 1993; 37, 411-414.

Oppenheimer-Shaanan, Y., Steinberg, N., Kolodkin-Gal, I. Small molecules are natural triggers for the disassembly of biofilms. *Trends Microbiol.,* 2013; 21, 594-601.

O'Riordan, K., Lee, J. C. *Staphylococcus aureus* capsular polysaccharides. *Clin. Microbiol. Rev.*, 2004; 17, 218-234.

Ottman, N., Smidt, H., de Vos, W. M., Belzer, C. The function of our microbiota: who is out there and what do they do? *Front. Cell. Infect. Microbiol.,* 2012; 2, 104-114.

Palmer, J. D. An introduction to biological rhythms. London, UK: Academic Press, Inc.; 1976.

Parm, U., Metsvaht, T., Sepp, E., Ilmoja, M. L., Pisarev, H., Pauskar, M., Lutsar, I. Risk factors associated with gut and nasopharyngeal colonization by common Gram-negative species and yeasts in neonatal intensive care units patients. *Early Hum. Dev.,* 2011; 87, 391-399.

Parviainen, I. Gastric tonometry in the assessment of splanchnic perfusion: Methodological aspects and evaluation of simultaneous regional blood flow measurements and gastric tonometry after coronary artery bypass grafting. Kuopio University Publications D. Medical Sciences 123. 1997. 87 p.

Parviainen, I., Ruokonen, E., Takala, J. Dobutamine-induced dissociation between changes in splanchnic blood flow and gastric intramucosal pH after cardiac surgery. *Br. J. Anaesth.*, 1995; 74, 277-282.

Pastell, H. Preparation, structural analysis and prebiotic potential of arabinoxylo-oligosaccharides. Academic Dissertation. University of Helsinki, EKT-series 1463. Helsinki, Finland: Helsinki University Press, 2010.

Pennisi, E. Microbiology. Gut bacteria lend a molecular hand to viruses. *Science,* 2011; 334, 168.

Pesola, J., Hakalehto, E. Enterobacterial microflora in infancy - a case study with enhanced enrichment. *Indian J. Pediatr.,* 2011; 78, 562-568.

Pesola J., Hakalehto, E. Importance of intestinal microbiota on immunocompromised pediatric patients. In: Hakalehto, E., editor. *Alimentary microbiome - a PMEU approach.* New York, NY, USA: Nova Science Publishers, Inc.; 2012; pp. 161-178.

Pesola, J., Vaarala, O., Heitto, A., Hakalehto, E. Use of portable enrichment unit in rapid characterization of infantile intestinal enterobacterial microbiota. *Microb. Ecol. Health Dis.,* 2009; 21, 203-210.

Pesola, J., Paakkanen, H., Hakalehto, E. Enhanced diagnostics of pyelonephritis – a case study. *Int. J. Med. Med. Sci.,* 2012; 2, 273-277.

Pitkänen, T., Bräcker, J., Miettinen, I., Heitto, A., Pesola, J., Hakalehto, E. Enhanced enrichment and detection of thermotolerant *Campylobacter* species from water using the Portable Microbe Enrichment Unit (PMEU) and realtime PCR. *Can. J. Microbiol.,* 2009; 55, 849-858.

Rao, B., Zhang, L. Y., Sun, J., Su, G., Wei, D., Chu, J., Zhu, J., Shen, Y. Characterization and regulation of the 2,3-butanediol pathway in *Serratia marcescens. Appl. Microbiol. Biotechnol.*, 2012; 93, 2147-2159.

Rhen, M., Mäkelä, P. H., Korhonen, T. K. P-fimbriae of *E. coli* are subject to phase variation. *FEMS Microbiol. Lett.,* 1983; 19, 267-271.

Rossi-George, A., Urbach, D., Colas, D., Goldfarb, Y., Kusnekov, A. W. Neuronal, endocrine, and anorexic responses to the T-cell superantigen staphylococcal enterotoxin A: Dependence on tumor necrosis factor-α. *J. Neurosci.*, 2005; 25, 5314-5322.

Russell, D. W., Setchell, K. D. Bile acid biosynthesis. Biochemistry, 1992; 31, 4737-4749.

Segre, J. A. What does it take to satisfy Koch's postulates two centuries later? Microbial genomics and *Propionibacteria acnes. J. Invest. Dermatol.,* 2013; 133, 2141-2142.

Sha, S., Liang, J., Chen, M., Xu, B., Liang, C., Wei, N., Wu, K. Systematic review: faecal microbiota transplantation therapy for digestive and nondigestive disorders in adults and children. *Aliment. Pharmacol. Ther.*, 2014; 39, 1003-1032.

Smirnov, A. Y., Mourokh, L. G., Nori, F. Electrostatic models of electron-driven proton transfer across a lipid membrane. *J. Phys. Condens. Matter.*, 2011; 23, 234101. Smyth, C. J., Möllby, R., Wadström, T. Phenomenon of hot-cold hemolysis: Cheletor-induced lysis of sphingomyelinase-treated erythrocytes. *Infect. Immun.,* 1975; 12, 1104-1111.Spector, S. A. Vitamin D and HIV: letting the sun shine in. *Top. Antivir. Med.*, 2011; 19, 6-10.

Spitz, D. R., Dornfeld, K. J., Krishnan, K., Guis, D., editors. Oxidative Stress in Cancer Biology and Therapy. New York, USA: Springer Science + Business Media; 2012.Steiner, C., Holleboom, A. G., Karuna, R., Motazacker, M. M., Kuivenhoven, J. A., Frikke-Schmidt, R., Tybjaerg-Hansen, A., Rohrer, L., Rentsch, K. M., von Eckardstein, A. Lipoprotein distribution and serum concentrations of 7alpha-hydroxy-4-cholesten-3-one and bile acids: Effects of monogenic disturbances in high density lipoprotein metabolism. *Clin. Sci. (Lond.),* 2012; 122, 385-396.

Tilly, K., Rosa, P.A., Stewart, P.E. Biology of infection with *Borrelia burgdorferi. Infect. Dis. Clin. North Am.*, 2008; 22, 217-234.

Torcato, I. M., Huang, Y. H., Franquelim, H. G., Gaspar, D. D., Craik, D. J., Castanho, M. A., Henriques, S. T. The antimicrobial activity of Sub3 is dependent on membrane binding and cell-penetrating ability. *Chembiochem.*, 2013; 14, 2013-2022.

Trock, D. H., Bollet, A. J., Markoll, R. The effect of pulsed electromagnetic fields in the treatment of osteoarthritis of knee and cervical spine. Report of randomized, double blind, placebo controlled trials. *J. Rheumatol.*, 1994; 21, 1903-1911.

Turnbaugh, P. J., Ley, R. E., Mahowald, M. A., Magrini, V., Mardis, E. R., Gordon, J. I. An obesity-associated gut microbiome with increased capacity for energy harvest. *Nature,* 2006; 444, 1027-1031.

Ubeda, C., Taur, Y., Jenq, R. R., Equinda, M. J., Son, T., Samstein, M., Viale, A., Socci, N. D., van den Brink, M. R., Kamboj, M., Pamer, E. G. Vancomycin-resistant *Enterococcus* domination of intestinal microbiota is enabled by antibiotic treatment in mice and precedes bloodstream invasion in humans. *J. Clin. Invest.,* 2010; 120, 4332-4341. Uzel, G., Kleiner, D. E., Kuhns, D. B., Holland, S. M. Dysfunctional LAD-1 neutrophils and colitis. *Gastroenterology,* 2001; 121, 958-964.

Vermeer, C., Braam, L. Role of K vitamins in the regulation of tissue calcification. *J. Bone Miner. Metab.*, 2001; 19, 201-206.Vrieze, A., Holleman, F., Zoetendal, E. G., de Vos, W. M., Hoekstra, J. B., Nieuwdorp, M. The environment within: how gut microbiota may influence metabolism and body composition. *Diabetologia*, 2010; 53, 606-613.

Walker, H. H. Carbon dioxide as a factor affecting lag in bacterial growth. *Science,* 1932; 76, 602-604.

Walker, W. A. Initial intestinal colonization in the human infant and immune homeostasis. *Ann. Nutr. Metab.,* 2013; 63 (Suppl. 2), 8-15.

Watson, D. L. Ovine opsonins for *Staphylococcus aureus* cell wall and pseudocapsule. *Res. Vet. Sci.,* 1989; 46, 84-89.

Wilson, B. A., Salyers, A. A., Whitt, D. D., Winkler, M. E., editors. Bacterial pathogenesis: a molecular approach, 3rd edition. Washington, DC, USA: ASM Press; 2011.

Wu, G. D., Chen, J., Hoffmann, C., Bittinger, K., Chen, Y. Y., Keilbaugh, S. A., Bewtra, M., Knights, D., Walters, W. A., Knight, R., Sinha, R., Gilroy, E., Gupta, K., Baldassano, R., Nessel, L., Li, H., Bushman, F. D., Lewis, J. D. Linking long-term dietary patterns with gut microbial enterotypes. *Science,* 2011; 334, 105-108.

Xuan, C., Shamonki, J. M., Chung, A., DiNome, M. L., Chung, M., Sieling, P. A., Lee, D. J. Microbial dysbiosis is associated with human breast cancer. *PLoS ONE,* 2014; 9, e83744. Zhao, Y., Tomas, C. A., Rudolph, F. B., Papoutsakis, E. T., Bennett, G. N. Intracellular butyryl phosphate and acetyl phosphate concentrations in *Clostridium acetobutylicum* and their implications for solvent formation. *Appl. Environ. Microbiol.*, 2005; 71, 530-537.

Zipfel, P. F., Mihlan, M., Skerka, C. The alternative pathway of complement: a pattern recognition system. *Adv. Exp. Med. Biol.*, 2007; 598, 80-92.

In: Microbiological Clinical Hygiene
Editor: Eino Elias Hakalehto
ISBN: 978-1-63463-428-1

Chapter 15

Monitoring *Clostridium difficile*

Markus Hell[1] and Elias Hakalehto[2]
[1]Zentrum für Krankenhaushygiene und Infektionskontrolle der SALK, Universitätsklinikum Salzburg, Paracelsus Medical University, Salzburg, Austria
[2]Department of Environmental Sciences, University of Eastern Finland, Kuopio, Finland

Abstract

The excessive use of antibiotics for safeguarding our health against infections or communicable microbial diseases has, quite paradoxically, lead to the emerging of new groups of harmful microbes such as antibiotic resistant bacteria, yeasts, or *Clostridium difficile*. The removal of normal microflora has given room for these tedious microbes, which conquer space from the balanced symbiotic microbiota. Moreover, they could intrude the body system with their toxins causing life-threatening illnesses. One reason for their strong abilities to produce diseases could be deriving from their origin. Members of Clostridium sp. are typically soil bacteria. Another reason of course is their capability of sporulation. Their spores can persist in the environment for decades and they resist any antibiotics in the human gut and many disinfectants in the environment.

1. Introduction

As discussed elsewhere in this book (Chapters 16 and 21), the antibiosis is a common phenomenon in soil where the microbes have to compete against each other for the relatively scarce nutrients. On the contrary, in the human bodies, or in the alimentary tract, most strains strive for cooperation. Any monocultures would be detrimental for the host as living organism, and thus counterproductive for the common members of the normal flora.

We have been using the PMEU technologies for mapping the microflora in different samples, and for simulating their joint influences and molecular communication (Hakalehto et al., 2010; Hakalehto, 2011). An example related to the bacterial interactions is the growth promoting signal effect of lactobacilli on the clostridial strains in the PMEU which is mediated by the CO_2 in the intestinal environment (Hakalehto and Hänninen, 2011). This effect is provoking the onset of growth of the anaerobic culture of the *Clostridium* sp.

In the intestinal environment, this activity of the mixed microflora could thus keep these strains in the active state which, in turn, could prevent them from colonizing the gut walls, or producing endospores.

In case of the CDI (*C. difficile* infections) the causative agents (strains) are mostly monophasic (Hell et al., 2011a). This is an indication of the flourishing of one pathogenic strain in the background of the illness. This behavior of the clostridial strains is a consequence of destroyed BIB (Bacterial Intestinal Balance). The routes of the infection need to be further studied on in particular cases of CDI. It needs to be investigated also the proportion of healthy carriers among the population and CDI exposed healthy health care workers.

In both groups it seems to be very low at the moment (Hell et al., 2011b) but further investigation at a larger scale is needed.

This emerging pathogen has caused severe threats for the healthcare system. It is typically belonging to the hospital acquired infections, whether originating from contaminated surfaces adjacent to the patient or from the patient directly. Therefore, this new widely spread pathogen should be mapped amongst the population (Spigaglia et al., 2011). Since 2005 The European institutions have made similar experience like the north American ones with several hospital outbreaks related to new, probably selected so called hypervirulent strains such as the NAP 1/ PCR Ribotype 027 related with higher morbidity and mortality among hospitalized patients (Kuijper et al., 2006).

But more over CDI has become also a community problem nowadays in some cases related to the food chain esp. pork and ground meat (Rodriguez-Palacios et al., 2007).

So epidemiology has taken a dynamic global development and made these new strains successful pathogens.

2. Clostridium Infections

There are several species of the genus *Clostridium* causing diseases in man. These bacteria are obligate anaerobic spore-formers. The endospores facilitate their survival in soil, from where they mostly spread into humans.

Infections by clostridia always mean infection via toxins and therefore one could also talk about "intoxification" related to these organisms. Even if the classical clostridial infections such as gas gangrene by *C. perfringens*, botulism by *C. botulinum* or tetanus by *C. tetani* are very dangerous and still associated with a high fatality in clinical outcome they very rare at least in the developed countries where vaccination programs are implemented and people are vaccinated (e.g., *C. tetani*).

All these come from soil, and are very dangerous. They should not belong to the normal microbiota of man, at least not to the permanent/resident flora.

Beside the most common species *Clostridium difficile* within the genus *Clostridia* there are also emerging species in health care setting like *Clostridium sordellii* which leads to myonecrosis and severe shock syndrome among previously healthy persons which has been described recently in a small number of *C. sordellii* cases, most often associated with gynecologic infections in women and infection of the umbilical stump in newborns (Aldape et al., 2006).

3. Clostridium Difficile: Epidemiology

The most common type of infection is *C. difficile* infection (CDI), which emerged and re-emerged the last ten years globally. Some experts are even talking about a *C. difficile* pandemic.

This phenomenon is not only due to antibiotic-overuse during the last decades in the health care setting but also food related, esp. linked to meat (ground meat). So CDI has also become a community associated infection and not only a hospital-acquired infection any longer. But these cases are still rare compared to the antibiotic-related cases at least in Europe. Within North America there are an estimated 25, 000 deaths each year linked to Clostridium difficile infections (CDI). The economic burden of CDI is estimated to be $10B per year with the C difficile control sector market being in the order of $7B and growing. Traditionally C difficile was considered to be exclusively linked to hospital-acquired infections primarily affecting the elderly or those with weakened immune system being administered antibiotics. Here, the antibiotics disrupt the gastrointestinal tract microflora thereby enabling the drug resistant C difficile- spores to proliferate and produce toxins leading to potentially fatal pseudomembranous colitis. Over the last 3 years there has been an increasing occurrence of Community Acquired C difficile infections and are thought to account for over 40% of all CDI reported. The case definition of Community Acquired CDI is patients who have no recent contact with health care facilities or taking antibiotics. There are many aspects of Community Acquired CDI that remain unknown and especially with relation to sources of the pathogen but there is evidence for foodborne, environmental and zoonotic transfer of *C. difficile* (Rupnik, 2007). In the hospital setting CDI is occurring only when the patient's normal flora and its balance has been destroyed by excessive antibiotic treatments. Patients who have other illnesses or conditions requiring prolonged use of antibiotics, and the elderly, are at greater risk of acquiring this disease. The bacteria are found in the feces.

People can become infected if they touch items or surfaces that are contaminated with feces and then touch their mouth or mucous membranes. Healthcare workers can spread the bacteria to patients or contaminate surfaces through hand contact.

Clinical symptoms of CDI range from a single episode of diarrhea, to watery and bloody diarrhea, to pseudomembranous colitis with systemic signs of severe infection. Complications from a perforation of the colon to a toxic megacolon, which usually needs surgical intervention (i.e., subtotal hemicolectomy).

C. difficile infections and the distribution of strains and types as described in recent pan-european study (Bauer et al., 2011). In this prevalence study it was demonstrated that there is not one prevalent strain all over Europe but nation by nation specific clusters of strains by classifying through PCR-ribotyping, one of the most popular typing method in Europe (Bidet et al., 2000). The so called hypervirulent strains like PCR-ribotype 027 or 078 or 001 remain still unclear if they maybe were overestimated in the potential of hypervirulence.

Transmission

Transmission of *C. difficile in Health care facilities*: *Clostridium difficile* is shed in feces. Any surface, device, or material (e.g., toilets, bathing tubs, and electronic rectal thermometers) that becomes contaminated with feces may serve as a reservoir for the *Clostridium difficile* spores. *Clostridium difficile* spores are transferred to patients mainly via the hands of healthcare personnel who have touched a contaminated surface or item. *Clostridium difficile* can live for long periods on surfaces (up to 6 months).

Prevention of *C. Difficile*

In order to properly understand the nature of the CDI, the hospital hygiene personnel should be able to get first hand information on the problem. Research facilities should be provided for every larger hospital unit in order to facilitate early warning and effective countermeasures in time.

People who are hospitalized or on antibiotics are most likely to become ill. For safety precautions you may do the following to reduce the chance of acquiring *C. difficile* or spreading to others:

- Wash hands with soap and water, especially after using the restroom and before eating.
- Clean surfaces in bathrooms, kitchens, and other areas on a regular basis with household detergent/disinfectants.
- By thoroughly cleaning of hands and cleaning of surfaces adjacent to the patient with spore-active or non-active detergents/disinfectants transmission of spores can be prevented. The most important concept is the mechanical removal of the bacterial spores.

Transmission of *C. difficile* within hospitals has been observed through time-space clustering of new cases with identical strains and a greater risk of acquisition of *C. difficile* from exposure to roommates or other patients in close proximity who have positive cultures *C. difficile* spores have been found to contaminate the hands of healthcare workers and the hospital environment frequently.

Because alcohol-based hand sanitizers do not inactivate the spores of *C. difficile*, concern over their role in transmission of *C. difficile* have been raised. However, hospitals using alcohol-based hand rubs as their primary means of hand hygiene have not seen increases in the incidence of CDI associated with their introduction due to the theoretical advantage of hand washing over alcohol-based hand sanitizers, hand washing with a non-antimicrobial soap or antimicrobial soap and water should be considered after removing gloves in the setting of a CDI outbreak or if ongoing transmission cannot be controlled by other measures.

Patients with CDI should be placed on contact precautions and housed in single rooms with private bathrooms or, if unavailable, cohorted in rooms with other patients with CDI. Single-use disposable or patient-dedicated noncritical equipment should be used. Wearing gloves is one measure that has been proven to reduce the spread of *C. difficile* in hospitals.

Gowns and gloves should be donned prior to entering the room of a patient with CDI and removed followed by hand hygiene before leaving the room.

Although all hospital cleaning agents can inhibit the growth of *C. difficile* in culture, only chlorine-containing agents inactivate *C. difficile* spores.

In the most definitive study evaluating environmental cleaning, the use of a 1:10 dilution of a 6% hypochlorite solution for daily room cleaning of CDI patients in a bone marrow transplant unit decreased the CDI rate significantly but had no effect on units with lower baseline CDI rates. Therefore, the use of hypochlorite might be most effective in units where CDI is highly endemic. The drawbacks of hypochlorite solutions are that most of them must be prepared fresh daily and they can be caustic and damaging to hospital equipment.

Antimicrobial use restrictions are another potential mechanism of controlling and preventing *C. difficile*. As with environmental cleaning, the exact role of antimicrobial restrictions is undefined due to the presence of confounding factors in most studies. However, several studies support the use of formulary restrictions promoting the use of narrow-spectrum antibiotics to reduce the incidence of CDI.

Formulary substitutions of 8-methoxyfluoroquinolones for levofloxacin have also been proposed to control CDI outbreaks caused by the BI/NAP1/027 strain. While this appeared to be effective in one study it was ineffective in another, most likely because the overall use of fluoroquinolones in the hospital was not controlled.

Since resistance of the BI/NAP1/027 strain to fluoroquinolones is a class effect resulting in higher minimum inhibitory concentrations (MICs) to all fluoroquinolones the incidence of disease caused by such resistant strains is not likely to be reduced without controlling fluoroquinolone use in general.

In conclusion the increasing incidence and severity of CDI in North America and Europe present major challenges for control and management of this disease. Continued gathering of data on the epidemiology of *C. difficile* through disease surveillance both within and outside of healthcare facilities, and on the efficacy of prevention and treatment strategies is essential to reduce the burden of this disease. Meanwhile, all clinicians and especially critical care physicians should maintain awareness of the changing epidemiology of CDI and undertake measures to reduce the risk of disease in their patients (Gould and McDonald, 2008).

Therefore specific guidelines/position papers were developed like the following European guideline (Vonberg et al., 2008):

4. Infection Control Measures to Limit the Spread of *Clostridium Difficile*

The “TEN commandments” of Good practice in Infection Control for CDI:

1 Early diagnosis
2 Surveillance: get an idea about what is going in your institution?
3 Training of health care personnel: How to convince your colleagues to adhere to the rules?
4 Isolation precautions: How to implement isolation techniques under limited patient room resources?

5 Hand hygiene: alcoholic handrubs do not work against *C. difficile* spores!
6 Protective clothing: How much is safe enough?
7 Environmental cleaning: cleaning with mechanical removal of spores or sophisticated sporicidal surface disinfection?
8 Medical devices: are bedpans and flexible endoscopes and their reprocessing a risk for transmission of *C. difficile*?
9 Antibiotics: restriction of antibiotics = the single most efficient measure to reduce CDI!
10 Specific measures in outbreaks: do as much as you can.

1. Early Diagnosis

The main purpose of screening cultures is to identify carriers of pathogens at the most early stage before inter-patient-spread can occur. For CD, the prevalence in asymptomatic and otherwise healthy adults stool cultures is less than 5%. In contrast, the rate of CD carriers among hospitalized patients varies significantly and may be as high as 25%. More than half of the CD strains from symptom-free individuals are toxinogenic.

Although screening cultures of CD have been performed in some nosocomial epidemics, there are no data showing that active screening of non-diarrhoeal patients in order to identify CD carriers will contribute to the reduction of the endemic baseline rate of CDI. Instead one should focus on diarrhoeal patients as they represent the major reservoir for CD transmission. Because recurrence of CDI after a symptom-free interval is not uncommon (up to 25-30% of cases), diagnostic testing for CD should also be performed at a new onset of diarrhoea.

Besides reducing the risk of pathogen spread, the second rationale of screening cultures is to identify carriers who are at risk to develop endogenous nosocomial CDI. However, in a prospective observational study on long-stay patients Johnson at al. could show that symptom-free excretors of CD even had a slightly decreased risk of subsequent CDI (0 of 51 patients) compared to 7 of 229 (3.1%) cases of CDI in patients who had been initially culture negative. Shim at al. also observed that there were 22 cases of CDI in 618 previously non-colonized patients (3.6%) compared with 2 of 192 (1.0%) in symptom-free carriers (p=.021). Additionally, treatment of asymptomatic carriers has been shown ineffective in eradicating CD. Hence, symptom-free CD colonization may actually be protective for subsequent symptomatic disease, but it is possible that asymptomatic carriers may still contribute to transmission of the organism. Screening of the environment is not generally recommended, but can be used to document environmental contamination or poor cleaning and disinfection.

2. Surveillance

Generally active surveillance of CDI has been recommended. Surveillance is useful to detect an increase in the CDI incidence, or its severity, at an early stage, or to identify risk factors for CDI acquisition, and should include the identification of deaths to which CDI is either the primary cause or contributory. The significance of surveillance is not limited to outbreaks. In the endemic setting it may reveal high baseline rates, or significant variations between locations that require interventions. At least stool testing for CD toxins should be performed in the case of nosocomial diarrhoea that cannot be unexplained otherwise, and for all patients that have been admitted to the hospital for severe non-nosocomial diarrhoea. Microbiological laboratories should consider testing for CD systematically in all stool specimens from patients hospitalized for more than 3 days ("3-day testing rule").

If possible, culture and typing of CD toxin positive samples should be performed. In practice this is best achieved by storing (aliquots of) toxin positive faecal samples, so that these can be examined retrospectively to aid CD cluster/outbreak management, if necessary by a reference laboratory.

A threshold incidence or prevalence of CDI should be defined locally that would trigger implementation of additional control interventions.

The alert level should be based on the incidence, severity of disease, institutional priorities, whether the patient population has conditions that would facilitate transmission or is at increased risk of adverse outcomes following CDI acquisition, and whether there is suspected or proven transmission within the facility.

Besides the surveillance of the number of CDI cases by infection control staff in a hospital notification system, surveillance of the antibiotic use in the hospital by the hospital's pharmacist in close cooperation with the medical microbiologist is also recommended. One future option could be the use of PMEU (Portable Microbe Enrichment Unit) technology for screening the CDI. In previous trials even the smallest concentrations of this bacterium were detected in less than 19 hours by the PMEU (Hell et al., 2010).

An additional option could be the use of the volatiles sensing version, PMEU Scentrion®, for the rapid testing. Such "electronic noses" have been recommended also elsewhere to be developed for ultra-fast bacterial monitoring (van Belkum et al., 2013).

In the case of the PMEU Scentrion® this gas detection technology has been combined with the enhanced enrichment option (Hakalehto and Heitto, 2012; Pesola et al., 2012).

3. Training of Health Care Personnel

Education of staff has shown to be one of the most effective measures to limit CD spread. This should include information about the basic pathogenetic mechanism of CD, its potential reservoirs, the route of transmission, contamination of the environment, and possible substance for decontamination of hands and surfaces. Training of staff should include not only the medical personnel (e.g., nurses or physicians), but should also be carried out on non-medical personnel – especially the staff involved in cleaning.

Education of visitors of patients with CDI is also necessary to prevent contamination of the environment by CD spores. Visitors should be encouraged to obey basic infection control measures with emphasis on appropriate hand hygiene. Visitors should not meet other patients after they have visited a patient with CDI. Individuals suffering from acute diarrhoea themselves should generally be discouraged to visit patients in a hospital.

4. Isolation Precautions

Isolation of patients colonized or infected with infectious agents in single rooms or in cohorts is one of the basic hygiene measures to limit pathogen spread. With few exceptions isolation of symptomatic patients with CDI is a key measure to control nosocomial CD outbreaks.

Occasionally even closure of a complete ward or department is necessary to control an outbreak.

Zafar et al. reported a 60% decrease from a mean of 155 cases per year to 67 per year by a combination of isolation enforcement, CDI surveillance, education of staff, phenolic disinfection of the environment, hand washing with soap containing 0.03% triclosan, and centralized re-processing of devices.

Struelens et al. observed a CDI incidence decline from 1.5 to 0.3 per 1,000 admissions (73% reduction) by early isolation precautions, active initial CDI surveillance, sufficient environmental surface disinfection, and early therapy of patients with CDI.

Additionally, re-isolation of patients presenting with diarrhoea at subsequent re-admission who were previously known to suffer from CDI may reduce attack rate of new nosocomial CDI cases, reducing the overall healthcare cost.

If daily clinical practice does not allow isolating symptomatic patients in single rooms on a regular ward, cohorting several patients or even on a separate cohort/isolation ward may be implemented. Staffs on CDI cohort wards may be better experienced in caring for such cases, cleaning protocols for CDI are easier put into operation in separate areas, materials used on a cohort ward are usually not used elsewhere, and there are less people entering a cohort ward unnecessarily. Another positive effect of cohorting is to localize environmental contamination to a small part of the hospital environment. This is different from having isolation rooms used for CDI dispersed throughout a hospital in numerous locations. Each failure of hygiene in these locations represents a high risk of extended local contamination and secondary cases. The overall effect may be to significantly reduce the burden of environmental contamination to a single focus (the cohort ward), where it is recognized and containable.

Apart from isolation procedures it is essential that patients suffering from any form of diarrhoea have a dedicated toilet or commode (i.e., should not be allowed to use general toilet facilities). Diarrhoeal stool samples should be processed as soon as possible to diagnose CDI. For practical purposes, patients with CDI can be sub-divided into risk groups, e.g., whether they are requiring treatment for CDI. This differentiation can be applied on both "regular wards" and on "CDI cohort wards".

One critical issue is how long isolation and other control measures need to be continued. Few data are available on the excretion of vegetative cells and spores during CDI. The consensus is that nosocomial outbreaks can be terminated if precautions are kept in place until bowel motion has returned to a normal level for at least 48 hours.

The environment of symptomatic patients with CDI is more frequently contaminated than that of asymptomatic CD carriers (49% vs. 29%; $p<.05$).

However, even after adequate therapy of CDI and return to normal bowel movements, patients may still show detectable CD toxins in faeces and continue to excrete CD. It is possible that 3% to 30% of stool samples remain toxin positive in patients treated with vancomycin or metronidazole and a correlation between stool cytotoxin levels and severity of gastrointestinal symptoms may not be present in all cases.

There is, however, no clinical value in retesting CDI cases once symptoms resolve, and therefore the carriage status of patients will usually be unknown.

Thus, the exact role of asymptomatic carriers for the spread of CD is currently unknown. Basic hygiene measures must therefore be an integral part of normal practice.

Furthermore, for most other pathogens alcohol-based hand hygiene is recommended, unless a major contamination of hand has occurred, and thus guidance must be provided locally when this method should be recommenced (see below).

5. Hand Hygiene

Standard hand hygiene practice is based on alcohol-based products, unless hands are in contact with body fluids or are visually contaminated. When hands are clearly contaminated, decontamination by soap-based washing has to be performed (possibly prior to hand disinfection). It is clear that the hands of health care workers (HCWs) are likely to become contaminated when caring for patients with positive CD cultures. Unfortunately, bacterial spores are not killed by alcohol, and indeed alcohol is used in the laboratory setting to select for CD spores. In an experimental study using hands of volunteers contaminated by CD, Barbut et al. have shown that 4% polyvidone soap was significantly more effective in reducing CD count than chlorhexidine or non-medicated soap, and these products were also more effective than alcohol-based products. In a recent observational study alcohol-based hand rub did not decrease the incidence of nosocomial CDI (mean 3-year incidence per 10,000 patient days before implementation of alcohol-based had rub: 3.24; mean 3-year incidence after: 3.38; p=.78), but one has to keep in mind that multiple factors are important for the successful prevention of CD transmission. In addition, Boyce et al. (2006) showed that a 10-fold increase in the use of alcohol-based had rub (3 to 30 l per 1,000 patient days; p<.001) within 4 years did not alter the incidence of CDI (1.74, 2.33, 1.14, and 1.18 per 1,000 patient days) in the corresponding time period. Bacterial spores can be removed from hands by the physical action of washing and rinsing hands, using either non-antimicrobial liquid soap or antiseptic substances such as chlorhexidine gluconate. In a cross-over study no differences in residual counts of CD on bare hands were observed comparing these the two agents, while others found a significantly improved removal of spores in 6/7 (86%) health care workers who used soap containing chlorhexidine gluconate in comparison with 2/16 (13%) using non-disinfectant soap (p<.01). Leischner et al. recently found that alcohol gels were significantly less effective at removing CD spores from the hands of volunteers when compared with hand washing with chlorhexidine (p<.009). However, there was a higher than expected reduction of spore counts following use of alcohol gels.

The role of the patient remains uncertain in the transmission of CD, although direct person-to-person transmission has been proposed. Endogenous infections can also occur in principle, even though there are some data suggesting that CD carriage is relatively protective for CDI. Thus hand washing by patients should be encouraged as usual especially after a toilet visit and before eating.

6. Protective Clothing

The use of gloves to protect the hands of health care workers from contamination is generally recommended by the HICPAC as a part of infection control standard precautions. In a prospective controlled trial of vinyl glove use to prevent CD spread, the incidence of CDI decreased significantly from 7.7 to 1.5 per 1,000 patient discharges within a six month intervention period. In another observational study, hands of all 4 members of staff using gloves remained free of CD spores.

This contrasts with a hand contamination rate of 7/15 (47%) for staff that did not use gloves and did not perform further hand hygiene measures (although the overall number of screened individuals was too low to reach statistical significance in this study; p=.13).

Of course, contaminated gloves need to be removed prior touching non-contaminated surfaces. Contamination of hands may occur during removal of contaminated gloves. Therefore, hand washing and drying remains important regardless of previous glove use.

The use of gowns or aprons represents an additional measure of infection control standard precautions to prevent contamination of the regular working cloths by infectious agents, and should therefore be used when caring for known CDI cases. Only few data exist on the use of gowns to specifically prevent inter-patient spread of CD. Perry et al. compared the level of contamination of nurses´ uniforms before and after duty in 57 different staff on different ward areas and working shifts. Although the authors recommend wearing appropriate plastic aprons to reduce the levels of contamination on a uniform in principle, it remains unclear to what extend this was performed during the study time period. Because a professional laundry service was unavailable in that hospital, uniforms were laundered by staff at home. Unfortunately, there is no further information on storage conditions of cleaned uniforms or on possible ironing of uniforms when dry. CD was cultured from uniforms of 4 nurses after work that had been CD negative before duty. However, clothes of 7 additional nurses were CD positive before duty already. If such difficulties arise, one may also consider using disposable clothing instead or using an external professional hospital-laundry service. However, it should be emphasised that recovery of CD from uniforms could simply represent either direct or indirect contamination (e.g., for the environment) and does not necessarily implicate such fomites in transmission. Optimal hand hygiene and barrier precautions will counteract any risk that may be associated with CD contamination of uniforms.

7. Environmental Cleaning

It is well-documented that environmental contamination occurs during CDI especially if patients suffer from large amounts of liquid stool or stool incontinence. Remarkably heavy contamination takes place on floors, commodes, toilets, bed pans, and bed frames. The actual degree of spore recovery from environmental swabs may directly correlate with the incidence of CDI, although a recent molecular epidemiological study was unable to determine whether environmental contamination is the consequence of CDI rather than the source of infection, primarily because of the often clonal nature of nosocomial CDI.

Once released in the environment, CD spores may persist for long periods (months or years) due to their resistance to drying, heat, and disinfection substances.

There is good evidence that environmental contamination can play a role in CD transmission. Wet cleaning using detergents only may be insufficient for decontamination purpose, and there is a need for effective and user-friendly sporocidal products.

Various disinfection substances are available to inactivate CD spores but the choice of substance may influence formation of spores e.g., non-chlorine based products may enhance sporulation. Sporulation levels of outbreak strains such as type 027 or type 001 may also exceed those of other CD strains. In the current CDC/HICHPAC guidelines no specific disinfection agent for standard environmental control of CD is recommended (i.e., in the absence of known CDI cases).

Hypochlorite-based disinfectants are recommended by the HICPAC in patient-care areas where CDI surveillance indicates ongoing CD transmission and are frequently used in many hospitals.

Of potential importance, chlorine-based products are significantly less likely to enhance sporolation of CD strains in vitro. Compared to cleaning with a detergent only, hypochlorite use at a concentration of 1,000 parts per million (ppm) was associated with a significant reduction in the incidence of CDI. The use of phosphate-buffered hypochlorite (1,600 ppm available chlorine) may be more effective against CD spores than unbuffered hypochlorite solution (500 ppm chlorine). A possible disadvantage that needs to be considered in the choice of disinfection substance is the corrosive nature of hypochlorite on metal surfaces. Also, hypochlorite alone products are not suitable for removing organic matter. Products containing a combination of hypochlorite and a detergent may overcome this problem.

Quaternary ammonium (QA) solutions have also been used for environmental CD decontamination. However, while no differences in the CDI incidence were observed in patient care areas with low CDI incidences (neurosurgical intensive care unit: 3.0 per 1,000 patient days and general medicine ward: 1.3 respectively), the change from QA to unbuffered 1:10 hypochlorite led to a significant reduction in the CDI incidence (8.6 to 3.3 per 1,000 patient days) in bone marrow transplant patients; the incidence of CDI increased to 8.1 per 1,000 patient days after reverting back to QA cleaning.

Hydrogen peroxide vapour recently showed efficacy for environmental CD eradication. However, this method is expensive and involves having to vacate and seal clinical areas.

Glutaraldehyde is a disinfection substance known to be effective in inactivation of CD spores and has been used for that purpose in nosocomial CD outbreaks. However, due to its risks to human health and for environmental safety grounds it should not be used freely for environmental decontamination. Peracetic acid 0.2% (Perasafe®) is more active in vitro than chlorine-releasing agents such as sodium dichloroisocyanurate (NaDCC) at 1,000 ppm available chlorine. This high-level disinfection substance may also be a substitute for glutaraldehyde and has also shown better effectiveness than tertiary amines although long contact times of 15 to 20 minutes are required. Peracetic acid has not been used for environmental decontamination. An alternative concept was shown recently using a liquid ready to use oxygen releaser as continous application in a high endemic CDI area within a hospital department. Hell et al. compared the usual daily use of a quaternary ammonia compound with additional oxygen-releasing sporocide –manual preparation-for targeted disinfection with a daily service decontamination of all services with an oxygen-releasing sporocide. They could reduce the *C. difficile* prevalence, especially in patients over 70 years old. The explanation is that the continuous disinfection might lower the environmental contamination by *C. difficile*. This concept is interesting and could replace the concept of targeted disinfection in this context.

When performing environmental decontamination of CD spores, one has also to keep in mind that the maximum permissible concentration of certain disinfection substances (e.g., chlorine) for environmental disinfection may differ depending upon diverse national regulations. Each organization responsible for cleaning of the hospital should have specific protocols for the treatment of rooms of CDI patients.

At least once a day all objects with frequent contact to hands of patients and staff, such as tables, chairs, or telephones, should become disinfected.

In clinical practice it has been shown to be essential to educate the cleaning personnel on regular basis; especially emphasizing the difference in cleaning and disinfection of areas used by CDI patients, in contrast to those for cases colonised/infected by MRSA or other multi drug resistant pathogens.

8. Medical Devices

Use of disposable equipment whenever possible to limit spread of pathogens that lead to heavy environmental contamination such as CD has proven effective to control CDI outbreaks. Due to the intestinal habitat of CD, rectal thermometers seem likely to play an important role in bacterial transmission. Although electronic thermometers do not necessarily need to become CD contaminated, there are numerous investigations in which positive CD cultures were obtained from these devices. For example, Samore et al. showed that 3 of 38 (7.9%) thermometers became contaminated by CD during use. Shared rectal thermometers should therefore be replaced by individual thermometers, or alternatively consider a change to tympanic thermometers by which a 40% risk reduction for CDI has been achieved. An even greater risk reduction (56%; p=.26) was accomplished by the use of disposable thermometers instead of shared electronic in a randomized crossover study.

There have been no reports of endoscopes transmitting CD in the hospital setting. However, Hughes et al. found that 10 of 15 (67%) of endoscopes were CD culture positive immediately after use. Since single use is not an option for such expensive equipment, endoscopes need to be re-processed adequately before further use. Disinfection of endoscopes by alkaline glutaraldehyde solution 2% or by peracetic acid was capable of CD spores inactivation at an exposure time of 5 to 10 minutes after thorough cleaning.

Therefore endoscopes have to be properly cleaned with adequate sporocidal disinfectants or by automated chemo-thermal reprocessing, as it should be the standard in most hospitals nowadays.

Additional devices that have been found CD positive may comprise blood pressure cuffs or oximeters. Although tested negative in one investigation, equipment for enemas may also count as a critical medical device in this context. Generally, instruments and equipment including stethoscopes and blood pressure cuffs should be used patient specific and cleaned carefully.

9. Antibiotics

Antibiotic therapy or prophylaxis alters the colonic flora and allows *C. difficile* to flourish and cause diarrhoea. Antibiotics are the most important predisposing factor for CDI. However, a systematic review of the studies that have examined the risk of CDI associated with different antibiotics concluded that most are flawed because of failure to control for potential confounding factors. Exposure to CD, antimicrobial polypharmacy and duration of antibiotics are frequently not addressed as causes of bias. Also, host humoral immunity to CD toxin(s) and the antibiotic susceptibility of the CD strain are likely to influence the risk of

CDI development. It is not surprising therefore that there are conflicting studies in respect of the risk of CDI associated with specific antibiotics or classes.

Almost any antibiotic may caused CDI, but broad spectrum cephalosporines (in particular third spectrum cephalosporins), broad spectrum penicillins and clindamyin are most frequently implicated. Since 2000, fluoroquinolones have also been identified as possible risk factors for CDI, including CDI caused by the new hypervirulent fluoroquinolones resistant PCR ribotype 027. Conversely, ureidopenicillins (with or without beta lactamase inhibitors) appear to have low propensity to induce CDI.

In many hospital patients receive combinations of antibiotics or multiple antibiotic courses. A cochrane analysis indicated that antibiotic use is unnecessary or inappropriate in as many as 50% of cases and that interventions to improve antibiotic prescribing can reduce hospital acquired infections, and most notably CDI. The exact duration of risk to develop CDI after antibiotic exposure still needs to be determined, but it is has been demonstrated that the duration of therapy also influences this risk. Aggressive antibiotic restriction of high risk antibiotics, reducing polypharmacy, prevention of long duration of therapy and avoiding inappropriate prescribing are the first steps to decrease a high incidence rate of CDI. Some measures to achieve this goal comprise automatic stop dates, electronic prescribing, banning of certain antibiotic classes, prescriber education and production of guidelines or policies. There is also a need for continuous training of medical staff on appropriate antimicrobial use and feedback of success, since systematic reviews have shown the positive effect of audit and feedback in helping healthcare workers implement evidence based practice. In a controlled interrupted prospective trial on a geriatric ward Fowler et al. showed that feedback on improved antibiotic prescribing can be successful in reducing the use of broad spectrum antibiotics (amoxicillin/clavulanic acid and cephalosporins) in favour of more narrow spectrum antibiotics (benzyl penicillin, trimethoprime, and amoxicillin). In consequence, this changed antimicrobial treatment regimen led to a significant decrease in CDI ($p=.009$). A definition of so-called "alert antimicrobials", drugs that need a patient-specific feedback by an authorized person (e.g., the hospital's pharmacist), may also be useful to further improve antibiotic use in the hospital.

Use of antibiotics is believed to lead to disturbance of the normal gastrointestinal flora. In consequence, this status may predispose for diarrhoea after bacterial selection of CD. Probiotics (bacteria and yeasts) are thought to restore the balance of the gut flora when delivered orally to the patients. At present, only few data exist on the interference of probiotics and CDI. There are some randomized controlled trials that show a significant reduction in the risk of antibiotic-associated diarrhoea by the use of *Saccharomyces boulardii*, but newer studies using *S. boulardii* or *Lactobacillus GG* failed to confirm these findings. Two recently published systematic reviews did not show sufficient evidence for the general recommendation of the use of probiotics for CDI prevention or treatment.

10. Specific Measures in Outbreaks

The key to reducing infection risk is prevention of transmission of CD. When an increased number of cases of CD are identified, infection control strategy should be informed by risk assessment that takes into account the background epidemiological pattern and the risk category of the patients involved. Outbreak situations require immediate action to control the situation.

Usually, this is associated with a combination of different infection control measures. Hence, the effectiveness of each individual measure is hard to determine. First of all, of all recommendations that apply in the endemic setting, adherence needs to be strengthened. These measures include strict separation of symptomatic patients, education of staff, increased awareness of CDI, and restricting use of risk-antibiotics such as broad spectrum penicillins, third generation of cephalosporines, clindamycine and fluoroquinolones. In addition, there are specific measures that may be helpful in a nosocomial CD epidemic.

Cohort nursing of confirmed CDI patients, and isolation of suspected CDI cases before laboratory test results are available have been shown to be effective during a CD outbreak. In a recently published nosocomial epidemic of CD on a geriatric ward Cherifi et al. reported that cohorting of infected patients on one ward with a single medical team was a key way of limiting the spread of infection. The potential to establish a dedicated nursing team for CDI patients will need to be considered alongside competing pressures locally.

Similarly, the measures used in outbreaks may depend on the wards involved and on the clinical severity of cases. However, a written local protocol must exist so that early adoption and/or review of control measures occur when CDI cases are identified.

5. Treatment of *C. Difficile* Infection: Current and Future Strategies

Recommendations for the Treatment of CDI (Bauer et al., 2009)

In the case of mild CDI (stool frequency < 4 times daily; no signs of severe CDI), clearly induced by the use of antibiotics, it is acceptable to stop the inducing antibiotic and observe the clinical response, but patients must be followed very closely for any signs of clinical deterioration and placed on therapy immediately if this occurs.

Antiperistaltic and opiate agents should be avoided, especially in the acute setting. There is no evidence that switching to 'low-risk' antibiotics when the antibiotic treatment that triggered the episode of CDI cannot be stopped or stopping gastric acid suppressants is effective. It seems rational, however, to always strive to use antibiotics covering a spectrum no broader than necessary. When the inciting antibiotic cannot be stopped, antibiotic treatment for CDI cannot be avoided.

In all other cases than mild CDI medical treatment for CDI should be started. Antibiotics may be started awaiting diagnostics when there is sufficient clinical suspicion. We recommend treatment of an initial episode of CDI with the following antibiotics, according to disease severity (implementation category between brackets; coding opened in Table 1), when oral therapy is possible:

- non-severe: metronidazole 500 mg tid orally for 10 days (A-I)
- severe: vancomycin 125 mg qid orally for 10 days (A-I)

CDI is judged to be severe when one of the markers of severe disease mentioned under 'definitions' is present.

When oral therapy is impossible, we recommend the following antibiotics, according to disease severity (implementation category between brackets):

- non-severe: metronidazole 500 mg tid intravenously for 10 days (A-III)
- severe: metronidazole 500 mg tid intravenously for 10 days + (A-III)
- retention enema: vancomycin 500 mg in 100 ml of normal saline every 4–12 h (or vancomycin 500 mg qid by nasogastric tube (C-III))

Oral vancomycin may be replaced by teicoplanin 200 mg bid, if available.

There is no evidence that various genotypes of *C. difficile* should be treated differently if disease severity does not differ.

Recommendations for Surgical Treatment of CDI

Colectomy must be performed to treat CDI in any of the following situations:

- perforation of the colon
- systemic inflammation and deteriorating clinical condition not responding to antibiotic therapy; this includes the clinical diagnoses of toxic megacolon and severe ileus

Since mortality from colectomy in patients with advanced disease is high, it is recommendable to operate in less severe stage. No strict recommendations as to the timing of colectomy can be given. Serum lactate may, inter alia, serve as a marker for severity, where one should attempt to operate before the threshold of 5.0 mmol/l.

Recommendations for Medical Treatment of Recurrent CDI

Observational data (Pépin et al., 2006) suggest that the incidence of a second recurrence after treatment of a first recurrence with oral metronidazole or vancomycin is similar. Therefore, we recommend treating a first recurrence of CDI as a first episode, unless disease has progressed from non-severe to severe. We recommend treatment of recurrent CDI with the following antibiotics (implementation category between brackets):

First recurrence:
See Recommendations for medical treatment of initial CDI.

Second recurrence and subsequent recurrences:

If oral therapy is possible:

- vancomycin 125 mg qid orally for at least 10 days (B-II)
- fidaxomicin 200mg bid orally for 10 days (B-II) (recurrence rate is proven to be lower compared to vancomycin)

If oral therapy is impossible:

- metronidazole 500 mg tid intravenously for 10 – 14 days + (A-III)
- retention enema: vancomycin 500 mg in 100 ml of normal saline every 4 – 12 h (C-III) or vancomycin 500 mg qid by nasogastric tube (C-III)

Recommendation for Prophylaxis of CDI

Currently, there is no evidence that medical prophylaxis for CDI is efficacious and therefore we do not recommend prophylactic antibiotics. Of course, other preventive measures should be taken, such as hand hygiene of hospital personnel, prompt isolation of patients suspected of having CDI and prudent use of antibiotics.

6. Future Strategies and Trends

New Pharmacological Agents

Due to the emergence of the highly virulent NAP1/BI/027 strain over the past few years, the response to metronidazole is decreased (Musher et al., 2005; Louie et al., 2007) leading to an interest in new treatments. The greatest promise is with agents used to interrupt relapses.

In this category ramoplanin, rifaximin, nitazoxanide, fidaxomicin, toxin-binding agents (tolevamer), probiotics (*Saccharomyces boulardii* and *Lactobacillus ramosus*), immune agents (toxoid vaccine and hyperimmune globulin) and fecal transplantation have all shown activity against CDI. The summary regarding the new treatment strategies of CDI is shown in Table 2.

Ramoplanin

Ramoplanin is a lipoglycodepsipeptide antibiotic manufactured by Oscient Pharmaceuticals that acts by blocking peptidoglycan synthesis by binding to lipid II. It has shown bactericidal activity against aerobic and anaerobic gram-positive bacteria such as *Enterococcus* app. and *Clostridium difficile* (Farver et al., 2005; Fulco and Hedge, 2005). Freeman et al. (2005) observed similar efficacy between vancomycin and ramoplanin but with more efficacy in killing spores both in citron and in vivo in hamster gut.

In a phase II multi centric trial the authors were able to establish a reasonable efficacy with limited side effects but the trial had insufficient power to establish non-inferiority to vancomycin (Musher et al., 2005).

Table 1. Strength of recommendation and quality of evidence according to the Canadian Task Force on the Periodic Health Examination

Strength of recommendation:
a. good evidence to support a recommendation
b. moderate evidence to support a recommendation
c. poor evidence to support a recommendation
Quality of evidence:
I. evidence from ≥ 1 properly randomized, controlled trial
II. evidence from ≥ 1 well-designed clinical trial, without randomization; from cohort or case-controlled analytic studies (preferably from ≥ centre); from multiple time-series; or from dramatic results from uncontrolled experiments
III. evidence from opinions of respected authorities, based on clinical experience, descriptive studies, or reports of expert committees

The doses were used were 200mg or 400 mg ramoplanin twice a day or vancomycin 125 mg four times a day for 10 days. The rate of cure at the end of therapy was 83-85% in the ramoplanin group versus 86% in the vancomycin group. The rate of relapses being 26.1% (ramoplanin 200mg), 21.7% (ramoplanin 400mg) and 20.8% (vancomycin 125mg). Mortality rates were similar in all groups and not attributable to the medicines. Larger trials are needed to gather evidence for establishing the role of this antibiotic in treatment of CDI.

Rifaximin

Rifaximin is a nonabsorbed (bioavailability <0.4%) rifamycin that concentrates in the intestinal tract and acts by inhibiting bacterial RNA synthesis. (Jiang et al., 2000) The drug appears to be particularly useful in treating and preventing recurrent CDI related to in-vitro activity of the drug against strains of *C. difficile* or the high drug concentrations available in the colon or both. In an open-label study, Boero et al. (1990) compared rifaximin 200 mg 3 times daily for 10 days with oral vancomycin 500 mg twice daily for 10 days in 20 patients. Rifaximin was found to be effective in 90%, while vancomycin was successful in all (100%) patients who received it.

In order to prevent the recurrence of CDI, rifaximin can be given 2 weeks after completion of standard therapy (Garey et al., 2009; Johnson et al., 2007). Johnson et al. (2009) later reported post-vancomycin strategies with rifaximin treatment in six patients with multiple recurrences of CDI. Four of the six patients (67%) had no further diarrhea episodes, but two patients failed shortly after or during the rifaximin treatment. *C. difficile* isolates from one of the two patients who failed treatment had an MIC of >256 ug/ml to rifampin. Authors concluded that serial therapy with vancomycin, followed by rifaximin remains an option for some patients with multiple CDI recurrences. Polymorphous forms of rifaximin, processes for their production and use in medicinal preparations are successfully described in US Patent 7045620 (Viscomi et al., 2006). However, emergence of resistance may be a problem.

Rifalazil, a newer benzoxazinorifamycin, is another potent rifamycin with fewer clinical data reported. The MIC_{50} and MIC_{90} for a total of 141 isolates range from 0.002 to 0.0075 μg/ml and 0.004 to 0.03 μg/ml, respectively (Hecht et al., 2007). The drug has a prolonged half-life permitting once-daily administration.

Nitazoxanide

Nitazoxanide is a new thiazolide antiparasitic agent that has excellent activity in treating both interstitial protozoal and helminthic infection. It interferes with pyruvate-ferredoxin oxidoreductase (PFOR) enzyme dependent electron transport reaction, which is necessary for anaerobic metabolism. The drug acts by blocking anaerobic metabolism.

In vitro, nitazoxanide has shown excellent activity against *C. difficile*. In one study, the 90% MIC (MIC_{90}) of the toxigenic strains of *C.* difficile was 0.5 μg/ml for nitazoxanide, which was identical to the MIC_{90} of metronidazole and vancomycin (McVay and Rolfe, 2000). Other investigators have reported lower MICs, ranging from 0.06 to 0.125 μg/ml (Dubreuil et al., 1996).

In a larger, prospective, randomized, double-blind study, nitazoxanide was compared with metronidazole in treatment of hospitalized patients with *C.* difficile colitis (Musher et al., 2006). In this study 44 patients received metronidazole 250 mg 4 times daily for 10 days, 49 received nitazoxanide 500 mg twice daily for 7 days, and 49 received nitazoxanide 500 mg twice daily for 10 days.

The per-protocol results showed an 82.4% response rate in the metronidazole group compared with 89.5% in the nitazoxanide 7- and 10-day groups combined ($p = 0.20$). This study also evaluated for recurrence rate for 31 days after the start of treatment. A sustained response rate was demonstrated in 19 of 33 (57.6%) patients who received metronidazole for 10 days compared with 25 of 38 (65.8%) patients who received 7 days of nitazoxanide and 26 of 35 (74.3%) patients who received 10 days of nitazoxanide.

In another randomized double blind study, Nitazomanide was compared against vancomycin in CDI. Sustained response rates were 78% (18 of 23 patients) for the vancomycin group, and 89% (16 of 18 patients) for the nitazoxanide group (Musher et al., 2009).

These studies support nitazoxanide compared with metronidazole and vancomycin as a superior drug for both initial and sustained treatment of CDI in hospitalized patients. However, the efficacy of nitrazoxanide used specifically in chemotherapy related CDI is unknown. US Patent no 20080254010 describes above described methods including nitrazoxande in treating CDI associated diarrhea (Sasser and Cousin, 2008).

Fidaxomicin (Tiacumicin B, OPT-80, PAR-101)

Fidaxomicin (OPT-80) is an18-membered macrolide antibiotic. This antibiotic has demonstrated in vitro and in vivo activity against *C. difficile* and has a favorable pharmacokinetic profile for its potential use in CDI as demonstrated in a hamster model. Swanson et al. (1991) found the MICs against 15 strains of *C. difficile* were 0.12 to 0.25 μg/ml for fidaxomicin and 0.5 to 1 μg/ml for vancomycin and achieved high concentrations in the cecum, but not the serum, of hamsters after oral administration) (Louie et al., 2006).

Fidaxomicin, unlike metronidazole and vancomycin, does not affect the normal colonic flora which provides colonization resistance against Clostridium difficile. The drug is well tolerated with oral administration and showed promising results in a phase 1 trial with a dose of 400 mg/d. Furthermore, the risk of relapse with fidaxomicin therapy is far less (only 5%) compared to either metronidazole or vancomycin (Swanson et al., 1991). Louie et al. (2011)] reported the results of the phase III trial of the drug, funded by Optimer pharmaceutical in February, 2011. A total of 629 patients were evaluated in a randomized trial treated for CDI with either fidaxomicin 200mg twice daily for 10 days or vancomycin 125mg four times a day for 10 days. The rates of cure with fidaxomicin were non-inferior to vancomycin in both modified intention-to-treat analysis (88.2% vs 85.8%) and the pre-protocol analysis (13.3% vs 24.0% p=0.004). There was lower rate of recurrence seen in patients with non-NAP1/027 strains when treated with fidaxomicin (7.8% vs 25.5%). Furthermore significantly higher rates of resolution of diarrhea in a shorter time span was seen with fidaxomicin as opposed to vancomycin (74.6% vs 64.1% p=0.006; 58 hours for resolution of symptoms for fidaxomicin versus 78 hours in vancomycin). The side effect profile was similar for the two agents.

Toxin Binding Agents-Tolevamer

Tolevamer is a high molecular weight, styrene sulfonate polymer. It is given orally for the treatment of CDI. Tolevamer covalently binds and neutralizes toxins A and B. By this mechanism, it may prevent CDI-associated injury to the gastrointestinal tract without disrupting the reestablishment of normal bacterial growth (Chiu et al., 2008). The efficacy of Tolevamir was evaluated in a multicenter, multinational, double-blind phase 2 study [37] in patients with mild to moderately severe CDI associated diarrhea.

Patients were randomized to 1 of 3 arms: tolevamer 3 g/day (n = 97), tolevamer 6 g/day (n = 95), or oral vancomycin 500 mg/day (n = 97) for 14 days. In the per-protocol analysis, with the primary endpoint being resolution of diarrhea, tolevamer 6 g/day was not inferior to vancomycin, with 58 of 70 (83%) patients achieving the primary endpoint versus 73 of 80 (91%) patients in the vancomycin-treated group. However, the 3 g/day dose of tolevamer was found to be inferior to vancomycin treatment. Interestingly, Louie et al. also found a trend toward lower recurrence rate in patients treated with tolevamer 6 g/day versus those who received vancomycin, 10% vs 19%, respectively; p = 0.19. In patients with metastatic disease where immune function is already compromised, tolevamir may be a much-needed alternative to antibiotic treatment. However, in two subsequent phase 3 trials, tolevamer was inferior to vancomycin and metronidazole for initial therapy (Chiu et al., 2008). In early 2008, a non-inferiority study versus vancomycin or metronidazole found that about half of the patient in the tolevamer group did not complete the treatment, versus 25% in the vancomycin and 29% in the metronidazole groups. Clostridium difficle infection recurrence in patients reaching clinical success was reduced significantly by tolevamer (6% recurrence rate), vancomycin (18%) and metronidazole (19%). However, the significant reduction in recurrence rate seen in the tolevamer group may in part be attributed to its high drop-out rate. The development of the agent was halted since tolevamer did not reach its primary endpoint in this study.

Immunotherapy

In *C. difficile* infections, patients who develop serum antitoxin A immunoglobulin G (IgG) titers in response to exposure tend to be 48 times less likely to develop diarrhea than those who do not mount a response (Owens, 2006). In immunodeficient patients, intravenous immunoglobulins (IVIG) introduce a level of passive immunity. In a study of 5 children with relapsing *C. difficile* colitis and low baseline serum levels of antitoxin A IgG, Leung et al. (1991) found that administration of IVIG 400 mg/kg every 3 weeks for 4-6 months was associated with a marked increase in serum antitoxin antibody and resolution of recurrent diarrhea. McPherson et al. (2006) published a retrospective review of 14 patients given adjunctive IVIG (150-400 mg/kg once or twice, with the second dose given 3 weeks later) in addition to conventional treatment and found a response to treatment by stool normalization in 64% (n = 9) of patients with severe, refractory, or recurrent disease.

Table 2. Summary of new treatments for *Clostridium difficile* infection

	Mechanism of Action	Clinical Activity	Results
Ramoplanin	Inhibits peptidoglycan synthesis by binding to Lipid II, an intermediate required for membrane formation.	Produces bactericidal effect against aerobic and anaerobic gram positive bacteria	Current trial has had insufficient power to establish non-inferiority to vancomycin. *Rate of Cure (at the end of therapy):* 200/400 mg ramoplanin: 83-85% 125 mg vancomycin: 86% *Rate of Relapse:* 200 mg Ramoplanin: 26.1% 125 mg Vancomycin: 20.8% *Mortality Rate:* Similar in all groups Larger trials need to be conducted in order to establish effectiveness of this drug.
Rifaximin	Inhibits bacterial RNA synthesis	Treats and prevents recurrent CDI related to in-vitro activity of the drug against strains of *C. difficile*	Rifaximin (200 mg, 3 times daily, 10 days): 90% effective Vancomycin (500 mg, 2 times daily, 10 days): successful in all (100%) patients who received it
Nitazoxanide	Inhibits pyruvate-ferredoxin oxidoreductase, an enzyme (necessary for anaerobic metabolism)	In vitro, nitazoxanide has shown excellent activity against *C. difficile*	Metronidazole (250 mg, 4 times daily, 10 days): 82.4% response rate Nitazoxanide (500 mg, 2 times daily, 7/10 days) 89.5% response rate ($p = 0.20$) *Recurrance rate (31 days):* Metronidazole (10 days): 57.6% sustained response rate *Nitazoxanide (10 days):* 74.3% (26/35) sustained response rate 89% (16/18) sustained response Vancomycin Results support nitazoxanide as a superior drug for both initial and sustained treatment of CDI in hospitalized patients.

	Mechanism of Action	Clinical Activity	Results
Fidoxomicin (Tiacumicin B, OPT-80, PAR-101)	Inhibits bacterial RNA synthesis by RNA polymerase	Demonstrates in vitro/ in vivo activity specific to C. difficile Does not affect normal colonic flora	Oral administration tolerated well Randomized trial [n=629] Fidaxomicin 200mg twice daily versus Vancomycin 125mg orally four times daily Rate of cure non-inferior to vancomycin Lower recurrence rate in patients with non-NAP1/027 strains, treated with fidaxomicin (7.8% vs. 25.5%) Higher rate of resolution of diarrhea in shorter time span Side effects similar to vancomycin
Tolevamer	Tolevamer covalently binds and neutralizes toxins A and B	Prevent CDI-associated injury to the gastrointestinal tract without disrupting the reestablishment of normal bacterial growth 80	Phase II study showed Tolevamer 6 g/day was not inferior to vancomycin. Patients with metastatic disease where immune function is already compromised, Tolevamir may be an alternative to antibiotic treatment. However, Since tolevamer did not reach its primary endpoint the development was halted.
Immunotherapy	Intravenous immunoglobulins (IVIG) introduce a level of passive immunity.	Binds to toxin A and Toxin B to neutralize toxin effects. Additive advantage when use with antibiotics	IVIG 400 mg/kg every 3 weeks for 4-6 months was associated with a marked increase in serum antitoxin antibody and resolution of recurrent diarrhea Favorable outcomes with use of monoclonal antibodies in addition to metronidazole or vancomycin in patients with CDI. There was a reduced risk of recurrence seen with combined administration of CD A1 and CD B1 monoclonal human antibodies (7% in study group vs 25% in placebo group $p < 0.001$).

Although some isolated reports have suggested a benefit of IVIG therapy in refractory cases or in severe cases in patients who are unable to develop an immune response alone or as adjunct to traditional therapy, less consistent results have been reported regarding the use of intravenous immunoglobulin to treat patients with severe, refractory infection who had not had a response to standard therapy and for whom colectomy was being considered.

A recent phase II trial comprising 200 screened patients has reported favorable outcomes with use of monoclonal antibodies in addition to metronidazole or vancomycin in patients with CDI. There was a reduced risk of recurrence seen with combined administration of two monoclonal antibodies against toxin A (CD A1) and and toxin B (CD B1) (7% in study group vs 25% in placebo group $p < 0.001$).

In many cases the patients susceptible to Clostridium difficile infections are suffering from lowered defense capabilities such as young or old age, lowered immunocompetence, or severe diseases such as malignancies. The latter situation is often encountered by the physicians dealing with severely sick patients.

The survey on C. difficile infections in Czech and Slovak Republics is giving the following ideas on the progression of the diseases where the malignancy is enforced by the bacterial infection (Weinbergerova, 2014).

Further considerations on the immunocompromised patients and their susceptibilities to bacterial infections is in the Chapter 14.

The combined administration of CDA1 and CDB1 human monoclonal antibodies in addition to antibiotics significantly reduced the recurrence of *C.* difficile infection. Larger studies are needed to confirm the findings of this phase II trial according to the authors (Martin et al., 2011). US patient no 6680168 describes the method of passive immunization against *C. difficile* infection (Thomas Jr. et al., 2004).

The published data regarding the efficacy of active immunization against *C. difficile* are even more sparse. Clinical trials using a toxoid vaccine (Acambis; Phase I) and monoclonal antibodies to toxin A and toxin B (Medarex; Phase II) are ongoing for prevention of *C. difficile* colitis. The vaccine is given in 3 doses (days 1, 8, and 30) and has a favorable side effect profile. Previous studies were done among healthy volunteers, and much of the data available supporting the use of intravenous immune globulin is from limited to uncontrolled studies and therefore at present it is not clear whether the vaccine will be effective in elderly, debilitated patients.

In addition to the toxoid vaccine against toxins A and B, research is being done to develop a carbohydrate conjugate vaccine against the NAP1/027 strains as well as immunization with recombinant Bacillus subtilis spores (Permpoonpattana et al., 2011).

US patents described active and passive immunizations methods for CDI in detail (Thomas et al., 2006). More recently, a vaccine for the treatment or prophylaxis of *C. difficile* associated disease comprises a *C. difficile* gene or a *C. difficile* peptide/polypeptide or a derivative or fragment or mutant or variant thereof which is immunogenic in humans has been made for prophylaxis. The gene encodes a *C. difficile* surface layer protein, SlpA or variant or homologue thereof. The peptide/polypeptide is a *C. difficile* surface layer protein, SlpA or variant or homologue thereof. The vaccine may comprise a chimeric nucleic acid sequence.

US patent application 20030054009 describes application of *C. difficile* vaccine for prophylaxis (Windle et al., 2003).

Fecal Transplantation: For Severe – and Severe Recurrent Cases

Finally, case reports and case series have shown success with administration of donor stool or 'synthetic stool' (bacterial mixtures), either by naso-gastric tube or colonoscopy. Very recently Els van Nood et al. reported a successful treatment in recurrent patients by comparing three treatment groups. Of 16 patients in the infusion group, 13 (81%) had resolution of *C. difficile*–associated diarrhea after the first infusion.

The 3 remaining patients received a second infusion with feces from a different donor, with resolution in 2 patients. Resolution of *C. difficile* infection occurred in 4 of 13 patients (31%) receiving vancomycin alone and in 3 of 13 patients (23%) receiving vancomycin with bowel lavage ($P<0.001$ for both comparisons with the infusion group).

No significant differences in adverse events among the three study groups were observed except for mild diarrhea and abdominal cramping in the infusion group on the infusion day. After donor-feces infusion, patients showed increased fecal bacterial diversity, similar to that in healthy donors, with an increase in *Bacteroidetes* species and clostridium clusters IV and XIVa and a decrease in *Proteobacteria* species.

The authors concluded that the infusion of donor feces was significantly more effective for the treatment of recurrent *C. difficile* infection than the use of vancomycin.

But there are no reported studies yet comparing fidaxomicin with fecal transplant and the future will show if experts in the field are able to establish well accepted protocols both for a broad range of institutions and health authorities and regulatory authorities in Europe and the US.

7. Probiotics As Adjunctive Therapy

Adjunctive therapies for refractory disease include efforts to replenish colonic flora with the use of orally administered probiotics, usually *Lactobacillus* species or *Saccharomyces boulardii*. A recent systematic review of randomized controlled trials to evaluate the efficacy of probiotic therapies identified only two treatment studies that showed some benefit of *S. boulardii*, although the benefit was restricted to subgroups of patients with severe or recurrent CDI A more recent randomized, controlled study found some benefit of a yogurt containing *Lactobacillus* spp. and *Streptococcus thermophilus* in the prevention of antibiotic-associated diarrhea and CDI in patients over 50 years of age, although the applicability of the study has been questioned due to highly selective exclusion and inclusion criteria. With respect to the future of probiotics for CDAD, Hell et al. (2013) have provided some good insights, as well as interesting initial clinical data. They postulated that a multi-strain probiotic, resembling a healthy human microbiota, would be most effective for treating CDAD (Hell et al., 2013). Therefore, these investigators developed a probiotic mixture (Ecologic® AAD) comprised of several *Bifidobacterium* and *Lactobacillus strains*, as well as *Enterococcus faecium*. In a small series of 10 patients (five with recurrent disease) excellent results were obtained in all evaluable patients with *C. difficile* infection, following combined treatment with the multi-strain probiotic plus vancomycin (Hell et al., 2013). This type of therapeutic paradigm seems to represent a logical future scientific approach for probiotic treatment in CDAD.

But there is still a concern over the safety of probiotics in severely ill or immunocompromised patients with several reports of *S. boulardii* fungemia and less frequent reports of sepsis due to *Lactobacillus* spp. In general, there is growing evidence to support the routine use of probiotics to prevent or treat adjunctively CDI.

Conclusion: Future Strategies in Prevention

1 Antibiotic resistance and *C. difficile* epidemic strains often show a typical resistance pattern but are in general not resistant against the most important drugs used for treatment like oral vancomycin and metronidazol. Fidaxomicin is the most promising substance due to its highly selective mechanism against *C. difficile* and its very low potential of resistance induction.

2 Controlling the usage of antibiotics with continuous CDI monitoring: in general no ban against specific antibiotics but against the general amount of all antibiotics consumed in hospitals; in some specific situation like CDI outbreaks with one hypervirulent strain like the PCR ribotype 027 it makes sense to ban the quinolones for a certain time period.

3 Hygienic measures: Infection control measures in the hospitals still have to be developed but the most important thing is keeping to the simple rules of thoroughly cleaning your hands after direct and indirect contact with symptomatic patients and thoroughly cleaning the surfaces adjacent to the patient twice a day. If hospital staff is sticking to these rules in most circumstances is not necessary to use routine or targeted sporicidal disinfection of the surfaces around the patients.

References

Aldape, M. J., Bryant, A. E., Stevens, D. L. *Clostridium sordellii* infection: epidemiology, clinical findings, and current perspectives on diagnosis and treatment. *Clin. Infect. Dis.* 2006 Dec. 1;43(11), 1436-1446.

Bauer, M. P., Kuijper, E. J., van Dissel, J. T. European Society of Clinical Microbiology and Infectious Diseases. European Society of Clinical Microbiology and Infectious Diseases (ESCMID): treatment guidance document for *Clostridium difficile* infection (CDI). *Clin. Microbiol. Infect.* 2009 Dec.;15(12), 1067-1079.

Bauer, M. P., Notermans, D. W., van Benthem, B. H., Brazier, J. S., Wilcox, M. H., Rupnik, M., Monnet, D. L., van Dissel, J. T., Kuijper, E. J. ECDIS Study Group. *Clostridium difficile* infection in Europe: a hospital-based survey. *Lancet.* 2011 Jan. 1;377(9759), 63-73.

Bidet, P., Lalande, V., Salauze, B., Burghoffer, B., Avesani, V., Delmée, M., Rossier, A., Barbut, F., Petit, J. C. Comparison of PCR-ribotyping, arbitrarily primed PCR, and pulsed-field gel electrophoresis for typing *Clostridium difficile*. *J. Clin. Microbiol.* 2000 Jul.;38(7), 2484-2487.

Gould, C. V., McDonald, L. C. Bench-to-bedside review: *Clostridium difficile* colitis. *Crit. Care.* 2008;12(1), 203.

Boero, M., Berti, E., Morgando, A., Verme, G. Treatment for *Clostridium difficile*: Results of a randomized open study with rifaximine vs. vancomycin. *Microbiol. Medica* 1990; 5, 74-77.

Boyce, J. M., Ligi, C., Kohan, C., Dumigan, D., Havill, N. L. Lack of association between the increased incidence of *Clostridium difficile*-associated disease and the increasing use of alcohol-based hand rubs. *Infect. Control Hosp. Epidemiol.*, 2006;27, 479-483.

Braunlin, W., Xu, Q., Hook, P., Fitzpatrick, R., Klinger, J. D., Burrier, R., Kurtz, C. B. Toxin binding of tolevamer, a polyanionic drug that protects against antibiotic-associated diarrhea. *Biophysical J.* 2004; 87, 534-539.

Chiu, Y.-H., Che, T. M., Romero, A., Ichikawa, Y., Shue, Y.-K. *Polymorphic crystalline forms of tiacumicin B-Patent* 7378508; 2008.

Dubreuil, L., Houcke, I., Mouton, Y., Rossignol, J. F. In vitro evaluation of activities of nitazoxanide and tizoxanide against anaerobes and aerobic organisms. *Antimicrob. Agents Chemother.* 1996; 40, 2266-2270.

Farver, D. K., Hedge, D. K., Lee, S. C. Ramoplanin a lipoglycodepsipeptide antibiotic. *Ann. Pharmacother.*, 2005; 39, 863-868.

Freeman, J., Baines, S. D., Jabes, D., Wilcox, M. H. Comparison of ramoplanin and vancomycin in vitro and in vivo models of clindamycin induced *Clostridium difficile* infection. *J. Antimicrob. Chemother.*, 2005; 56, 717-25.

Fulco, P., Wenzel, R. P. Ramoplanin - a topical lipoglycodepsipeptide antibacterial agent. *Expert Rev. Anti. Infect.* 2006; 4, 939-945.

Garey, K. W., Jiang, Z. D., Bellard, A., DuPont, H. L. Rifaximin in treatment of recurrent *Clostridium difficile*-associated diarrhea: an uncontrolled pilot study. *J. Clin. Gastroenterol.* 2009; 43, 91-3.

Hakalehto, E. Simulation of enhanced growth and metabolism of intestinal *Escherichia coli* in the Portable Microbe Enrichment Unit (PMEU). In: Rogers, M. C., Peterson, N. D., editors. *E. coli infections: causes, treatment and prevention.* New York, US: Nova Publishers; 2011.

Hakalehto, E., Heitto, L. Minute microbial levels detection in water samples by Portable Microbe Enrichment Unit Technology. *Environment and Natural Resources Research,* 2012; 2, 80-88.

Hakalehto, E., Hänninen, O. Gaseous CO_2 signal initiate growth of butyric acid producing *Clostridium butyricum* both in pure culture and in mixed cultures with *Lactobacillus brevis. Can. J. Microbiol.,* 2012; 58, 928-931.

Hakalehto, E., Hell, M., Bernhofer, C., Heitto, A., Pesola, J., Humppi, T., Paakkanen, H. Growth and gaseous emissions of pure and mixed small intestinal bacterial cultures: Effects of bile and vancomycin. *Pathophysiology,* 2010; 17, 45-53.

Hecht, D. W., Galang, M. A., Sambol, S. P., Osmolski, J. R., Johnson, S., Gerding, D. N. In vitro activities of 15 antimicrobial agents against 110 toxigenic *Clostridium difficile* clinical isolates collected from 1983 to 2004. *Antimicrob. Agents Chemother.,* 2007, 51; 2716-2719.

Hell, M., Bernhofer, C., Huhulescu, S., Indra, A., Allerberger, F., Maass, M., Hakalehto, E. How safe is colonoscope-reprocessing regarding *Clostridium difficile* spores*? The Journal of Hospital Infection* Vol. 76, Supplement 1: Abstracts, 8th International Congress of the Hospital Infection Society, 10-13 October 2010, Liverpool, UK, S21-22.

Hell, M., Permoser, M., Chmelizek, G., Kern, J. M., Maass, M., Huhulescu, S., Indra, A., Allerberger, F. Clostridium difficile infection: monoclonal or polyclonal genesis? *Infection*, 2011; 39, 461-465.

Hell, M., Sickau, K., Chmelizek, G., Kern, J. M., Maass, M., Huhulescu, S., Allerberger, F. Absence of *Clostridium difficile* in asymptomatic hospital staff. *Am. J. Infect. Control,* 2012; 40, 1023-4.

Hell, M., Bernhofer, C., Stalzer, P., Kern, J. M., Claassen, E. Probiotics in *Clostridium difficile* infection: reviewing the need for a multistrain probiotic. *Benef. Microbes,* 2013; 4, 39-51.

Hell, M., Schmid, D., Simons, E., Bernhofer, C., Voith, M., Wagner, A., ... & Allerberger, F. Improved control of nosocomial *C. difficile* transmission by daily use of an oxygen-releasing sporicidal disinfectant. *International Journal of Infection Control*, 2014; *10*(2).

Jiang, Z. D., Ke, S., Palazzini, E., Riopel, L., Dupont, H. In vitro activity and fecal concentration of rifaximin after oral administration. *Antimicrob. Agents Chemother.,* 2000; 44, 2205-2206.

Johnson, S., Schriever, C., Galang, M., Kelly, C. P., Gerding, D. N. Interruption of recurrent *Clostridium difficile*-associated diarrhea episodes by serial therapy with vancomycin and rifaximin. *Clin. Infect. Dis.* 2007; 44, 846-848.

Johnson, S., Schriever, C., Patel, U., Patel, T., Hecht, D. W., Gerding, D. N. Rifaximin Redux: treatment of recurrent *Clostridium difficile* infections with rifaximin immediately post-vancomycin treatment. *Anaerobe,* 2009; 15, 290-291.

Juang, P., Skledar, S. J., Zgheib, N. K., Paterson, D. L., Vergis, E. N., Shannon, W. D., Ansani, N. T., Branch, R. A. Clinical outcomes of intravenous immune globulin in severe *clostridium difficile*-associated diarrhea. *Am. J. Infect. Control.* 2007; 35, 131-7.

Kuijper, E. J., Coignard, B., Tüll, P. The ESCMID Study Group for Clostridium difficile (ESGCD), EU Member States, and the European Centre for Disease Prevention and Control (ECDC). Emergence of *Clostridium difficile* -associated disease in North America and Europe. *Clin. Microbiol. Infect.* 2006;Vol. 12(Suppl. 6), 2-18.

Leung, D. Y., Kelly, C. P., Boguniewicz, M., Pothoulakis, C., LaMont, J. T., Flores, A. Treatment with intravenously administered gamma globulin of chronic relapsing colitis induced by *Clostridium difficile* toxin. *J. Pediatr.* 1991; 118, 633-7.

Louie, T. J., Miller, M., Donskey, C., et al. Safety, pharmacokinetics and outcomes of PAR-101 in healthy subjects and patients with *Clostridium difficile*-associated diarrhea [abstract LB2–29], *Program and abstracts of the 45th Interscience Conference on Antimicrobial Agents and Chemotherapy (Washington DC)* volume. 226, American Society for Microbiology, Washington, DC; 2005.

Louie, T. J. Peppe, J., Watt, C. K., Johnson, D., Mohammed, R., Dow, G., Weiss, K., Simon, S., John, J. F. Jr, Garber, G., Chasan-Taber, S., Davidson, D. M. Tolevamer, a novel nonantibiotic polymer compared with vancomycin in the treatment of mild to moderately severe *Clostridium difficile*-associated diarrhea. *Clin. Infect. Dis.* 2006; 43, 411-20.

Louie, T., Gerson, M., Grimard, D. Results of a phase III trial comparing tolevamer, vancomycin and metronidazole in patients with *Clostridium difficile* -associated diarrhea (CDI). *Abstract presented at the 47th International Conference on Antimicrobial Agents and Chemotherapy Meeting* at Chicago IL September 17-20, 2007.

Louie, T. J., Miller, M. A., Mullane, K. M., Weiss, K., Lentnek, A., Golan, Y., Gorbach, S., Sears, P., Shue, Y. K. OPT-80-003 Clinical Study group. Fidaxomicin versus vancomycin for *Clostridium difficile* infection. *N. Engl. J. Med.* 2011; 364, 5.

Lowy, I., Molrine, D. C., Leav, B. A., Blair, B. M., Baxter, R., Gerding, D. M., Nichol, G., Tomas Jr. W. D., Leney, M., Sloan, S., Hay, C. A., Ambrosino, D. M. Treatment with monoclonal antibodies against *Clostridium difficile* toxins. *N. Eng. J. Med.* 2010; 362(3), 197-205.

Martin, C. E., Weishaupt, M. W., Seeberger, P. H. Progress toward developing a carbohydrate-conjugate vaccine against *Clostridium difficile* ribotype 027: synthesis of cell-surface polysaccharide PS-I repeating unit. *Chem. Commun.* 2011; 47, 10260-10262.

McPherson, S., Rees, C. J., Ellis, R., Soo, S., Panter, S. J. Intravenous immunoglobulin for the treatment of severe, refractory, and recurrent *Clostridium difficile* diarrhea. *Dis. Colon Rectum* 2006; 49, 1-6.

McVay, C. S., Rolfe, R. D. In vitro and in vivo activities of nitazoxanide agents against *Clostridium difficile*. *Antimicrob. Agents Chemother.* 2000; 44, 2254-2258.

Musher, D. M., Aslam, S., Logan, N., Nallacheru, S., Bhalia, I., Borchert, F., Hamill, R. J. Relatively poor outcome after treatment of *Clostridium difficile* colitis with metronidazole. *Clin. Infect. Dis.* 2005; 40, 1586-1590.

Musher, D. M., Logan, N., Hamill, R. J., Dupont, H. L., Lentnek, A., Gupta, A., Rossignol, J. F. Nitazoxanide for the treatment of *Clostridium difficile* colitis. *Clin. Infect. Dis.* 2006; 43, 421-427.

Musher, D. M., Logan, N., Bressler, A. M., Johnson, D. P., Rossignol, J. F. Nitazoxanide versus vancomycin in *Clostridium difficile* infection: a randomized, double-blind study. *Clin. Infect. Dis.* 2009; 48, e41-46.

Owens, R. C. *Clostridium difficile*-associated disease: an emerging threat to patient safety. *Pharmacotherapy,* 2006; 26, 299-311.

Pépin, J., Routhier, S., Gagnon, S., Brazeau, I. Management and outcomes of a first recurrence of *Clostridium difficile*-associated disease in Quebec, Canada. *Clin. Infect. Dis.* 2006 Mar. 15;42(6), 758-764.

Permpoonpattana, P., Hong, H., Hetcharaburanin, J., Huang, J. M., Cook, J., Fairweather, N. F., Cutting, S. M. Immunization with *Bacillus* spores expressing toxin A peptide repeats protects against infection with *Clostridium difficile* strains producing toxins A and B. *Infect. Immun.* 2011; 79, 2295-302.

Pesola, J., Paakkanen, H., Hakalehto, E. Enhanced diagnostics of pyelonephritis – a case study. *Int. J. Med. Sci.,* 2012; 2, 273-277.

Rodriguez-Palacios, A., Staempfli, H. R., Duffield, T., Weese, J. S. Clostridium difficile in retail ground meat, Canada. *Emerg. Infect. Dis*. 2007. 13, 485-487.

Rupnik, M. Is *Clostridium difficile* -associated infection a potentially zoonotic and foodborne disease? *Clin. Microbiol. Infect*. 2007. 13, 457-459.

Sasser, J. M., Cousin, K. S. Controlling Clostridium difficile-associated disease in the gastrointestinal tract. US20080254010; 2008.

Spigaglia, P., Barbanti, F., Mastrantonio, P. European Study Group on Clostridium difficile (ESGCD). Multidrug resistance in European Clostridium difficile clinical isolates. *J. Antimicrob. Chemother.* 2011 Oct.;66(10), 2227-34.

Swanson, R. N., Hardy, D. J., Shipkowitz, N. L., Hanson, C. W., Ramer, N. C., Fernandes, P. B., Clement, J. J. In vitro and in vivo evaluation of tiacumicins B and C against *Clostridium difficile. Antimicrob. Agents Chemother,* 1991; 35, 1108-1111.

Thomas, Jr. W. D., Giannasca, P. J., Zhang, Z., Lei, W., Monath, T. P. Passive immunization against Clostridium difficile disease. *US patent no: 6680168; 2004.*

Van Belkum, A., Durand, G., Peyret, M., Chatellier, S., Zambardi, G., Schrenzel, J., Shortridge, D., Engelhardt, A., Dunne, W. M. Jr. Rapid clinical bacteriology and its future impact. *Ann. Lab. Med.*, 2013; 33, 14-27.

Viscomi, G. C., Campana, M., Braga, D., Confortini, D., Cannata, V., Severini, D., Righi, P., Rosini, G. Polymorphous forms of rifaximin, processes for their production and use thereof in medicinal preparations. *US Patent 7045620; 2006.*

Vonberg, R. P., Kuijper, E. J., Wilcox, M. H., Barbut, F., Tüll, P., Gastmeier, P. European C difficile-Infection Control Group; European Centre for Disease Prevention and Control (ECDC), van den Broek, P. J., Colville, A., Coignard, B., Daha, T., Debast, S., Duerden, B. I., van den Hof, S., van der Kooi, T., Maarleveld, H. J., Nagy, E., Notermans, D. W., O'Driscoll, J., Patel, B., Stone, S., Wiuff, C. *Clin. Microbiol. Infect.* 2008 May;14 Suppl. 5, 2-20. Review.

Weinbergerova, B. Clostridium difficile infections in patients with hematological malignancy in Czech and Slovak Republic – a retrospective analysis (Poster). In: *19th Congress of European Hematology Association*, June 12-15, 2014, Milan, Italy.

Windle, H., Doyle, R., Kelleher, D., Walsh, J., Eidhin, D. N. Clostridium difficile vaccine. *US patent application: 20030054009; 2003.*

In: Microbiological Clinical Hygiene
Editor: Eino Elias Hakalehto
ISBN: 978-1-63463-428-1

Chapter 16

Aspects of Skin Infection

Osmo Hänninen[1], Ilkka Pesola[2], Robert Armon[3] and Elias Hakalehto[4]

[1]Department of Physiology, University of Eastern Finland, Kuopio, Finland
[2]Dental Clinic, Kuopio, Finland
[3]Faculty of Civil & Environmental Engineering, Technion, Haifa, Israel
[4]Department of Environmental Sciences, University of Eastern Finland, Kuopio, Finland

Abstract

Skin is our largest organ and a boundary towards biological, chemical and physical agents. It owns defense mechanisms to encounter all these agents. People have had traditional methods for prevention and care of skin diseases.. For example: saunas and hot water serve as practical patterns. Those means have been shown to be even recently applicable and often overrun current antibiotic regular approach that has a serious weaknesses: development of resistances that became a very serious common problems. Skin is a site of hormone synthesis and also influenced by them as well by drugs circulating within our body. Skin can show unexpected reactions to several drugs and other chemicals in use. Skin has a remarkable capacity to renew as expressed in wound healing.

Skin area is one of the most important of infection routes for the whole body system. Simultaneously skin has a very potent capacity to handle foreign antigens trying to break in the bloodstream and deeper tissues. This is the case especially when for example some trauma has injured the skin epithelial structure. Although several cures have been known traditionally for a long time, some skin infections are severe and often fatal, such as those caused by Group A streptococci, which can spread into various tissues. Long periods of time are required for the development of borreliosis from a tick bite but it usually starts with symptoms on the skin (erythema migrans). Skin tests, such as tuberculin test, have been developed for detecting various serious microbial infections.

Newborn wounds can heal scarless while at older ages this characteristic is lost. Skin also reflects the health of an individual as a whole. Skin is the tissue where allergic reactions can be visible. Skin carries a rich microflora, but also may carry pathogens although not necessarily causing disease in healthy individuals.

1. Introduction

Herodotos, father of historians, have written some 3000 years ago that Persians were aware of clean water need. They warned not to introduce dirt of their hands to river water. Herodotos also writes that Skythians used saunas. In these saunas, Skythians used wood saw dust to clean their skin to get it fresh and beautiful. Saw dust contains polyphenols which have been used to cure skin problems. Saunas have been common all over, although less common nowadays except in Finland, where they still are very widespread. In Herodotos' times these Finnish habits were well known. Sauna or similar examples are known both in the east (Japan) and west (both Americas). However, it should be kept in mind that both of those geographical sites have been populated by people originating from northern Asia and Europe.

The Hungarian Ignaz Semmelweis was the first one to understand the hazard of germs carried by physicians from autopsies to delivering mothers thus infecting them with puerperal fever with a disastrous outcome both for mothers and newborns (Hakalehto, 2006). However, Semmelweis had difficulties among his own professional colleagues and even in his own University, Viennese Medical Clinic. He apparently died due to this disease as his colleagues still did not understand the nature of his infection. Unfortunately Semmelweis had a very small number of supporters. One of those was Pippinskiöld, then professor of obstetrics at the University of Helsinki, Finland. (Hänninen et al., 2006, Monos et al., 2002).

Scottish surgeon Joseph Lister (1827-1912) observed that lay people used carbolic acid, tar water, in taking care of the wound of their cattle. He adopted this method, and on the basis of Lister's own findings and demonstrations, the era of antiseptic surgery was born. This eventually took place after he had demonstrated the efficacy of this therapy in his public operations in the imperial capital London.

During the same time period, in Finland babies were delivered in smoke saunas. They were practically sterile due to heat and smoke as boiled water was also abundantly available. Thus in the 1800's the loss of newborns and their mothers was lower than in many other countries and even much later on. Nowadays, most Finns are born in hospitals, but ever since Semmelweis' and Pippinskiöld's days preventive measures have been developed.

In sauna bathing people use birch tree twigs and their leaves (as well other trees like oaks) soaking them in water and whipping their skins. Birch leaves are rich in polyphenols which are spread on the sweating skin and later washed out resembling the Skythians' procedure with saw dust in their sauna bathing.

2. Skin Structure and Functions

The surface area of human skin is some 1.5-2 square meters. Skin protects the tissues underneath. Loss of skin in burns can still even now have poor outcome, although the cultivation of patients own skin cells is now well-known technology (Chrapusta et al., 2014).

The growth of these cells has been used in specialized clinics to cover the areas lost in the burns (Lewis et al., 2014). This technology has been a major step in patient care. The outmost epidermic layer is only about 0.5 – 1.5 mm thick. Mechanical load usually determines its thickness. Keratin is an important protein component of the skin. Children have thin and soft skin. In old age skin turns again thinner (Mizukoshi et al., 2014).

Skin has important functions as sensory organ, which is useful especially in the fingers. Pain sensors help to avoid damage and wounds (Southall et al., 2003). Thermal receptors are important to avoid both too hot and too cold exposures. Such conditions can endanger the body system. In the Department of Physiology, University of Eastern Finland, special clothing has been developed for maintaining thermal balance of patients and wearable sensors in underwear to help in his or her thermal regulation (Myontech^{R}, Finland).. Skin is an important natural contributor to temperature control.

Skin also serves as blood storage which is important to take into account in accidents. When patients are exposed to cold, the blood circulation is diminished as blood escape inside organs, and skin consequently turns pale.

Skin is also important in the synthesis of vitamin (actually the right title would be hormone) D (Holick et al., 2007). After prolonged exposure to sunshine also white people tan when the melanin synthesis is increased. Since melanin in dark-skinned people hinders the skin to make vitamin D this means that also their vitamin D supplementation is necessary at least when they sojourn in areas with low sunlight exposure.

Skin is one of the major components of the human body and it constitutes for some 5% of our body weight, but up to 15-25% if also the subcutis is counted. Subcutis contains adipose tissue of variable thickness, especially in hips, buttocks and waist (Chudecka et al., 2014). These tissues protect other tissues against damage, but the main purpose is to serve as energy storage during possible famine.

Thickness of skin varies. This variation depends on the thickness of the keratin layer that responds to the use of *e.g.,* hands. Thickness is greatest in soles as expected, where mechanical load is also the greatest, especially when walking with bare foot. People are also running this way. In the outer layers of skin the cells dye and the dead cells are lost in the washing. The thinnest skin is in flexor side areas of joints.

Epidermis, outermost layer of dead cells prevents the drying out of the body. Some 0.5 l of water is, however, lost without sweating through the skin. Skin oils are produced by special skin glands to prevent the water escape, but oil soluble fluids go through this layer. The fatty acids released in skin help also to control the microflora, and too intensive skin washing causes its oil loss.

Hairs and nails are keratinized skin structures. Hairs help the thermoregulation as they increase the air preserved close to skin. Nails protect the fingers and toe tips. They are sources of microbes and they may be infected. Especially fungi causing nail infections are resistant against desinfectants and may need some medication (Shemer et al., 2014).

Skin contributes to thermoregulation by evaporation and sweating. Sweat is dilute salt solution, and it can be formed in quantities i.e., up to 12 liters. In hot environments while a person is at rest, its volume is minimally about 0.5–1 liter. Human skin is very rich in small sweat glands (Kurata et al., 2014). In armpits and groins there are large sweat glands, which give us our personal odor. Actually milk glands are also large sweat glands. Sweat helps to moisture the skin and helps to handle various items in hands and walking on rocks.

Skin has a huge microbiome and different techniques have been assessed for its evaluation: swabs, scrabes or punch biopsies (Grice et al., 2008). Castelino et al. (2014) suggest that the bacterial skin microbiome may be a potent link in the etiology of psoriatic arthritis.

Many skin diseases manifest also on the mucosal areas in the body. Skin diseases like lichen ruber planus (Davari et al., 2014), pemphigoid or pemphigus (Hayakawa et al., 2014), erythema multiforme (Yager, 2014), dermatitis herpetiformis (West et al., 2014) and LED (lupus erythematosus discoides), (Nico et al., 2014), manifest quite often also on the oral mucosa. Typical lesions are reddish, lightly painful ulcers, which mimic clinically somewhat oral aphtous ulcers. Wide plaques, scars and long lasting bulla formations indicate that a histopathological examination from biopsy specimen would be needed. Histopathological diagnosis may be behind such mucosal symptoms of some skin diseases. Sometimes it may also happen, that oral lesions are first visible on oral epithelia. Symptoms in skin area may occur even months later.

Staphylococci are common bacterial inhabitants of the skin (Scott, 1989). From that surface they are often introducing into the body system via wounds or medical devices (Nielsen et al., 1998). After all the penetration capabilities of infective bacterial strains are subjected to the challenge by the host defenses and possible medications. In order to evaluate the treatment correctly, a proper real-time view on the microbiological situation would be helpful.

The importance of skin health is well documented by orthopedic surgeons (Banerjee et al., 2014). Especially nasal *Staphylococcus aureus* is one of most important pathogens that may cause nosocomial infections to surgical patients (Skramm et al., 2014). In future it is a great challenge to decrease or eliminate nasal staphylococcal carriage perioperatively. In orthopedic hospitals it is usual that even minor traumas or scars on the skin area on the target tissue can make an obligatory reason for cancelling the operation. In a way it is a catastrophy if skin lesion containing infective agent, causes postoperative infection in joint prosthesis, for example. In the most severe cases it may disable the patient for the rest of his or her life.

3. Tuberculin Test

The late 19th and the beginning of 20th centuries was the "golden era" of microbiology. During this period, the major catastrophic disease agents have been identified opening the area of antibiotic offensive. Among those pestilences one can find: anthrax, diphtheria, tuberculosis, tetanus, cholera, syphilis, etc. Among these bacteria, tuberculosis withstand for its specific features. The genus *Mycobacterium* contains many species among which *M. tuberculosis*, *M. bovis*, *M. africanum*, *M. canetti*, *M. microti* and *M. africanum* (van Soolingen et al., 1997) are potential human pathogens. *Mycobacterium tuberculosis* complex (MBTC) members are causative agents of human and animal tuberculosis. Species in this complex include: *M. tuberculosis*, the major cause of human tuberculosis, *M. bovis*, *M. bovis BCG*, *M. africanum*, *M. canetti*, *M. caprae*, *M. microti and M. pinnipedii*. For the fast recognition of *Mycobacterium* sp. with the PMEU (Portable Microbe Enrichment Unit) see Hakalehto (2013) and Hakalehto et al. (2014). See also the Chapther 9 of this book.

Mycobacterium genus is a class of Gram-positive bacteria (due to lack of outer membrane) difficult to classify as such based only on the simple Gram staining due to poor retention of crystal violet dye. The unique characteristics of its cell wall are thickness in comparison with other bacteria, hydrophobicity, waxy, rich in mycolates and the polysaccharide arabinogalactan that interconnect the mycolate and the peptidoglycan layers. This distinctive structure has a substantial contribution to this bacterium resistance to environmental stresses, *e.g.,* desiccation.

Global Distribution

As can be seen in Figure 1, the prevalence of tuberculosis is worldwide with few exceptions. Many African countries are among the countries that annual information is poorly documented, therefore left as "no cases". However Figure 2 represents the real incidence rates revealing main foci located mostly in African countries (below the equatorial line) and South-East Asia.

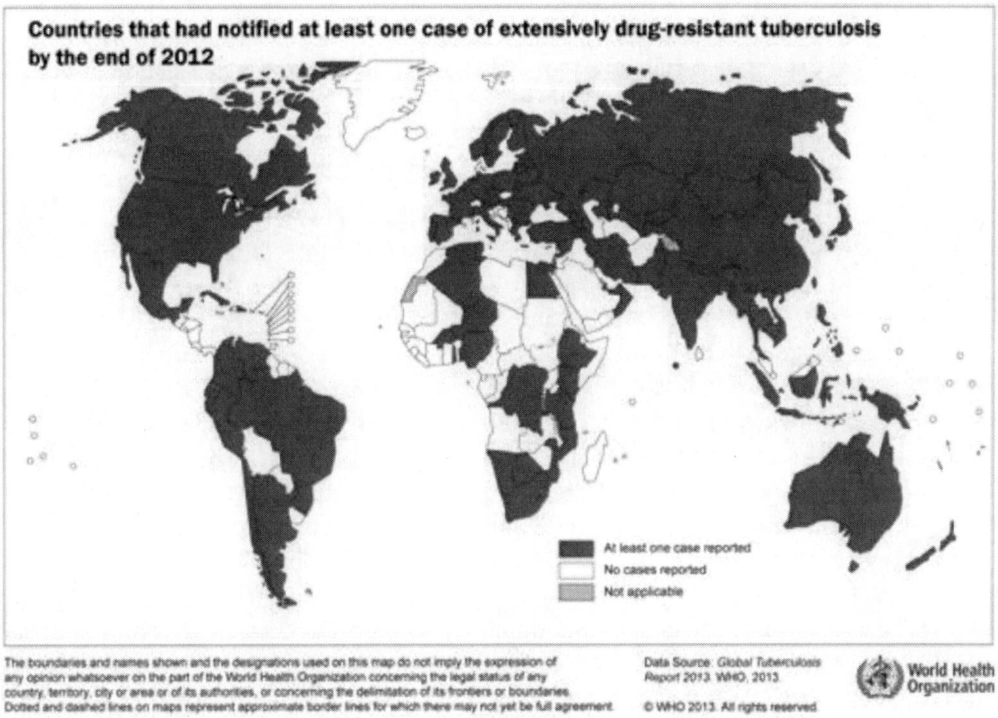

Figure 1. Countries that had notified at least one case of extensively drug-resistant tuberculosis by end of 2012 (WHO, Global tuberculosis Report, 2013).

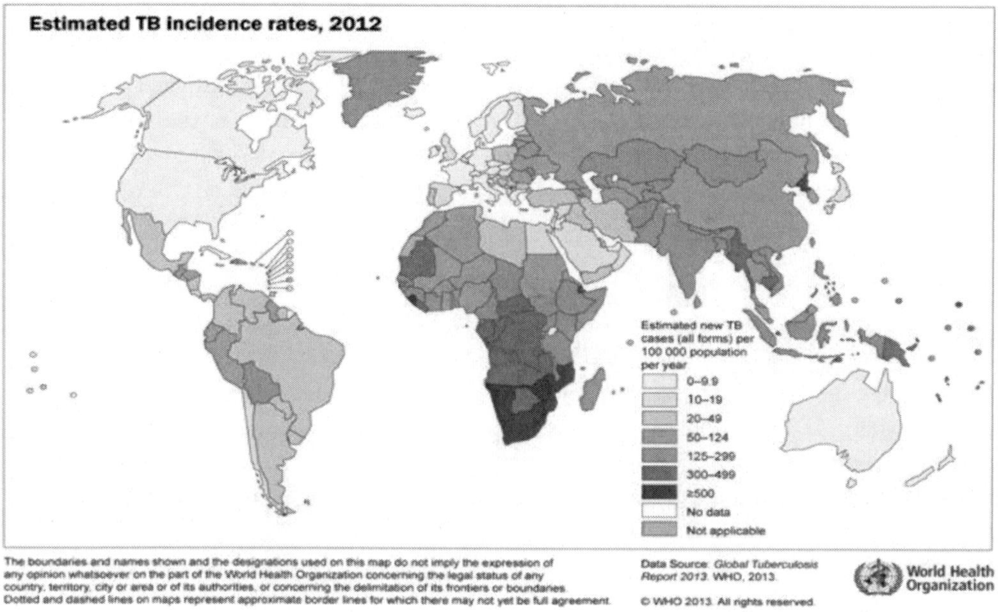

Figure 2. Global estimated TB incidence rates, 2012 (WHO, Global tuberculosis Report, 2010.

4. Tuberculin (Mendel-Mantoux Test) As Indicator of Exposure

Tuberculin test has been first described by the prominent microbiologist Robert Koch in 1890 (Koch, 1882). Later Dr. Felix Mendel and Charles Mantoux (1908) developed the test in order to identify potential contact/exposure to *M. tuberculosis*. Tuberculin is a glycerol extract of *Mycobacterium tuberculosis*, *M. bovis*, or *M. avium* used in skin testing. It is also known as PPD (Purified protein derivative) tuberculin, a precipitate of species-nonspecific molecules obtained from filtrates of sterilized, concentrated cultures. An exposed person to *M. tuberculosis* or other species is expected to mount an immune response in the skin inoculated with tuberculin complex. The more intense precedent exposure will be coupled by a stronger the immune reaction (CDC, 2000). Commonly, a physician or nurse will read the reaction (48 and 72 hours after administration) by measuring the diameter of induration across the forearm in millimeters. No induration, is recorded as "0 mm", while erythema should not be considered (Table 1). Other skin tests for detecting infectious diseases are presented in Table 2.

5. Streptococcus Pyogenes (Group A Streptococcus)

This Gram-positive bacterium is a pathogen often found on human skin, able to cause localized skin infection ("impetigo"). The bacterium displays streptococcal group A antigen on its cell wall. *S. pyogenes* belongs to Group A (beta-hemolytic) *Streptococcus* (in short *GABHS*). The incubation period is ~1 to 3 days under optimal conditions.

Table 1. Tuberculin test interpretation (adapted from CDC site, http://www.cdc.gov/tb/publications/factsheets/testing/skintesting.htm)

	Induration size (positivity)	
≥ 5 mm	**≥10 mm**	**≥15 mm**
-HIV-infected persons -A recent contact of a person with TB disease -Persons with fibrotic changes on chest radiograph consistent with prior TB -Patients with organ transplants -Persons who are immunosuppressed for other reasons (*e.g.*, taking the equivalent of >15 mg/day of prednisone for 1 month or longer, taking TNF-α antagonists)	Recent immigrants (< 5 years) from high-prevalence countries -Injection drug users -Residents and employees of high-risk congregate settings -Mycobacteriology laboratory personnel -Persons with clinical conditions that place them at high risk -Children < 4 years of age - Infants, children, and adolescents exposed to adults in high-risk categories	In any person, including persons with no known risk factors for TB. However, targeted skin testing programs should only be conducted among high-risk groups.

Table 2. Some Intradermal Injection Tests in Skin Used in the Diagnosis of Infection

Disease	Test
Tuberculosis	Mantoux Multiple punctures
Brucellosis	Brucellin
Leprosy	Lepromin
Fungous diseases: -Dermatophytes -Histoplasmosis -Coccidioidomycosis	 Trichophytin Histoplasmin Coccidioidin
Hydatid disease	Casoni
Leishmaniasis	Leishman antigen
Virus diseases: -Lymphogranuloma venereum	 Frei
Cat-scratch fever	Cat-scratch antigen
Diphtheria	Schick Direct susceptibility test to diphtheria toxin. Positive result denotes susceptibility.

When present inside the throat the infection is defined as pharyngitis ("strep throat"). More severe cases are manifested as: scarlet fever, cellulitis, necrotizing fascitis, toxic shock syndrome, etc.. In these severe cases, the antibiotic of choice is penicillin for at least 10 days or more (Falagas et al., 2008). Since 1985, many reports mentioned *S. pyogenes* tolerance to penicillin; therefore in such cases macrolides, chloramphenicol, and tetracyclines can be used instead, if sensitivity has been proved (Kim and Kaplan, 1985). In pharyngeal or skin infections, oral or parenteral penicillin should be administered for 10 days, while in cases of penicillin allergy, alternative treatment for 5 to 10 days could be with oral cephalosporin or macrolide, revealing good results (Ratgeber Infektionskrankheiten, 2000).

In severe cases, clindamycin should be administered in addition to parenteral penicillin. Interestingly, people with rheumatic fever should take prophylactic penicillin against relapse for more than 5 years or lifelong after a relapse.

6. Controversial Views on the Influences of Bacterial Infection

Lichen ruber planus is a quite common skin disease that affects both skin and oral and genital mucosa. It is postulated that lichen is an autoimmune disease like many other general diseases in the body system. In recent years it has been showed that symptoms of oral lichen can be healed effectively with immunomodulatory medicin tacrolimus (Resende et al., 2013). Tacrolimus is a potent medicine in atopic dermatitis. That medicine was discovered in 1984 in Japan, when there was screened large amounts of isolated soil samples. The purpose of the search was to find new immunosuppressive and bioactive metabolites. Soil bacteria sample was identified on Mount Tsukaba. The product strongly inhibited the MLR (mixed lymphocyte reaction) but did not damage the cells in culture (Ruzicka and Reitamo, 2004). The bacterium of that product has been called *Streptomyces tsukubaensis* according to the site of discovery.

Later on it has been found that tacrolimus has very potent effect on the symptoms of oral ulcerative, erosive oral lichen planus. The effect of that medicine disappears almost in every patient if the medication is ceased.

It could be assumed that lichen planus is most likely an autoimmune disease that has its bacteriological origin and causes that maintain mucosal symptoms. Tacrolimus resembles an antibiotic medicine as deduced by its effects on the oral epithelia since the symptoms disapper usually after 1-2 weeks local therapy. In atopic dermatitis the effect on the skin lesions is almost as effective as in the case of lichen planus. As a positive effect this medicine does not make the skin thinner like steroids, which have been recommended for wider use (Reitamo and Remitz, 2014).

7. Insects Carry Skin Invaders

Borrelia burgdorferi, which also often becomes an intracellular pathogen (Stanek et al., 2012), is causing tedious long-term infections, whose treatments are often controversial. The treatment for a long-term borreliosis is currently under debate. Two lines of treatment are somewhat conflicting with each other, namely the recommendation of ILADS (International Lyme and Associated Diseases Society) for using long-lasting antibiotic treatments, and those of IDSA (The Infectious Diseases Society of America) focusing on the actual appearance of the disease. The vague treatment policies have caused confusion among the suffering patients, who are sometimes relieved by special clinics, such as the Augsburg Borreliosis Clinic in Germany or the Antioxidant Clinic in Finland.

Some other common infectious diseases intruding through skin damages are the bacterium *Yersinia pestis* (causative agent of plague) and *Plasmodium falciparum* (protozoan cause of malaria), which are disseminated through a flea or mosquito bite, respectively. A more comprehensive list of arthropod-borne zoonoses is presented in Kreuss et al. (2003). Sometimes the insects are even functioning as vectors for transmission from a hospital room to another (Hakalehto, 2006).

8. Saunas – Sweat Lodges

Finns and their related nations have had saunas at least as long we have had written documents. The living traditions tell that people have been accustomed to visit saunas on regular, at least weekly basis i.e., have been exposed to heat and smoke containing waters from their very first moments after their birth as they were also actually born in saunas. Therefore the child deaths have been low in number due to hygienic matters. The heat and also the smoke killed the bacteria. Therefore saunas have been practically sterile. The expecting mother could be wasted with rich amounts of warm water. So was also the newborn baby cleaned with water. In old days the saunas were warmed in log cabins without chimneys. There for the waters were exposed to smoke and became bactericidal. Today's saunas seldom have the old heating system, but still the high hygiene tradition continues. Babies are born in hospitals.

In sauna bathing people have been using birch twigs with leaves to stimulate their skin circulation and sweating. Birch leaves have polyphenols which are bacteriocidic.

Skin bacteria have adapted to live in human skin where pH is slightly acidic, i.e., even some pH 3-5 which also helps to control bacterial growth.

9. Wound Healing

Sauna bathing has been the basic measure to keep skin clean. In old times and even nowadays the Finnish farms have had spruce tree(s) near to the homes. These trees can have wounds to provide resin for wound healing of humans and animals. By mixing with fat one could make ointments for the wounds. These resins contain bactericidal polyphenols. Not only humans but also animals were successful treated. As spruce provided resin all seasons such ointments could be made ant time of year.

In Finland one commonly used soap liquid as also solid pieces of soap contains pine polyphenols.

10. Cattle Health

Recently pine oil components have been found to stimulate cattle growth and thus pine polyphenols can be used to promote the health of farm animals. This helps to control intestinal microflora and decreases the use of antibiotics in animal care. In Finland the use of antibiotics was not allowed from 1999 onwards to be used in farm animal care. Neither the European Union permits to use antibiotics in animal feeds to control the MRSA bacteria. In Denmark already almost 90 % of pigs are said to carry these bacteria. In the Netherlands the farmers cannot enter hospitals without quarantee of not being a carrier of MRSA. In case of battling against antibiotic resistance, wood industry will thus possibly have new markets in farm animal production with manufacturing of antimicrobial polyphenols.

11. Wild Plants

People have used also the leaves of several wild plants available near their homes. *Plantago major* has been called iron leaf. Also cabbages have been successfully used in traditional wound treatments.

12. Berries As Healthy Food Supplements

Common wild berries contain several kinds of polyphenols. These effects have been studied in the University of Eastern Finland, and they are known by old folks to be helpfull in infections like the respiratory infections (Kärenlampi and Törrönen, results not shown here). Black current is still famous as grandmothers' drink. Its has been the key component of nectars to prevent respiratory infections (Tompuri and Hänninen, results not shown here). Granberries are known in the cure of urinary infections.

Adaptogens are compounds which many plants contain and help the body resist viral and also other harmful microbial agents.

13. Sour Milk

Not very far back in time the refrigerators were not available in homes. Milk had to be preserved as fermented. The lactic acid increased the life span, and the nutritional value of the milk was also maintained. In order to keep sour milk in slow motion people used to add living frogs to sourmilk. We know now that frog skin excretes antibiotic peptides (Samgina et al., 2012).

Conclusion

Egyptians expected that their dead kings and other eminent people had new life afterwards and mummified their bodies using the resins of plants and their mixtures in a lengthy process. Several other nations have their own methods to do the same. These plants could also be used as remedies for control infections of living people and cattle. The skin infections are manifold, and both traditional cures and methods of modern medicine are needed for controlling them. Besides, the skin tests are useful in diagnosis of several diseases, such as tuberculosis.

References

Banerjee, S., Kapadia, B. H., Mont, M. A. Preoperative skin disinfection methodologies for reducing prosthetic joint infections. *J. Knee Surg.*, 2014; 27, 283-288.

Castelino, M., Eyre, S., Upton, M., Ho, P., Barton, A. The bacterial skin microbiome in psoriatic arthritis, an unexplored link in pathogenesis: challenges and opportunities offered by recent technological advances. *Rheumatology (Oxford),* 2014; 53, 777-784.

CDC. Targeted tuberculin testing and treatment of latent tuberculosis infection. *MMWR, 2000;* 49, No. RR-6.

Chrapusta, A., Nessler, M. B., Drukala, J., Bartoszewicz, M., Mądry, R. A comparative analysis of advanced techniques for skin reconstruction with autologous keratinocyte culture in severely burned children: own experience. *Postepy. Dermatol. Alergol.*, 2014; 31, 164-169.

Chudecka, M., Lubkowska, A., Kempińska-Podhorodecka, A. Body surface temperature distribution in relation to body composition in obese women. *J. Therm. Biol.*, 2014; 43, 1-6.

Davari, P., Hsiao, H. H., Fazel, N. Mucosal lichen planus: an evidence-based treatment update. *Am. J. Clin. Dermatol.,* 2014; 15, 181-195.

Falagas, M. E., Vouloumanou, E. K., Matthaiou, D. K., Kapaskelis, A. M. Effectiveness and safety of short-course vs long-course antibiotic therapy for group a beta hemolytic streptococcal tonsillopharyngitis: a meta-analysis of randomized trials. *Mayo Clin. Proc.,* 2008; 83, 880-889.

Grice, E. A., Kong, H. H., Renaud, G., Young, A. C., NISC Comparative Sequencing Program, Bouffard, G. G., Blakesley, R. W., Wolfsberg, T. G., Turner, M. L., Segre, J. A. A diversity profile of the human skin microbiota. *Genome Res.,* 2008; 18, 1043-50.

Hakalehto, E. Enhanced mycobacterial diagnostics in liquid medium by microaerobic bubble flow in Portable Microbe Enrichment Unit. *Pathophysiology,* 2013; 20, 177–180.

Hakalehto, E. Semmelweis' present day follow-up: Updating bacterial sampling and enrichment in clinical hygiene. *Pathophysiology,* 2006; 13, 257-267.

Hakalehto, E., Heitto, A., Heitto, L., Rissanen, K., Pesola, I., Pesola, J. Enhanced recovery, enrichment and detection of *Mycobacterium marinum* with the Portable Microbe Enrichment Unit (PMEU). *Pathophysiology,* 2014; 21, 231-235.

Hänninen, O., Farago, M., Monos, E. Semmelweis‘ innovations and its Finnish follow-up. *Acta Physiologica Hungarica,* 2003; 90, 83-95.

Hänninen, O., Monos, E., Farago, M. Semmelweis' discovery and its Finnish follow-up. *Communicationes de Historia Artis Medicinae,* 2006; 194-195, 20-28.

Hayakawa, T., Furumura, M., Fukano, H., Li, X., Ishii, N., Hamada, T., Ohata, C., Tsuruta, D., Shimozato, K., Hashimoto, T. Diagnosis of oral mucous membrane pemphigoid by means of combined serologic testing. *Oral Surg. Oral Med. Oral Pathol. Oral Radiol.*, 2014; 117, 483-496.

Holick, M. F., Chen, T. C., Lu, Z., Sauter, E. Vitamin D and skin physiology: a D-lightful story. *J. Bone Miner. Res.*, 2007; 22 (Suppl. 2), V28-33.

Kim, K. S., Kaplan, E. L. Association of penicillin tolerance with failure to eradicate group A streptococci from patients with pharyngitis. *J. Pediatr.,* 1985; 107, 681-684.

Koch, R. "Die Aetiologie der Tuberculose" (The etiology of tuberculosis). *Berliner Klinische Wochenschrift (Berlin Clinical Weekly)*, 1882; 19, 221-230.

Kurata, R., Futaki, S., Nakano, I., Tanemura, A., Murota, H., Katayama, I., Sekiguchi, K. Isolation and characterization of sweat gland myoepithelial cells from human skin. *Cell. Struct. Funct.*, 2014; Sep 5.

Lewis, C. J., Mardaryev, A. N., Sharov, A. A., Fessing, M. Y., Botchkarev, V. A. The Epigenetic Regulation of Wound Healing. *Adv. Wound Care (New Rochelle)*. 2014; 3, 468-475.

Mizukoshi, K., Yonekura, K., Futagawa, M., Nakamura, T., Hirayama, K., Takahashi, K. Changes in dermal papilla structures due to aging in the facial cheek region. *Skin Res. Technol.*, 2014; Aug 23.

Monos, E., Farago, M., Hänninen, O., Semmelweis ja Suomi. *Hippokrates,* 2002; 19, 43-55.

Nico, M. M., Bologna, S. B., Lourenço, S. V. The lip in lupus erythematosus. *Clin. Exp. Dermatol.,* 2014; 39, 563-569.

Nielsen, J., Ladefoged, S. D., Kolmos, H. J. Dialysis catheter-related septichaemia. Focus on *Staphylococcus aureus* septichaemia. *Nephr. Dial. Transplant.*, 1998; 13, 2847.

Ratgeber Infektionskrankheiten 19. Folge: Scharlach und andere Infektionen durch *Streptococcus pyogenes*. (In German). *Epidemiologisches Bulletin,* 2000; 43, 343-345. (http://www.rki.de/INFEKT/EPIBULL/EPI.HTM)

Reitamo, S., Remitz, A. An update on current pharmacotherapy options in atopic dermatitis. *Expert. Opin. Pharmacother.,* 2014; 15, 1517-1524.

Resende, J. P., Aarestrup F. M., Aarestrup, B. V., Olate, S., Netto, H. D. Oral lichen planus treated with tacrolimus 0.1%. *Int. J. Clin. Exp. Med.*, 2013; 6, 917-921.

Ruzicka, T., Reitamo, S., editors. Tacrolimus ointment: A topical immunomodulator for atopic dermatitis. Development of Tacrolimus Ointment. New York, USA: Springer-Verlag; 2004; pp. 81-98.

Samgina, T., Vorontsov, E., Gorshkov, V., Hakalehto, E., Hänninen, O., Zubarev, R., Lebedev, A. Composition and antimicrobial activity of the skin peptidome of Russian brown frog *Rana temporaria. J. Proteome Res.,* 2012; 11, 6213-6222.

Scott, M. A. Bacterial skin infections. *Prim. Care.*, 1989; 16, 591-602.

Shemer, A., Gupta, A., Farhi, R., Daigle, D., Amichai, B. When is onychomycosis, onychomycosis? *Br. J. Dermatol.*, 2014; Sep 5.

Skråmm, I., Fossum, Moen A. E., Arøen, A., Bukholm, G. Surgical site infections in orthopaedic surgery demonstrate clones similar to those in orthopaedic *Staphylococcus aureus* nasal carriers. *J. Bone Joint Surg. Am.*, 2014; 96, 882-888.

Southall, M. D., Li, T., Gharibova, L. S., Pei, Y., Nicol, G. D., Travers, J B. Activation of epidermal vanilloid receptor-1 induces release of proinflammatory mediators in human keratinocytes. *J. Pharmacol. Exp. Ther.*, 2003; 304, 217-222.

Stanek, G., Wormser, G. P., Gray, J., Strle, F. Lyme borreliosis. *Lancet*, 2012; 379, 461-473.

van Soolingen, D., Hoogenboezem, T., de Haas, P. E., Hermans, P. W., Koedam, M. A., Teppema, K.S., Brennan, P. J., Besra, G. S., Portaels, F., Top, J., Schouls, L. M., van Embden, J. D. A novel pathogenic taxon of the *Mycobacterium tuberculosis* complex, Canetti: characterization of an exceptional isolate from Africa. *Intern. J. System. Bacteriol.,* 1997; 47, 1236–1245.

West, J., Fleming, K. M., Tata, L. J., Card, T. R., Crooks, C. J. Incidence and prevalence of celiac disease and dermatitis herpetiformis in the UK over two decades: population-based study. *Am. J. Gastroenterol.,* 2014; 109, 757-768.

Yager, J. A. Erythema multiforme, Stevens-Johnson syndrome and toxic epidermal necrolysis: a comparative review. *Vet. Dermatol.,* 2014; Jul 3 [Epub ahead of print].

In: Microbiological Clinical Hygiene
Editor: Eino Elias Hakalehto

ISBN: 978-1-63463-428-1

Chapter 17

Tendencies in Probiotic Treatments

Elias Hakalehto[1], Kaarlo Jaakkola[2], Jouni Pesola[3], Anneli Heitto[4], Markus Hell[5] and Osmo Hänninen[6]

[1]Department of Environmental Sciences, University of Eastern Finland, Kuopio, Finland
[2]Kruunuhaka Medical Center, Helsinki, Finland
[3]Department of Pediatrics, Kuopio University Hospital, Kuopio, Finland
[4]Finnoflag Oy, Kuopio, Finland
[5]Zentrum für Krankenhaushygiene und Infektionskontrolle der SALK, Universitätsklinikum Salzburg, Salzburg, Austria
[6]Department of Pathology, University of Eastern Finland, Kuopio, Finland

Abstract

On the basis of accumulating results of modern research on probiotic functions, it has become increasingly clear that not any single strain can cause best achievable impacts on the GI health alone. Instead, an individually designed combination of several strains (or mixed cultures) together with prebiotics are needed for the optimization of the effect. At best this effect has been shown to prevent diseases, or dysbiosis, as well as to interrupt vicious circles toward ill health. Since the bacterial and other microbial metabolic activities in the intestinal chyme are in motion as a "movable feast" which takes place in a close control of the host defensive and epithelial hormonal factors, there is a need to form an online view on the events taking place inside the digestion. One option for optimizing the probiotic functions is the simulation of microbial interactions *in vitro*. It is also possible to develop probes and sensors to recover various intestinal activities along the gut.

Intestinal environment is providing several niches for a big variety of micro-organisms. These strains are generally striving for balanced collaboration due to the fact that the alimentary microbiome is an entity as such, rather than a track of competition between the microbes. The survival of each strain is often dependent on the ability to maintain the balance by this particular micro-organism. In exceptional conditions, in connection with health or nutritional problems of the host, the microbiota may get severely disturbed. This gives an opportunity for some microbes to turn into pathogens, and distort the balance. Any incoming true pathogen may also get then a chance for invasion. In these undesired cases, and in order to avoid such situations, the implementation of probiotic strains is often needed.

Practices of probiotic treatments require further modernization, because more tools are required for the prevention of imbalances of the body and in its microbiome. Novel testing methods for validating the probiotic impacts are also needed.

Additional research is warranted, as well as vigorous testing of ideas; compatibilities of particular strains, relations between them etc.

These studies have been conducted also by the PMEU. In these simulation studies rather a realistic view on microfloral interactions could be acquired.

It is extremely important for our health to learn to take care of the microbial communities in our alimentary tract.

1. Introduction

Since the manifold positive influences of probiotic strains have been documented in the scientific literature focusing on human health parameters, it is a logical consequence to shift the major focus to the means of increasing, or optimizing, those effects (Hatakka et al., 2007a). Besides the direct intestinal delivery and impacts, it is documented that the probiotic effects could extend to the mouth and the respiratory tract.

In case of children in a Finnish day care center where 571 small children were using the probiotic *Lactobacillus rhamnosus* strain GG in milk, 17% less respiratory illnesses were observed, and 19% less antibiotics were used during one "infectious season" from October to April (Hatakka et al., 2001).

In an elderly people's home, probiotics reduced the prevalence of oral *Candida* sp. infections to 25% among 276 individuals in old age (Hatakka et al., 2007b). In immunosuppressed patients *Candida* sp. may cause severe or even fatal invasive infections and candidemias, in neonatal patients, for example (Brissaud, et al., 2011).

In a recent study, the PMEU method has been successfully applied for precisely and exactly measuring the probiotic "attenuation" effect on excessive intestinal bacterial growth, when the probiotics were used together with a prebiotic flax product (Hakalehto and Jaakkola, 2013).

In principle, two major misdirections of the past research have been that A. the emphasis has been almost solely on the large intestinal flora, and B. the one-sided idea on the competition of space on the mucosal membranes being the sole or main explanatory factor behind probiotic influences.

These issues are certainly a part of the entire picture of the intestinal microbial action. However, in the small bowel about 80% of our nutrients are absorbed. There the microbes are not necessarily situated exclusively on the epithelia, but merely in the moving chyme, where these strains also propagate and degrade the food components. Cooperation between different microbes, and between them and their host are essential and reciprocally beneficial (Hakalehto, 2012). The intestinal microbiota has also an important role in xenobiotic metabolism (Hänninen, et al., 1987).

Probiotics are applied widely also in the animal husbandry, where they can in some cases offer an alternative to the antibiotics. In case of the health protection of poultry, the probiotics have been documented as useful for a long period of time (Nurmi and Rantala, 1973).

The competitive exclusion principle with respect to e.g., campylobacteria has been developed for improving the poultry production (Aho et al., 1992).

Notwithstanding these established practices, we have been conceiving the intestinal (or alimentary) ecosystem comprising of a community, which contains numerous species in ever-changing concentrations.

2. Foundations of the Balance in the Microbiome

There is huge diversity in the intestinal microbiota (Eckburg, et al., 2005). However, there prevails a balance between the participating microbes that forms the basis for good health.

According to the PMEU simulation studies with *Escherichia coli* and *Klebsiella mobilis*, strains of these species kept the pH oscillating around 6 (Hakalehto et al., 2008; Hakalehto, 2011a, 2013). This value corresponds to the duodenal pH. These coliformic facultatively anaerobic species acted in an equal way, in a dualistic fashion also in the presence of other bacteria, such as *Bacillus cereus* and *Staphylococcus aureus* (Hakalehto et al., 2010).

Their dualistic balance could be the basis of the BIB (Bacterial Intestinal Balance), which is the foundation of our health and the basis of interactions between man and his microbes in the intestines (Hakalehto, 2011a, 2012). The concept of "alimentary microbiome" was defined in 2000 by Prof. Joshua Lederberg (Lederberg, 2000).This concept brings along the idea of microbes interacting with each other and with the host organism in order to form symbiotic balances (Hakalehto, 2012).In the scientific literature regarding the probiotic microbes, and especially the bacteria, mostly the large intestines have been taken into account when selecting the scope of the investigations (Quigley, 2010). However, it has been shown that even in the acidic gastric areas (Helander and Sundell, 1984) probiotic LAB (lactic acid bacteria) could survive considerable periods of time (Hakalehto et al., 2011; Hakalehto et al., 2012a). In the duodenal region with advantageous pH and plentiful of nutrients, occasional rapid growth and metabolism of bacterial strains is taking place (Hakalehto et al., 2008; Hakalehto et al., 2012b). The amount of these bacteria is most likely varying from rather low values into highly elevated levels in the intestinal chyme. Already in 1909 it was observed that nutritional factors divided the types of intestinal into saccharolytic and proteolytic communities (Kendall, 1909). The food given to apes was determining the residing microflora which then was able to flourish during bursts of incoming food substances. This nutritional division was found to be remarkably strict since the apes fed with carbohydrate food did not possess the proteolytic strains at all. It should be emphasized that this result was not a consequence of any competition between the strains. Instead, it derived from the necessities or rules formulating the intestinal ecosystems. This microbiota is in a crucial role in contributing to our health status via various interactions (Lyte et al., 2006; Jaakkola and Hakalehto, 2012; Hakalehto et al., 2012c).

Interestingly, signals from emitted gaseous compounds of the microbes are shaping this flora (Hakalehto and Hänninen, 2012). For example, the CO_2 produced by probiotic LAB is supposed to flush the large intestines in such a way that tedious obligate anaerobes e.g., clostridia cannot extensively root onto the gut epithelial walls.

PMEU enrichment of the gastric endoscopic samples have revealed that lactic acid bacteria are surviving remarkable periods of time on the stomach epithelia (Hakalehto et al., 2011). This observation was made in a study with 13 Finnish healthy middle-aged individuals. It also gives new views on the potential of probiotic treatments. By remaining on the mucosal membranes of the stomach, and also on the mouth cavities (Pesola et al., 2012), these bacteria begin the "molecular communication" with the host body. This mutually beneficial interaction is a prerequisite for the Bacterial Intestinal Balance (BIB) (Hakalehto, 2011a, 2012, 2013). Since it seems to be likely that in the intestines the microbes form a cooperative network instead of mainly competing with each other, it is of utmost importance that our immune system is familiar with the basic components of the microbiota. In case of lactic acid bacteria the rooting onto stomach surfaces could somewhat compensate their low presence in the bile-containing duodenal areas where facultatively anaerobic coliforms dominate (Kalliomäki et al., 2008; Hakalehto et al., 2010). From the epithelia of the upper GI tract the microbes inoculate the intestinal chyme. Our studies on the combined effects of prebiotics and probiotics strongly support their integrated use (Hakalehto and Jaakkola, 2013). The product (Acidophilus Forte™) of Biomed Oy (Helsinki, Finland) consisted of *Lactobacillus acidophilus* strains (cfu 20 billion) and *Bifidobacterium bifidum* (cfu 4 billion) was used together with prebiotic flax mixed with berries (Linomix™). The field of prebiotics and probiotics in nutrition has been widely reviewed (Watson and Preedy, 2010).

3. Microbes Effect the Whole Body System and Its Functions

Once the normal flora of the gastrointestinal tract has been established during the first years of life, it is supporting the balance between our body system and the microbiome (Bezirtzoglou and Stavropoulou, 2011). The normal flora is comprising largely of lactic acid bacteria, especially in the lower intestines (Collado et al., 2012). There it seems to keep up the metabolic activities of e.g., some anaerobic members of the microbiota by gas production (Hakalehto and Hänninen, 2012). This stimulative signal effect is preventing the putrefactive strains from occupying the space on the membranes. In this case of "biological ventilation", the CO_2 is supposed to have an active role in rooting out tedious obligate anaerobes. Also, the influences of other microbial exhaust gases on the microflora components and on our body system needs to be elucidated. For example, it has been postulated that gaseous hydrogen sulfide (H_2S) is penetrating the blood veins, and consequently lowering the blood pressure (Polhemus and Lefer, 2014). Similarly, it could be supposed that there are several other beneficial influences of the microbes on the various body balances.

On the contrary, there are numerous mechanisms of the human body whose purpose is to protectthe organs against invading microbes (Kelsall, 2008). In fact, many illnesses, such as autoimmune diseases could at least partially be caused by dysfunctional protective mechanism (Subramanian et al., 2006; Lidar et al., 2009). Imbalanced microbiota may lead or participate in the pathogenic process of autoimmune inflammatory bowel diseases (Hata et al., 2001). In these circumstances some bacterial strains of microbiota may cause a systemic antibody response (Saitoh, et al., 2002).

Therefore, it is also worth paying attention to the balancing function of the healthy normal flora (Hakalehto, 2012). The microbial components of balanced niches inside the gut and other cavities of the body are able to keep control over the regions without allowing too dramatic changes to be caused by newcoming organisms or changing conditions (Hakalehto et al., 2010). Therefore, the probiotic function could always be considered as an interaction between the host body and its micro-organisms which have established an ecosystem in or around the functional areas. The formation of the alimentary microbiome in the alimentary canal is a typical example of such development leading to interfaces between man and his microbes. Since the microbes are relatively small entities, the molecular communication exercised between them and the host could take place e.g., in relatively small niches or on transparent and often microscopic surface layers or biofilms. The duodenal microflora, for example, can have a remarkable probiotic influence on the body function regardless of its relatively small cell number on the epithelia in normal circumstances (Hakalehto et al., 2008).

Besides situating the mucosal surfaces as attached cells or microcolonies, the duodenal and other surface microbes liberate cells into the swarming state. Within the intestinal chyme they form a kind of moving submerged population which takes part in the degradation and refinement of the food materials and particles together with the enzymes originating from the host body, or the food itself. This involvement of the microbes both on the surfaces and inside the fluids or solid particles is an important function also for the host digestion. If the corresponding reactions benefit the host health and metabolism they could well be called probiotic, synergic actions.

More widely, during any encounter of the host with the microbes, the bodily neuronal, humoral and immunological mechanisms take part in the recognizing and buffering of any undesired side-effects of the microbial presence. On many surfaces and inside the body, in blood circulation and elsewhere, the microbes can also exploit the degradation products of adjacent strains. Moreover, peptides originating from the microbial cells may have an influence on the body (Hakalehto et al., 1997).

Microbial structures have been assumed to take part in the pathophysiology of several diseases and conditions, such as arthritis (Castelino et al., 2014), autism (Hornig, 2013) and obesity (Lyra et al., 2010).

Therefore, probiotics are needed also for "attenuating" the excessive microbial growth in the gut, which flora could then cause the formation and absorption of molecular residues.

4. Microbial Attachment on the Epithelial Surfaces

In order to fully exploit the different probiotics it is useful to learn about their surface structures. For example, many lactobacilli attach with their S-layer consisting of regularly shaped (RS) protein subunits. These proteins are quite easily detachable in the laboratory by relatively mild acid treatments (Hakalehto et al., 1984).

However, they could also provide some protection against harsh environmental conditions. This adsorption and attachment mechanism is different from that of many enteric pathogens which exploit rapidly synthesized surface organs (e.g., fimbriae) and adhesives for anchoring onto the gut walls (Hakalehto et al., 2000). Fimbriated bacteria are important clinical pathogens e.g., in newborn babies and other pediatric patients (Tullus et al., 1984;

Tullus and Sjöberg, 1986). The latter attachment "strategies" have the drawback that the protrudements are often cut off by the bacteria in short time if the nutrients are exhausted, or when the conditions get otherwise unfavorable. It is possible to make an assumption that the LAB are able to establish more stable colonies onto the walls in general.

Some lactobacilli have, however, shown to contain also pili (fimbriae). The widely used probiotic *Lactobacillus rhamnosus* GG was genetically compared with the similarly sized genome of *L. rhamnosus* LC705, an adjunct starter culture exhibiting reduced binding to mucus (Kankainen et al., 2009). Some pilin genes were detected only with the GG strain. Using anti-SpaC antibodies (against pilin protein), the physical presence of cell wall-bound pili was confirmed by immunoblotting. Also the adherence of the strain GG to human intestinal mucus was blocked by SpaC antiserum.

Consequently, it was concluded that the presence of SpaC is essential for the mucosal interaction of *L. rhamnosus* GG and likely explains its ability to persist in the human intestinal tract longer than any ordinary starter strain could remain active in there.

An illustration of interfacial phenomena between microbes and gut epithelia is presented elsewhere (Hell et al., 2013). It seems evident that the metabolic status and available carbon sources could influence the attachment of enteric bacteria on gut epithelia (Chang et al., 2004). In this study, gluconate appeared to be a major source for *E. coli* strain MG1655 to colonize the mouse intestine.

N-acetylglucosamine and N-acetylneuraminic acid were involved in the initiation, but not in the maintenance, of the attachment. On the contrary, glucuronate, mannose, fucose, and ribose appeared to be involved in maintenance but not initiation.

A well attached probiotic strain could at best keep the tight junctions of the intestinal epithelia really tight, and it is holding back the invasive, not wanted pathogens.A study showed that a *L. rhamnosus* strain GG was able to attach *in vivo* to colonic mucosal membranes and to remain for more than a week after discontinuation of the GG administration in whey drinks (Alander et al., 1999). The supplementation of *L. rhamnosus* GG has also shown to decrease the colonic hydrolytic and reductive enzyme activities (Ling et al., 1994).

The results from this study also demonstrated that the research on fecal samples alone is not sufficient for evaluating the colonization by a probiotic strain. This was deduced from the difference between results from the fecal and colonoscopic culture samples.

5. Probiotics and *Clostridium Difficile*

Positive results accumulate from probiotic trials and usage. Randomized placebo controlled trials have shown promising results for probiotics in the treatment of certain childhood conditions, including gastroenteritis, or stomach flu, and diarrhea. *Lactobacillus rhamnosus* strain GG, for example, has been shown to reduce by 18 hours the duration of acute diarrhea, particularly the one caused by rotavirus (Szajewska and Mrukowicz, 2001).

Antibiotic treatments cause remarkable changes in intestinal microbiota (Finegold, et al., 1987).Prophylactic *Lactobacillus* GG reduced antibiotic-associated diarrhea in children with respiratory infections (Arvola et al., 1999). In Austria, there have been in active clinical use different multistrain preparations, with 10 strains included in one supplement. These products have acutely helped in adjunctive therapy of severe CDI (*Clostridium difficile* infections) cases and reduced mortality significantly. In an Israeli trial at 14 day-care centers, the children taking probiotics (*B. lactis* and *L. reuteri*) had fewer episodes and shorter periods of diarrhea and less occurrence of fever (Van Niel, 2005). Along the small intestines, the probiotics can take action in balancing the food uptake and digestion (Hakalehto and Jaakkola, 2013).

Gould et al. (2008) have written about the concept of treating *Clostridium difficile* associated diseases. Moreover, the concept of treatments of *C. difficile* infections probiotics has been recently reviewed by Fitzpatrick (2013).

Some strains of this tedious and persistent pathogen are highly transmissible (Hell et al. 2008). They are enriched e.g., during antibiotic treatments, and could spread epidemically in the wards. Their eradication may constitute a hygienic problem.

Stool transfer is fashionable, but could in many cases have a "clean" alternative in a multi-strain probiotic product. In some cases stools from close relatives could include "native" strains for the particular individual, which could be a benefit. More research on this topic is warranted.

Also the tested disinfective substance with "on site oxidation" is according to a reasonable, practical line of thinking (Hell et al., 2014).

In fact, couldn't we combine this with some rooting of effective probiotics? The combined effect could be simulated in the PMEU (Hakalehto and Jaakkola, 2013).

Regarding the antibiotic treatments there should be openness for continuous development. Any antibiotic treatment should be possible to get combined and/or enforced by other procedures, such as joint pre- and probiotic treatments. In this context, a need for a multistrain probiotic has been recognized (Hakalehto et al., 2012c, Hell et al., 2013).

6. Probiotics and Human Efforts to Improve the Alimentary Microflora

Nowadays, common understanding on the importance of the alimentary microbes on our health has rapidly increased. The interest of producing bioactive foods by adding probiotics into foods has also increased (Farnworth and Champagne, 2010).

One author (Elias Hakalehto) was at 1986 the first scientist in a joint project between Helsinki University and the Finnish Dairy company Valio (then a cooperative, now Valio Oyj, the largest dairy corporation in Finland). At that time, 25 years ago, the aim of the investigation was to make a recommendation on ways for Valio to get involved in the probiotics business. The conclusion of the preliminary work was to suggest the acquisition of a microbial strain that was as profoundly researched as possible. The intention was to find a probiotic bacterium whose beneficial influences on human health had been scientifically widely documented. On this basis Valio then purchased the rights for the GG (*Lactobacillus rhamnosus*) strain (Goldin and Gorbach, 2008), whose trade name was to be Gefilus™ in Finland (Yli-Knuuttila et al., 2006).

The research behind, or on the basis of the Gefilus™, "good bacteria", has been further accumulated since then. Nevertheless, the research has mostly focused on the microbiota in the colon (and thus the fecal microbes). These are the most numerous populations of the normal flora. However, even more important ecosystems could exist within different parts of our alimentary tract. The microbes of the large intestines take a benefit of our metabolic waste materials, but the microflora in the duodenum, for example, takes part in the nutrient intake. When researching these microbial communities, we also have to make a clear distinction between the biofilms attached onto the surfaces and the suspended microbial growth in the fluidic contents of the alimentary tract. Inoculum for the latter one often originates (or gets detached) from the biofilm microflora. The mechanisms behind the population dynamics in these different niches need to be better understood, as well as their interactions.

7. Probiotic Bacteria and Mouth

The use of probiotics in regulation of the microbiota of the gastrointestinal tract has been studied for years and it is based on the assumptions and accumulating data on probiotics having a favorable influence to the intestinal functions and balance. A total amount of 1.5 kg of bacterial mass is permanently colonizing intestinal surfaces. Probiotic and antibiotic effects to that alimentary ecosystem are complex and diverse. Less is known about the effects of probiotics in the oral cavity. Thus, the influences of probiotics on the oral mucosa and other surfaces should be one focus of future studies. Patients with immunosuppressive status in oral mucosa or having x-ray therapy to head and neck region are examples of patient groups that could benefit from this line of research.

Long term effects of probiotic therapy of oral diseases have been studied inadequately. Probiotic bacteria have possible favorable effect in parodontal infection, but when dosing of probiotic bacteria will be stopped, oral biofilm returns back to its previous state in a couple of weeks. Reliable long term clinical knowledge and evidence of this issue is lacking (Teughels et al., 2011). In vitro data support the protective effects of the probiotics. When probiotics of yoghurt *(Lactobacillus bulgaricus, Streptococcus thermophilus, Lactobacillus acidophilus,* and *Bifidobacterium* sp.*)* were inoculated with parodontopathogens those probiotics prevented the growth of most important these pathogens (Zhu et al., 2010).

Growth of Gram-negative anaerobic parodontopathogens can be restricted with so called BALObacteria (Bdellovibrio and like organisms) at least *in vitro*.

Those bacteria isolated from intestinal or fecal samples have been used *in vitro* for the predation of e.g., *Aggregatibacter actinomycetemcomitans, Porphyromonas gingivalis and Prevotella intermedia, Fusobacterium nucleatum.* These predator bacteria could be promising tools for treatments for parodontal diseases in dental clinics in the future (Van Essche et al., 2011).

8. Probiotic Cure Considerations

So far the major probiotic organisms have belonged to the lactic acid bacteria (LAB) group, which contain widely spread genuses among intestinal organisms. They are either coccoid in form, or demonstrate rod-like cellular shape.

Most of the members of this group are facultative anaerobes. They grow well in good growth conditions but also tend to be somewhat demanding with respect to the prevailing circumstances. Especially this is true in case of lactobacilli.

These facultatively anaerobic organisms, nevertheless, have been demonstrated to exhibit several positive functions inside the human GI tract (Ahrne and Hagslatt, 2011; Daniluk et al., 2012; Hakalehto et al., 2012c). They have been shown to have an attenuating effect on other intestinal flora (Hakalehto and Jaakkola, 2013).

In an overall view on the intestinal microbial ecosystem the lactobacilli and other lactic acid bacteria have an important role in maintaining the balance in the entire GI tract. Their wide presence has been verified even in the gastric areas (Hakalehto et al., 2011). *Lactobacillus rhamnosus* GG has shown beneficial effects in case of infants with atopic dermatitis (Nermes et al., 2011) and acute viral gastroenteritis (Majamaa et al., 1995).

Besides the lactic acid bacteria, nowadays many other organisms have been used or suggested for the probiotic functions. The problem with many of these strains is that they belong to a microbial group which includes some pathogenic members, or their role in the GI tract has not been otherwise clear enough for official acceptance, so far. However, in real life, various microbial strains do inhabit the intestines and other alimentary tract in mixed cultures. Most essential for the health effect considerations is usually the sum effect on the overall microflora. In these surroundings, microflora is carrying out specific digestive functions which often are performed by different strains within different human host individuals. Therefore, in general considerations on microbial health effects, it is of crucial importance to take in to account the total contribution of all the strains on host health. This microbial action is functioning in association with several host functions such as humoral, neuronal and immunological activities of the host body system (Lyte, 2010; Trakhtenberg and Goldberg, 2011).

On the basis of the above-mentioned generalized view on human microbiota, it is often self-evident to recommend the use of mixed cultures or mixed flora products with several microbial strains as substitutes. However, according to the present ideology and practices these strains are investigated individually with respect to their characteristics and interactions with human body system. Therefore, any and all supplementations are subjected to acceptance by the authorities, which naturally is important for maintaining high qualities of the treatments and these supplementations.

One option has been to use the microbial strains which are isolated from the host self. In this case there are other options and points of view to be taken in to account. This might be an interesting option for preterm babies or other immunodeficient patients, for example. However, there is still some controversy in the use of probiotics in this population (Isolauri, 2007).

This option has been referred to in part 5 of this chapter. The effects of probiotic distribution could be followed even from environmental water samples (Heitto et al., 2006; Hakalehto, 2011a, 2014).

Often good results have been achieved by using probiotic strains belonging to genera of the family *Enterobacteriaceae* (Cary and Boullata, 2010; Jacobi and Malfertheiner, 2011). However, the problem with this family is their wide variance and the possibilities of transform of genetic material etc., all though the view on these potential limitations in probiotic use have not been clearly established.

In any case, the consequences of the treatment have to be validated on individual basis with respect to the condition of the individual patients. On the basis of the studies with the PMEU in our laboratory it has been noticed that enterobacterial strains can form a delicate balance between acid producing and neutral substances producing strains (Hakalehto et al., 2008). This dualistic balance is in away the base line for the BIB (bacteriological intestinal balance) (Hakalehto, 2011b, 2012, 2013).

In this context, it has been documented that any new stains invading or existing in the microbial community can find their niches under the "umbrella" of basic pH regulation and other functions inside the intestines. On the basis of all these considerations it is possible to understand the essential role of the enteric bacteria in controlling the balance in the chyme. These findings give a basis for the understanding on the functioning of the intestinal microflora as stated in Chapter 14. This microflora is participating in the digestive processes and the enterobacterial members and other bile tolerant members of the flora are inoculating the chyme already in the duodenum. The bile is an important selective agent participating in the maintenance of the healthy balance of the microbiota (Ejderhamn, et al., 1991).

Detection of enterobacterial strains, and recovery of any individual strains, was significantly improved by the use of PMEU methods (Pesola et al., 2009; Pesola and Hakalehto, 2011).

It has been shown that the adhesion of various pathogenic *E. coli* strains on the intestinal epithelia has been inhibited by strains of *Lactobacillus plantarum, Streptococcus thermophiles, L. acidophilus,* and by *L. helveticus* and some other lactobacilli (Lodemann, 2010). As discussed in Chapter 32, the different surface attachment mechanisms, and structures responsible for them, could explain the "attenuation" of the intestinal coliforms (Hakalehto and Jaakkola, 2013). However, the PMEU method turned out to be a potential tool for validating some probiotic influences on the other microflora in the presence of prebiotic supplementation. The prebiotic flax would possibly provide the LAB strains with platforms where they could exercise the attenuative mechanisms, whatever they actually were in closer inspection (Figure 1 a-b).

Some effects of probiotic *Saccharomyces boulardii* are based on their effects on secretion in the small gut, where the yeast is converting the cAMP-mediated chloride-ion secretion into absorption of these ions (Krammer and Karbach, 1993).

This indicates the importance for bacterial colonization of ionic strength and movements in the intestines and in other tissues. *S. boulardii* has also been shown to secrete a protease which cleaves *C. difficile* toxin A molecule (Castagliuolo et al., 1996).

This probiotic yeast also increases the mucosal polyamine concentrations (Buts et al., 1994). All the above-mentioned functions of a probiotic *S. boulardii* influence on the epithelial conditions in such a way that it helps the body system to resist the pathogens.

The examples also demonstrate that many of the probiotic effects are functional with in a network of molecular communication between host body and its microbes.

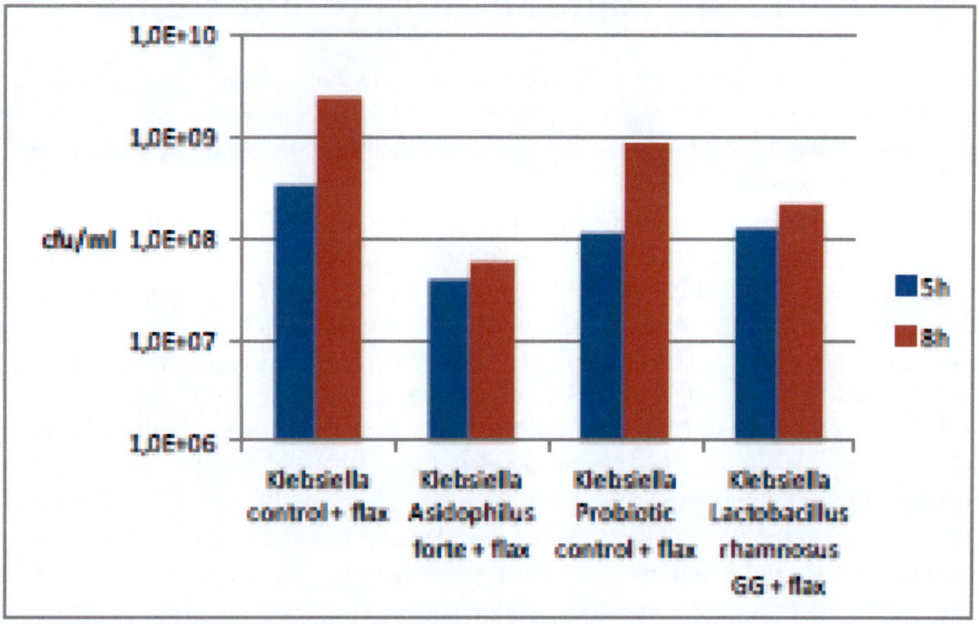

a

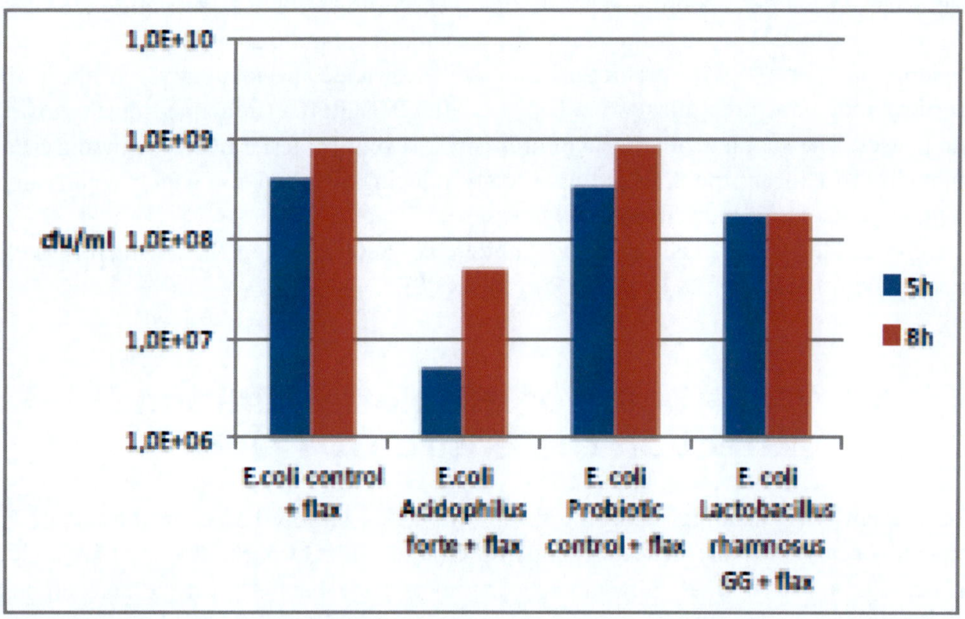

b

Figure 1. (a-b) Influences of three different probiotic products on the growth of a. *Klebsiella mobilis* and b. *Escherichia coli* with flax containing prebiotic supplementation in the PMEU Spectrion® (Modified from Hakalehto and Jaakkola, 2013).

9. Combined Prebiotic and Probiotic Effects

Different prebiotics and probiotics have been studied in therapy and prevention of gastrointestinal diseases (De Vrese and Marteau, 2007;–Salvatore and Vandenplas, 2010). Aim of this study was to test the probiotic effect in conditions simulating the duodenum with and without prebiotic addition.

In our study Acidophilus Forte™ including *Lactobacillus acidophilus, Bifidobacterium bifidum* and *B. lactis* was inoculated into mixed culture of facultative *Klebsiella mobilis* and *Escherichia coli* in the PMEU (Portable Microbe Enrichment Unit) (Hakalehto, 2012). Growth curves were determined by the PMEU Spectrion®, and by subsampling onto CHROMagar™ (Becton, Dickinson and Company, US) plates. Incubations at +37 °C with microaerobic gas (85% N_2, 10% CO_2, 5% O_2) resembled the duodenal conditions. Another probiotic product containing lactobacilli and bifidobacteria (probiotic control) was used as reference. For the best effect, a joint influence with Linomix™ with crushed flax seed (52%) and berries (24%) in buffer was required.

After 5 hours in the PMEU, Acidophilus Forte™ with prebiotics diminished the growth of *K. mobilis* by 88% and *E. coli* by 99%. Corresponding values for the probiotic control were 64% and 17%, respectively. After 8h cultivation (in the stationary phase), the culture with Acidophilus Forte™ was short of 98% and 94% of *K. mobilis* and *E. coli* cell numbers in the comparison with the zero control, respectively. These values for the probiotic control were 67% and 0%. Probiotics alone had not any significant effect on the growth.

Acidophilus Forte™ with prebiotic Linomix™ restricted the facultatives in the PMEU. Neither probiotics nor prebiotics alone had this effect. The effect remained during different growth phases. The supplementations could *in vivo* prevent bacterial overgrowth and balance the numbers of acid and neutral end-products producing facultatives, which could support food uptake (Kristensen and Jensen, 2011).

. *E. coli* and the klebsiellas formed a symbiotic co-culture in the PMEU which is likely to function in the small intestines (Hakalehto et al., 2008).

10. What Kinds of Probiotic Additions? Effect on the Entire GI Tract?

The present understanding regarding the probiotics is largely based on the use of LAB (lactic acid bacteria) as the active organisms (Goldin and Gorbach, 2008). This bacterial group belongs to our normal flora, and its members have been shown to have numerous positive effects on our health. They have even shown to inhibit Th2 cytokine production by mononuclear cells of allergic patients thereby reducing the deviation of the immune system towards allergy (Pochard, et al., 2002).

Perhaps even more importantly, this group is not containing any pathogenic strains, which makes the usage of the strains relatively safe. It has also been documented that the LAB strains are relatively well surviving in the GI tract, including the acidic gastric regions of healthy individuals (Hakalehto et al., 2011). However, if we wish to extend our understanding on the alimentary microbiology, as well as to increase the potential for curing and preventing the diseases using this knowledge, also other groups of microbes should be considered as vehicles for treatment. Non-lactic acid probiotics often work by increasing acidity in the intestine, thereby inhibiting the proliferation of bacteria, destroying undesirable microorganisms, and suppressing inflammation. In the future it should be a goal to produce such probiotics or their mixtures, which take into account the entire microbial community of the gut, and its interactions with the host.

In fact, it should be kept in mind that one part of the health effects of the lactic acid bacteria are related to the lactic acid itself. This was documented by Metchnikoff already more than one hundred years ago (Metchnikoff, 1907).

The regulatory mechanism on the probiotics usage should be flexible enough for achieving the goals of the supplementations. At the same time, the individuals have to be protected from any side-effects. Keeping this baseline in mind the restrictions of the current policies should be wisely simplified by the following ways:

1 The probiotic treatments with several simultaneous additions (by mixed cultures) should be made more easily achievable, and more research should be directed on them. The correct combinations of strains should be searched for.
2 The absolute amounts of the probiotic cells should be increased for the best effect.
3 The selection of the probiotic organisms should not be restricted to lactic acid bacteria (LAB) only.
4 The interactions of chosen formulae should be simulated on various foods and nutritive factors by using such tools as the PMEU (Portable Microbe Enrichment Unit) for the monitoring of these interactions.
5 Novel means for following up the positive health effects both in human populations and in the individual alimentary systems have to be designed.
6 Also other sites within the alimentary tract, besides the colon, have to be targeted. For example, in the PMEU studies there has been shown to exist a balanced symbiotic community of different enterobacterial species in the duodenum (Hakalehto et al., 2008, 2010; Hakalehto, 2011b). Most nutrient are absorbed in the small intestines.

In many studies, the joint effect of e.g., bifidobacteria with *Streptococcus thermophilus* has been documented (Saavedra et al., 1994, Thibault et al., 2004). In additions of mixed cultures it could be possible to achieve a long-lasting effect which is directed toward the various parts of the alimentary tract at the same time.

In the case of preventing antibiotic associated diarrhea (AAD) a mixture of strains: LGG, *Bifidobacterium lactis* (former *B. bifidus*), *Streptococcus thermophilus* and *Saccharomyces boulardii* reduced the risk from 28.5% to 11.9% (Szajewska et al., 2006). *S. boulardii* yeast also significantly reduced the risk of diarrhea on days 3, 6 and 7 (Szajewska et al., 2007). Also the risk of diarrhea lasting for more than seven days was significantly lowered.

In our recent studies, one probable mechanism of probiotic effects is the production of gaseous compounds such as the CO_2 by the LAB in the intestines (Hakalehto, 2011; Hakalehto and Hänninen, 2012). This substance is keeping the clostridia in an active growth phase, thus inhibiting their sporulation and spread or penetration onto the gut walls. It was observed in our experiments also that the 100% CO_2 as the gassing agent in the PMEU was well tolerated by *Clostridium difficile* and other clostridia (Hell et al., 2010). Also other bacteria such as *E. coli* have been shown to be provoked by some CO_2 but they generally also have an upper limit for CO_2 level (Hakalehto and Hänninen, 2012). The requirement for small carbon dioxide concentration for promoting the growth among eubacteria, was detected already a long time ago (Volley and Rettger, 1927). This phenomenon has not been explained so far. In our studies with the PMEU it is possible to investigate the precise effects of various gases on the microbial populations. Their gas generation has also been studied in several projects with the PMEU Scentrion® (Hakalehto, 2010, 2011b; Hakalehto et al., 2008, 2009, 2011; Pesola et al., 2012; Laitiomäki et al., 2014).

The probiotic addition could consist of several kinds of micro-organisms, not only of the LAB (lactic acid bacteria). For example the use of viruses, bacteriophages for the treatments in the gastrointestinal tract has been suggested (Lederberg, 1996). These components are numerous in the GI tract in any case, and being like parasites of the bacterial species, they could be used to control or block out some undesired strains. It is also imaginable that by the phages it could be possible to maintain, manipulate, and carry out the formulation of the microbial ecosystem. Another option and trial for a new kind of implementation of the probiotics has been the use of yeasts for outgrowing *Salmonella typhimurium* or *Clostridium difficile* in the mice intestines (Martins et al., 2005). The *Saccharomyces cerevisiae* yeasts isolated from natural sources were able to decrease mortality in a group of conventional mice challenged with *S. typhimurium* and to rule out the effects of *C. difficile* in germ-free gnotobiotic mice. However, these kinds of probiotic additions in humans require caution because the yeasts as such may constitute a risk of microbial overgrowth or dysbiosis in some conditions, and could thus have detrimental effects on the microbiome as a whole. It has been stated that "one factor impeding the introduction of effective probiotics has been our very limited understanding of the composition of the human microbiome, as well as the biological requirements for these organisms" (Dominguez-Bello and Blaser, 2008).

Probiotic strains that cannot survive in the gastric acidity could be protected e.g., by using microencapsulation method (Chen, et al., 2012). This could offer the possibility to use new interesting probiotic microbes.

For this purpose, it is not enough to study the metagenome of the micro-organisms in the various hosts, but to also increase knowledge of competition and cooperation between the microbes, and also that of the host-microbe signaling.

Only robust scientific basis makes it possible to develop further the probiotic strategies leading to clinical trials and commercialization of the novel products. The PMEU (Portable Microbe Enrichment Unit) offers one tool for testing the microbial interactions, and the influences of the gut environmental factors on the specific strains and the mixed cultures (Hakalehto, 2010, 2011b; Pesola and Hakalehto, 2011). This work should be extended as infection control to the nearest environments of the patients inside the hospital systems, and in the homes and working places (Hakalehto, 2006, 2010).

For example, such strains in the hospital equipment as the *Enterobacter cloacae* may develop more easily multi-resistant forms than the actual intestinal bacteria (Hakalehto, 2011a). The antibiotic resistance markers in them could then pose a risk for distribution and transfer to other strains, and to the pathogenic bacteria.

Lactobacillus and *Streptococcus* strains are found in mucosal membranes in all parts of the mouth cavity as predominant species. These strains had been used for the treatment of *Candida albicans* (Hakalehto, E, unpublished results). Many probiotics are lactic acid bacteria (LAB), which are believed to promote healing in the intestine by reducing gut permeability and enhancing intestinal immune responses. Lactic acid is the least absorbing organic acids in the alimentary tract. Its production by the bacteria is taking part of the nutrients out of the body's most instant reach and distributes the substrate for even the distal colonic bacteria (see also Chapter 14), thus the effect of the probiotic addition can extend its effect onto the entire length of the GI tract.

Conclusion

In probiotic treatment strategies various factors have to be studied simultaneously, namely:

- balancing ecosystem effects on the communities
- population dynamics in mixed cultures
- persistence in relation with bacterial cell surface structures
- metabolic action in the chyme
- immunomodulation by the strains
- gaseous signal effects within the biofilms and chyme populations
- host - microbe "molecular communication"
- relations with the host defenses
- development of human normal flora during the first years of age
- target tissues to be defined precisely, as well as the effects and efficacies of the treatments
- joint exploitation of pre- and probiotic functions

This generalized but still focused list hopefully could help in designing future probiotics, and in their improvement.

References

Aho, M., Nuotio, L., Nurmi, E., Kiiskinen, T. Competitive exclusion of campylobacters from poultry with K-bacteria and Broilact®. *Int. J. Food Microbiol.*, 1992; 15, 265-275.

Ahrne, S., Hagslatt, M. L. Effect of lactobacilli on paracellular permeability in the gut. *Nutrients*, 2011; 3, 104-117.

Alander, M., Satokari, R., Korpela, R., Saxelin, M., Vilpponen-Salmela, T., Mattila-Sandholm, T., von Wright, A. Persistence of colonization of human colonic mucosa by a probiotic strain, *Lactobacillus rhamnosus* GG, after oral consumption. *Appl. Environ. Microbiol.,* 1999; 65, 351-354.

Arvola, T., Laiho, K., Torkkeli, S., Mykkanen, H., Salminen, S., Maunula, L., Isolauri, E. Prophylactic *Lactobacillus* GG reduces antibiotic-associated diarrhea in children with respiratory infections: a randomized study. *Pediatrics,* 1999; 104, e64.

Bezirtzoglou E., Stavropoulou, E. Immunology and probiotic impact of the newborn and young children intestinal microflora. *Anaerobe*, 2011; 17, 369-374.

Brissaud, O., Tandonnet, O., Guichoux, J. Invasive candidiasis in neonatal intensive care units. *Arch. Pediatr.*, 2011; 18 (Suppl. 1), S22-32.

Buts, J. P., De Keyser, N., De Raedemaeker, L. *Saccharomyces boulardii* enhances rat intestinal enzyme expression by endoluminal release of polyamines. *Pediatr. Res.*, 1994; 36, 522-527.

Cary, V. A., Boullata, J. What is the evidence for the use of probiotics in the treatment of inflammatory bowel disease? *J. Clin. Nurs.*, 2010; 19, 904-916.

Castagliuolo, I., LaMont, J. T., Nikulasson, S. T., Pothoulakis, C. *Saccharomyces boulardii* protease inhibits *Clostridium difficile* toxin A effects in the rat ileum. *Infect. Immun.*, 1996; 64, 5225-5232.

Castelino, M., Eyre, S., Upton, M., Ho, P., Barton, A. The bacterial skin microbiome in psoriatic arthritis, an unexplored link in pathogenesis: challenges and opportunities offered by recent technological advances. *Rheumatology*, 2014; 53, 777-784.

Chang, D.-E., Smalley, D. J., Tucker, D. L., Leatham, M. P., Norris, W. E., Stevenson, S. J., Anderson, A. B., Grissom, J. E., Laux, D. C., Cohen, P. S., Conway, T. Carbon nutrition of *Escherichia coli* in the mouse intestine. *PNAS*, 2004; 101, 7427-7432.

Chen, S., Zhao, Q., Ferguson, L. R., Shu, Q., Weir, I., Garg, S. Development of a novel probiotic delivery system based on microencapsulation with protectants. *Appl. Microbiol. Biotechnol.*, 2012; 93, 1447-1457.

Collado, M. C., Meriluoto, J., Salminen, S. Role of commercial probiotic strains against human pathogen adhesion to intestinal mucus. *Lett. Appl. Microbiol.*, 2007; 45, 454-460.

Collado, M. C., Cernada, M., Bäuerl, C., Vento, M., Pérez-Martínez, G. Microbial ecology and host-microbiota interactions during early life stages. *Gut Microbes*, 2012; 3, 352-365.

Daniluk, U., Alifier, M., Kaczmarski, M. Probiotic-induced apoptosis and its potential relevance to mucosal inflammation of gastrointestinal tract. *Adv. Med. Sci.*, 2012; 57, 175-182.

De Vrese, M., Marteau, P. R. Probiotics and prebiotics: effects on diarrhea. *J. Nutr.*, 2007; 137, 803S-811S.

Dominguez-Bello, M. G., Blaser, M. J. Do you have a probiotic in your future? *Microbes Infect.*, 2008; 10, 1072-1076.

Eckburg, P. B., Bik, E. M., Bernstein, C. N., Purdom, E., Dethlefsen, L., Sargent, M., Gill, S. R., Nelson, K. E., Relman, D. A. Diversity of the human intestinal microbial flora. *Science*, 2005; 308, 1635-1638.

Ejderhamn, J., Rafter, J. J., Strandvik, B. Faecal bile acid excretion in children with inflammatory bowel disease. *Gut*, 1991; 32, 1346-1351.

Farnworth, E. R., Champagne, C. P. Production of probiotic cultures and their incorporation into foods. In: Watson, R. R., Preedy, V. R., editors. *Bioactive Foods promoting health: Probiotics and Prebiotics*: Academic Press/Elsevier Inc.; 2010; 3-17.

Finegold, S. M., Ingram-Drake, L., Gee, R., Reinhardt, J., Edelstein, M. A., MacDonald, K., Wexler, H. Bowel flora changes in humans receiving cefixime (CL 284,635) or cefaclor. *Antimicrob. Agents Chemother.*, 1987; 31, 443-446.

Fitzpatrick, L. R.. Probiotics for the treatment of *Clostridium difficile*–associated disease. *World J. Gastrointest. Pathophysiol.*, 2013; 4, 47-52.

Goldin, B. R., Gorbach, S. L. Clinical indications for probiotics: an overview. *Clin. Infect. Dis.*, 2008; 46 (Suppl. 2), S96-100; discussion S144-151.

Gould, C. V., McDonald, L. C. Bench-to-bedside review: *Clostridium difficile* colitis. *Crit. Care,* 2008; 12, 203-210.

Hakalehto, E. Semmelweis' present day follow-up: Updating bacterial sampling and enrichment in clinical hygiene. *Pathophysiology,* 2006; 13, 257-267.

Hakalehto, E. Hygiene monitoring with the Portable Microbe Enrichment Unit (PMEU). *41st R3 -Nordic Symposium. Cleanroom technology, contamination control and cleaning. VTT Publications 266.* Espoo, Finland: VTT (State Research Centre of Finland); 2010.

Hakalehto, E. Antibiotic resistant traits of facultative *Enterobacter cloacae* strain studied with the PMEU (Portable Microbe Enrichment Unit). In Press. In: Méndez-Vilas, A., editor. *Science against microbial pathogens: communicating current research and technological advances. Microbiology book series Nr. 3.* Badajoz, Spain: Formatex Research Center; 2011a; pp. 786-796.

Hakalehto, E. Simulation of enhanced growth and metabolism of intestinal *Escherichia coli* in the Portable Microbe Enrichment Unit (PMEU). In: Roger, M. C., Peterson, N. D., editors. *E. coli infections: causes, treatment and prevention.* New York, US: Nova Publishers; 2011b; pp. 159-175.

Hakalehto, E., editor. *Alimentary microbiome - a PMEU approach.* New York, NY, US: Nova Science Publishers, Inc.; 2012.

Hakalehto, E. Interactions of *Klebsiella* sp. with other intestinal flora. In: Pereira, L. A., Santos, A., editors. *Klebsiella Infections: Epidemiology, Pathogenesis and Clinical Outcomes*. New York, US: Nova Science Publishers, Inc.; 2013; pp. 1-33.

Hakalehto, E. Bacteriological indications of human activities in the ecosystems. In: Armon, R., Hänninen, O., editors. *Environmental indicators*. Germany: Springer Verlag; 2014. (In Print).

Hakalehto, E., Hänninen, O. Gaseous CO_2 signal initiate growth of butyric acid producing *Clostridium butyricum* both in pure culture and in mixed cultures with *Lactobacillus brevis. Can. J. Microbiol.,* 2012; 58, 928-931.

Hakalehto, E., Jaakkola, K. Synergistic effect of probiotics and prebiotic flax product on intestinal bacterial balance. *Clinical Nutrition,* 2013; 32 (Suppl. 1), S200.Hakalehto, E., Santa H, Vepsäläinen J, Laatikainen R, Finne J. Identification of a common structural motif in the disordered N-terminal region of bacterial flagellins. Evidence for a new class of fibril-forming peptides. *Eur J Biochem,* 1997; 250, 19-29.

Hakalehto, E., Haikara, A., Lounatmaa, K.,Enari, T.-M. Hydrochloric acid extractable protein patterns of *Pectinatus cerevisiophilus* strain, *Food Microbiol.,* 1984; 1, 209-216.

Hakalehto, E., Hujakka, H., Airaksinen, S., Ratilainen, J., Närvänen, A. Growth-phase limited expression and rapid detection of *Salmonella* type 1 fimbriae. In: Hakalehto, E., editor. *Characterization of Pectinatus cerevisiiphilus and P. frisingiensis surface components. Use of synthetic peptides in the detection fo some Gram-negative bacteria.* Kuopio, Finland: Kuopio University Publications C. Natural and Environmental Sciences 112; 2000.

Hakalehto, E., Humppi, T., Paakkanen, H. Dualistic acidic and neutral glucose fermentation balance in small intestine: Simulation in vitro. *Pathophysiology,* 2008; 15, 211-220.

Hakalehto, E., Pesola, J., Heitto, A., Deo, B. B., Rissanen, K., Sankilampi, U., Humppi, T., Paakkanen, H. Fast detection of bacterial growth by using Portable Microbe Enrichment Unit (PMEU) and ChemPro100i((R)) gas sensor. *Pathophysiology,* 2009; 16, 57-62.

Hakalehto, E., Hell, M., Bernhofer, C., Heitto, A., Pesola, J., Humppi, T., Paakkanen, H. Growth and gaseous emissions of pure and mixed small intestinal bacterial cultures: Effects of bile and vancomycin. *Pathophysiology,* 2010; 17, 45-53.

Hakalehto, E., Vilpponen-Salmela, T., Kinnunen, K., von Wright, A. Lactic acid bacteria enriched from human gastric biopsies. *ISRN Gastroenterol.,* 2011; 2011, 109183. doi: 10. 5402/2011/109183.

Hakalehto, E., Pesola, I., Jaakkola, K. Isolations of gastric microbes using the PMEU. In: Hakalehto, E., editor. *Alimentary microbiome - a PMEU approach.* New York, NY, US: Nova Science Publishers, Inc.; 2012a; pp. 47-60.

Hakalehto, E., Pesola, J., del Amo, E.M., Hänninen, O. Bacterial interactions in the small intestine and their contribution to host nutrient uptake. In: Hakalehto, E., editor. *Alimentary microbiome - a PMEU approach.* New York, NY, US: Nova Science Publishers, Inc.; 2012c; pp. 61-94.

Hakalehto, E., Hell, M., Hänninen, O. What should a future probiotic be like? In: Hakalehto, E., editor. *Alimentary microbiome - a PMEU approach.* New York, NY, US: Nova Science Publishers, Inc.; 2012c; pp. 233-245.

Hänninen, O., Lindström-Seppä, P., Pelkonen, K. Role of gut in xenobiotic metabolism. *Arch. Toxicol.,* 1987; 60, 34-36.

Hata, K., Andoh, A., Sato, H., Araki, Y., Tanaka, M., Tsujikawa, T., Fujiyama, Y., Bamba, T. Sequential changes in luminal microflora and mucosal cytokine expression during developing of colitis in HLA-B27/beta2-microglobulin transgenic rats. *Scand. J. Gastroenterol.,* 2001; 36, 1185-1192.

Hatakka, K., Savilahti, E., Pönkä, A., Meurman, J. H., Poussa, T., Näse, L., Saxelin, M., Korpela, R. Effect of long term consumption of probiotic milk on infections in children attending day care centres: double blind, randomised trial. *BMJ*, 2001; 322, 1327-1331.

Hatakka, K., Ahola, A. J., Yli-Knuuttila, H., Richardson, M., Poussa, T., Meurman, J. H., Korpela, R. Probiotics reduce the prevalence of oral candida in the elderly--a randomized controlled trial. *J. Dent. Res.*, 2007a; 86, 125-130.

Hatakka, K., Pitkäranta, A., Valtonen, V. Probiootit infektioiden ehkäisyssä (in Finnish) ("Probiotics in prevention of infections". *Duodecim*, 2007b; 15, 1795-1796.

Heitto, L., Heitto, A., Hakalehto, E. Tracing wastewaters with faecal coliforms and enterococci In: Simola H., editor. *Seminar on Large Lakes 2006*. Joensuu, Finland; 2006, 101-106.

Helander, H. F., Sundell, G. W. Ultrastructure of inhibited parietal cells in the rat. *Gastroenterology,* 1984; 87, 1064-1071.

Hell, M., Bernhofer, C., Huhulescu, S., Indra, A., Allerberger, F., Maass, M., Hakalehto, E. How safe is colonoscope-reprocessing regarding *Clostridium difficile* spores? *Supplement 1: Abstracts, 7th International Congress of the Hospital Infection Society;* 10-13 October 2010; Liverpool, UK; 2010.

Hell, M., Bernhofer, C., Stalzer, P., Kern, J. M., Claassen, E. Probiotics in *Clostridium difficile* infection: reviewing the need for a multistrain probiotic. *Benef. Microbes*, 2013; 4, 39-51.

Hell, M., Schmid, D., Simons, E., Bernhofer, C., Achleitner, D.-I., Stalzer, P., Allerberger, F. Improved control of nosocomial *Clostridium difficile* transmission by daily use of an oxygen-releasing sporicidal disinfectant. *Int. J. Infect. Control*, 2014; doi: 10.3396/IJIC. v10i2.014.14.

Hornig, M. The role of microbes and autoimmunity in the pathogenesis of neuropsychiatric illness. *Curr. Opin. Rheumatol.*, 2013; 25, 488-795.

Isolauri, E. Probiotics in preterm infants: a controversial issue. *J. Pediatr. Gastroenterol. Nutr.*, 2007; 45 (Suppl. 3), S188-189.

Jacobi, C. A., Malfertheiner, P. *Escherichia coli* Nissle 1917 (Mutaflor): new insights into an old probiotic bacterium. *Dig. Dis.*, 2011; 29, 600-607.

Jaakkola, K., Hakalehto, E. Intestinal imbalances and diseases of the digestive tract. In: Hakalehto, E., editor. *Alimentary microbiome - a PMEU approach.* New York, NY, US: Nova Science Publishers, Inc.; 2012; pp. 127-160.

Kalliomaki, M., Salminen, S., Isolauri, E. Positive interactions with the microbiota: probiotics. *Adv. Exp. Med. Biol.,* 2008; 635, 57-66.

Kankainen, M., Paulin, L., Tynkkynen, S., von Ossowski, I., Reunanen, J., Partanen, P., Satokari, R., Vesterlund, S., Hendrickx, A. P., Lebeer, S., De Keersmaecker, S. C., Vanderleyden, J., Hämäläinen, T., Laukkanen, S., Salovuori, N., Ritari, J., Alatalo, E., Korpela, R., Mattila-Sandholm, T., Lassig, A., Hatakka, K., Kinnunen, K. T., Karjalainen, H., Saxelin, M., Laakso, K., Surakka, A., Palva, A., Salusjarvi, T., Auvinen, P., de Vos, W. M. Comparative genomic analysis of *Lactobacillus rhamnosus* GG reveals pili containing a human- mucus binding protein. *Proc. Natl. Acad. Sci. US,* 2009; 106, 17193-17198.

Kelsall, B. L. Innate and adaptive mechanisms to control of pathological intestinal inflammation. *J. Pathol.,* 2008; 214, 242–259.

Kendall A. I. Some observations on the study of the intestinal bacteria. *J. Biol. Chem.*, 1909; 6, 499–507.

Krammer, M., Karbach, U. Antidiarrheal action of the yeast *Saccharomyces boulardii* in the rat small and large intestine by stimulating chloride absorption. *Zeitschrift für Gastroenterologie,* 1993; 31 (Suppl. 4), 73-77.

Kristensen, M., Jensen, M. G. Dietary fibres in the regulation of appetite and food intake. Importance of viscosity. *Appetite,* 2011; 56, 65-70.

Laitiomäki, E., Pesola, J., Hakalehto, E. *Projected improvement in the fast microbiological analysis of neonatal blood samples; 2014*. Submitted for publication.

Lederberg, J. Infectious history. *Science*, 2000; 288, 287-293.

Lederberg, J. Smaller fleas ... ad infinitum: therapeutic bacteriophage redux. *Proc. Natl. Acad. Sci. US,* 1996; 93, 3167-3168.

Lidar, M., Langevitz, P., Barzilai, O., Ram, M., Porat-Katz, B.S., Bizzaro, N., Tonutti, E., Maieron, R., Chowers, Y., Bar-Meir, S., Shoenfeld, Y. Infectious serologies and autoantibodies in inflammatory bowel disease: insinuations at a true pathogenic role. *Ann. N. Y. Acad. Sci.*, 2009; 1173, 640-648.

Ling, W. H., Korpela, R., Mykkänen, H., Salminen, S., Hänninen, O. *Lactobacillus* strain GG supplementation decreases colonic hydrolytic and reductive enzyme activities in healthy female adults. *J. Nutr.,* 1994; 124, 18-23.

Lodemann, U. Effects of probiotics on intestinal transport and epithelial barrier function. In: Watson, R. R., Preedy, V. R., editors. *Bioactive Foods in Promoting Health: Probiotics and Prebiotics*. London, UK: Academic Press; 2010; pp. 303-333.

Lyra, A., Lahtinen, S., Tiihonen, K., Ouwehand, A. C. Intestinal microbiota and overweight. *Benef. Microbes,* 2010; 1, 407-421.

Lyte, M. The microbial organ in the gut as a driver of homeostasis and disease. *Med. Hypotheses*, 2010; 74, 634-638.

Lyte, M., Li, W., Opitz, N., Gaykema, R. P., Goehler, L. E. Induction of anxiety-like behavior in mice during the initial stages of infection with the agent of murine colonic hyperplasia *Citrobacter rodentium*. *Physiol. Behav.,* 2006; 89, 350-357.

Majamaa, H., Isolauri, E., Saxelin, M., Vesikari, T. Lactic acid bacteria in the treatment of acute rotavirus gastroenteritis. *J. Pediatr. Gastroenterol. Nutr.,* 1995; 20, 333-338.

Martins, F. S., Nardi, R. M., Arantes, R. M., Rosa, C. A., Neves, M. J., Nicoli, J. R. Screening of yeasts as probiotic based on capacities to colonize the gastrointestinal tract and to protect against enteropathogen challenge in mice. *J. Gen. Appl. Microbiol.,* 2005; 51, 83-92.

Metchnikoff, E. Lactic acid inhibiting intestinal putrefaction. In: *The prolongation of life: optimistic studies*. London. W. Heinemann. pp. 161, 1907.

Nermes, M., Kantele, J. M., Atosuo, T. J., Salminen, S., Isolauri, E. Interaction of orally administered *Lactobacillus rhamnosus* GG with skin and gut microbiota and humoral immunity in infants with atopic dermatitis. *Clin. Exp. Allergy,* 2011; 41, 370-377.

Nurmi, E. V., Rantala, M. New aspects of *Salmonella* infection in broiler production. *Nature*, 1973; 241, 210.

Pesola, J., Vaarala, O., Heitto, A., Hakalehto, E. Use of portable enrichment unit in rapid characterization of infantile intestinal enterobacterial microbiota. *Microb. Ecol. Health Dis.,* 2009; 21, 203-210.

Pesola, J., Hakalehto, E. Enterobacterial microflora in infancy - a case study with enhanced enrichment. *Indian J. Pediatr.,* 2011; 78, 562-568.

Pesola, J., Paakkanen, H., Hakalehto, E. Enhanced diagnostics of pyelonephritis – a case study. *Int. J. Med. Med. Sci.,* 2012; 2, 273-277.

Polhemus, D. J., Lefer, D. J. Emergence of hydrogen sulfide as an endogenous gaseous signaling molecule in cardiovascular disease. *Circ. Res.,* 2014; 114, 730-737.

Pochard, P., Gosset, P., Grangette, C., Andre, C., Tonnel, A. B., Pestel, J., Mercenier, A. Lactic acid bacteria inhibit TH2 cytokine production by mononuclear cells from allergic patients. *J. Allergy Clin. Immunol.,* 2002; 110, 617-623.

Quigley, E. M. M. Prebiotics and probiotics; modifying and mining the microbiota. *Pharmacological Research*, 2010; 61, 213-218.

Saavedra, J. M., Bauman, N. A., Oung, I., Perman, J. A., Yolken, R. H. Feeding of *Bifidobacterium bifidum* and *Streptococcus thermophilus* to infants in hospital for prevention of diarrhoea and shedding of rotavirus. *Lancet,* 1994; 344, 1046-1049.

Saitoh, S., Noda, S., Aiba, Y., Takagi, A., Sakamoto, M., Benno, Y., Koga, Y. *Bacteroides ovatus* as the predominant commensal intestinal microbe causing a systemic antibody response in inflammatory bowel disease. *Clin. Diagn. Lab. Immunol.,* 2002; 9, 54-59.

Salvatore, S., Vandenplas, Y. Prebiotics and Probiotics in therapy and prevention of gastrointestinal diseases in children, In: Watson, R. R., Preedy, V. R., editors. *Bioactive Foods in Promoting Health: Probiotics and prebiotics.*: Elsevier Science; 2010; 181-204.

Subramanian, S., Campbell, B.J., Rhodes, J.M. Bacteria in the pathogenesis of inflammatory bowel disease. *Curr. Opin. Infect. Dis.,* 2006; 19, 475-484.

Szajewska, H., Mrukowicz, J. Z. Probiotics in the treatment and prevention of acute infectious diarrhea in infants and children: a systematic review of published randomized, double-blind, placebo-controlled trials. *J. Pediatr. Gastroenterol. Nutr.,* 2001; 33 Suppl. 2, S17-25.

Szajewska, H., Ruszczynski, M., Chmielewska, A., Wieczorek, J. Systematic review: racecadotril in the treatment of acute diarrhoea in children. *Aliment. Pharmacol. Ther.,* 2007; 26, 807-813.

Szajewska, H., Ruszczynski, M., Radzikowski, A. Probiotics in the prevention of antibiotic-associated diarrhea in children: a meta-analysis of randomized controlled trials. *J. Pediatr.,* 2006; 149, 367-372.

Teughels, W., Loozen, G., Quirynen, M. Do probiotics offer opportunities to manipulate the periodontal oral microbiota? *J. Clin. Periodontol.,* 2011; 38 Suppl. 11, 159-177.

Thibault, H., Aubert-Jacquin, C., Goulet, O. Effects of long-term consumption of a fermented infant formula (with *Bifidobacterium breve* c50 and *Streptococcus thermophilus* 065) on acute diarrhea in healthy infants. *J. Pediatr. Gastroenterol. Nutr.,* 2004; 39, 147-152.

Trakhtenberg, E. F., Goldberg, J. L. Neuroimmune Communication. *Science, Immunology,* 2011; 334, 47-48.

Tullus, K., Horlin, K., Svenson, S. B., Kallenius, G. Epidemic outbreaks of acute pyelonephritis caused by nosocomial spread of P fimbriated *Escherichia coli* in children. *J. Infect. Dis.,* 1984; 150, 728-736.

Tullus, K., Sjöberg, P. Epidemiological aspects of P-fimbriated E. coli. II. Variations in incidence of *E. coli* infections in children attending a neonatal ward. *Acta Paediatr. Scand.,* 1986; 75, 205-210.

Van Niel, C. W. Probiotics: not just for treatment anymore. *Pediatrics,* 2005; 115, 174-177.

Van Essche, M., Quirynen, M., Sliepen, I., Loozen, G., Boon, N., Van Eldere, J., Teughels, W. Killing of anaerobic pathogens by predatory bacteria. *Mol. Oral Microbiol.,* 2011; 26, 52-61.

Volley, G., Rettger, L. F. The influence of carbon dioxide on bacteria. *Journal of Bacteriology,* 1927; 14, 101-137.

Watson, R. R., Preedy, V. R., editors. *Bioactive Foods in Promoting Health: Probiotics and Prebiotics.* London, UK: Academic Press; 2010.

Yli-Knuuttila, H., Snall, J., Kari, K., Meurman, J. H. Colonization of Lactobacillus rhamnosus GG in the oral cavity. *Oral Microbiol. Immunol.,* 2006; 21, 129-131.

Zhu, Y., Xiao, L., Shen, D., Hao, Y. Competition between yogurt probiotics and periodontal pathogens in vitro. *Acta Odontol. Scand.,* 2010; 68, 261-268.

In: Microbiological Clinical Hygiene
Editor: Eino Elias Hakalehto

ISBN: 978-1-63463-428-1

Chapter 18

Personalized Medicine and Microbial Monitoring

Elias Hakalehto[1,*] ***and Jouni Pesola***[2,†]
[1]Department of Environmental Sciences, University of Eastern Finland, Kuopio, Finland
[2]Department of Pediatrics, Kuopio University Hospital, Kuopio, Finland

Abstract

During the modern era of several simultaneous microbiological influences and threats on the health of individuals, the symptoms of diseases become increasingly variable. This is placing the physicians into a challenging situation if they want to get the patients recovered. In order to achieve better treatment results, concept of personalized medicine needs to get implemented into recommendations on the practical level. In case of microbiological illnesses or complications, profound knowledge on patient's normal flora and its development history could aid the recovery remarkably. Acceptable hygienic circumstances around the patient are of crucial importance for successful cure and recovery.

One essential point in the follow up of the microbiological status of an individual patient is the care-taking personnel's ability to make prognosis of health development in any particular case. All the previously collected data from various cases could be combined into a library which then could assist in the confidential comparative analysis of various results. Also the personal history of a patient could be recorded on this confidential basis. This aspect is introduced more deeply in Chapter 1 of this book. This approach of personalized patient evalution and treatments, of course, could require several studies on his or her microflora with the PMEU method, for example. Statistical analysis could be helpful in the characterization of the personal microflora in relation to any pathological condition.

* Department of Environmental Sciences, University of Eastern Finland, FI-70211 Kuopio, Finland.
† Department of Pediatrics, Kuopio University Hospital, FI-70029Kuopio, Finland.

1. Introduction

The personalized medicine could be divided, as almost any healthcare function or field of medicine, into actual treatments and into monitoring of their effects. These dual functions need to complement each other and the follow up of the diseased patient should preferably be carried out simultaneously with the cure process. For each treatment, the physicians need to obtain correct up-to-date information for decision-making upon the current condition and the subsequent treatments. Inevitably, this leads to the spread of the concept of personalized medicine, and the practical implementation of such concepts as "Hospital at Home" (Williams, 2000) as well as "Bacteriological Intestinal Balance" (Hakalehto, 2011a, 2012, 2013a). The surroundings of the patient, and the overall hygienic quality in there, essentially influence the treatment results.

Rapid assessment of microbiological status of the samples is essential for reliably estimating the past, present and future developments of the object in question. This object can be a hospital space, equipment, or the patient in question. Several successive samples indicate directions of the development in case of any particular object. It is often recommendable to take a few samples also to the three dimensions of space in order to rule out the effects of local gradients or concentrated specimens from the microbiological considerations. Sampling microbes is actually a matter of space and time. Often the samples can also be pooled in order to get an overall estimate. The samples then need to get processed as soon as possible.

Since the emerging objects of study in each sample are often previously more or less unknown, the microbiologist needs to obtain clear views on sampling strategies on site before starting the investigation. Time is usually limited, and therefore some intuition plays a role in this matter. Then it comes to the question, what is the "microbiological intuition" on the characteristics and behavior of an unknown sample ecosystem. Virtually all cases somewhat resemble some past situations. Therefore, an experienced microbiologist should have an intuitive but evidence based approach in outlining the sampling and subsequent research steps.

If the results from the analysis come earlier, or their formation is possible to get followed on a continuous basis, these results are more likely to get in time in order to help the patient- even to save his or her life.

2. Estimating the Sampling Sites

If the microbes are supposed to have distributed into a variety of sample matrices, the challenges increase. For example, if we need to study, which parts of a human body are contaminated with a particular pathogen, or where a toxin producing microorganism has spread within the building structures, the tasks are demanding ones. In both of these instances, we need to understand the routes of contamination and the history of the microbial invasion. Enough samples are to be taken in order to get a picture on these aspects. Also, it is of crucial importance to investigate the potential of different materials which could have provided a platform for the contaminating strains. In this evaluation, in turn, we need to have a view on the cultivation mode, whether to carry out the research after taking samples aerobically, or microaerobically, or anaerobically. Often the microbiological niches are deprived from oxygen *in vivo*. Aspects of environmental and structural sampling of the hospitals are further elucidated in Chapters 6 and 5, respectively.

A generalized advice for choosing the correct relation of sample mass with its volume and surface area is: "Think about the effective size." In other words, which parts of the samples do have the potential to contain key microbes, and what are their concentration likely to be in a rough estimation. For example, tissue surfaces get contaminated relatively easily, whereas the microbial growth into tissues is time-consuming. Therefore, the surface vs. volume ratio is of importance in case of many specimens.

Another interesting sampling problem is related to the number of unit objects. For example, how many nuts are needed to be studied to be sure that 16 tons of nuts are free from salmonellas? In these questions we need to diversify our sampling methods. One recommendation is to use various methods, and compare the results of several analysis. Such evaluations could lead us to new paths in method development. Often we can pool a big number of samples in the preliminary search for e.g., the salmonellas, whether they are to be found in food or clinical samples.

Individual samples may consist of concentrated particles from the air, liquid or suspension. Filtering of the samples is often offering one potential alternative for sample quality improvement. The samples could also produce gas or liquid substances indirectly carrying information of the microbes. Typically these traces are consequences of metabolic activities of the microbes. They often specify some features of the studied microorganisms. For example, the bacteria from septic blood samples emit gases in enrichment cultures which eventually lead to their verification (Hakalehto et al., 2009). Similarly, we can detect microbial intervention into the body system by titrations of patient antibodies against the microbes. Then it has to be taken into account that a proper immune response comes usually after 2-3 weeks.

3. Enrichment Techniques

In a PMEU study several microbiological media could be used at the same time. For example, when the enterobacterial microflora of eight neonates was characterized, the results were obtained from an extensive research material based on analysis with numerous growth media, also other than those specifically intended for studying the members of the *Enterobacteriaceae*, in the background analysis (Pesola et al., 2009). In case of microbiological testing in a water distribution network, the use of different media is justified for obtaining better views on the hygienic situation (Hakalehto et al., 2011a). In the analysis of around 300 patients with microbiological problems in their biliary tract in an Austrian hospital, the investigation gave a clear idea on the dominating strains in these organic failures or disturbances (Hakalehto et al., 2010).

The foundation of health care is the good knowledge about the functions of our body and also on the interactions between the microbes living inside it or on its surfaces. Concerning the latter aspects some useful information has been collected by using the PMEU-system to simulate the microbial activity in the small intestines (Hakalehto et al., 2008). Accordingly, there has been conducted a survey with PMEU involving lactic acid bacteria of stomach biopsies (Hakalehto et al., 2011b), and the bacteria in the bile ducts in the intestinal tract (Hakalehto et al., 2010). In several studies the reasons of the spreading of the antibiotic resistance and the distribution of the resistant strains in the human body have been elucidated. See Chapter 19.

Such enrichment accelerations as the PMEU system have potential to be developed into frontline tool to monitor clinical hygiene, to follow microbiological health of a human being and his or her interactions with microbes, to treat and prevent diseases and to be an instrument for microbiological studies in health care (Hakalehto 2010, 2012, 2013..

In fact, in case of cultivable microorganisms one evident way for more precise characterization is the enrichment culture. In this case it isof crucial importance that the behaviour of studied microbes in the enrichment conditions is adequately understood. Otherwise the claims that the enrichment is altering the sample could increasingly find some ground which eventually hampers the utilization of the results. However, if the microbes in a sample remain unviable due to the lack of a suitable enrichment method, this is changing the sample outlook or status even more drastically as the strains remain unnoticed. In sample processing it is quite easy to neglect essential features, or leave some results out of consideration. Methodology development is of crucial importance.

The PMEU method was used for tracing pathogenic *Campylobacter* sp., *Yersinia* sp., and salmonellas in water, food, and clinical samples in Burkina Faso summer 2011 (Hakalehto et al., 2014a). For example, sampling was required for the irrigation water derived from sewage effluents which were collected into a pool, and then used for watering the vegetable fields. As a consequence, risk of bacterial infection was prominent. However, it was impossible by current methods to cultivate e.g., the *Campylobacter* species beneath the more abundant and fiercely growing strains of other fecal population. Patients in a nearby pediatric hospital were infected with some of the genotypes that were present in the chicken food samples from the nearby market.

Another example emphasizing the need for careful design of a PMEU enrichment process is the detection of *Salmonella* sp. These food pathogens were not readily separable from the closely related *Citrobacter* sp. strains growing equally well on many selective media for salmonellas at 37°C (Hakalehto, 2001; Hakalehto et al., 2000). However, when enrichment temperatures of 42-43°C were used, the selection of salmonellas was clear on such selective media as Rappaport-Vassiliadis broth. Surprisingly, the population growth speed was equally fast both in aerobic and in anaerobic conditions in the PMEU. Thus the anaerobiosis could be used as an additional selective marker ruling out aerobic competition in some cases (Hakalehto et al., 2007). However, the expression of such antigens as fimbrial type 1 antigen was faster and stronger in aerobic conditions. The salmonellas turned out to produce fimbrial protrudements detectable in electron microscopy in 3,5 hours which structures then disappeared in 7 hours as the nutrients were more or less exhausted. In case of using the PMEU as a pretreatment for the PCR (Polymerase Chain Reaction) it turned out that single *Salmonella* cells were found in detectable levels in 7 hours by this approach. By using the PMEU Scentrion® device with sensors for verifying the presence of a single *Salmonella* cell in tap water was accomplished in about 10 hours (Hakalehto et al., 2011a). The presence of *Salmonella* sp. in the enrichment broth could be confirmed by a simple dot blot test (Hakalehto et al., 2007).

In a survey of a small epidemic of salmonellosis among a touristic group, an old asymptomatic man (80 years of age) was reported to be a carrier of intestinal salmonellosis.

Due to the lack of any other typing method besides antibiotic resistance profiling, it was not known whether the pathogenic strain was identical with the isolates from other members of the tourist group, or if this man had been a carrier of the bacterium for a longer period of time. In any case, doctors recommended antibiotic medication for him using ciprofloxacin as the antibacterial medicine. However, considering his old age and the asymptomatic status of the patient it was concluded that no antibiotic treatment was to be started immediately. Instead, a probiotic bacterial product with prebiotic flax and antioxidants (Hakalehto and Jaakkola, 2013) was administered daily together with some herbal medicines. After one month of alternative or complementary treatment the patient was confirmed clean of any salmonellosis or salmonellas on the basis of repeated laboratory tests.

In order to separate closely related microbes with practical relevance from each other, the PMEU method has been applied for distinguishing water pollution originating from a paper and pulp plant from the effect of a municipal waste water treatment plant on the same lake area. In this case, the klebsiellas from the industrial source easily outnumbered and were growing out the related *Escherichia coli* mostly originating from the fecal sources. In order to develop a means for reliable detection of all indicator bacteria in the natural waters, a PMEU application was tested for this purpose. This environmental monitoring could bring essential improvement for general health. In this area of effluent outflows, one male worker had been taking part in a repair of a pier for two weeks working in aquatic environment, and got infected with a highly pathogenic *E. coli.* Another method for investigating (or source-tracking) the origin of the effluent microbial load in lake water, is the selective cultivation of *E. faecium* and *E. faecalis,* the latter being more typical for the fecal contamination ((Heitto, 2006; Heitto et al. 2006; Heitto et al., 2009; Heitto et al., 2012). If the PMEU technology is used as a pre-enrichment method for the enterococci, it is noteworthy that different strains react somewhat differently on various partial pressures of oxygen in the cultivation gas flow. This feature has to be taken into account when designing the experimental protocol.

Similarly, careful planning is required when various antimicrobial substances on antibiotics are added to the medium as selective factors in the PMEU cultivations. For example, in case of wood industry aerobic bacilli, the selective effect of polymyxin B was reached with approximately 25% antibiotic level of the normal concentration only (Mentu et al., 2009). During the experimentation of kaolin clay used in paper making, *Bacillus cereus* strains turned out to have cross-reactions with antibodies against bacterial isolates from sulcuses of dental patients. Resembling tendencies with respect to antibiotics as selective factors were found in case of *Campylobacter* sp. strains growing on the regular standard media (Pitkänen et al., 2009). Therefore, it is suggested that modifications of the composition of several broth media could be advantageous for the PMEU cultivation in order to achieve optimal growth results of the desired strains - together with adequate selection.

4. Effects of Culture Gas on PMEU Results

The application of gas flow in the PMEU is one of the most influential adjustments behind the speedy recovery and growth in this device (Hakalehto, 1998). It was documented that around 2.6 times more versatile enterobacterial microflora was recovered from neonatal fecal samples in the PMEU than by the traditional cultivation methods (Pesola et al., 2009).

We have noticed that amongst several groups of micro-organisms, the PMEU application is selecting more numerous and different strains when compared with the standard test tube culture or equivalent (Heitto et al., 2009). It is also possible to apply the measurement data on the liberated gases from the PMEU cultures as basis of detection and identification (Hakalehto et al., 2009).

If the gas flow from previous PMEU culture syringes has been directed into another growing population there has been observed stimulation in some cases (Hakalehto, 2011b, 2012, 2013b). This effect could by partially due to the boosting impact of CO_2 on bacterial onset of growth (Valley and Rettger, 1927). This phenomenon has been documented in all eubacteria. In case of *Clostridium* sp. we were able to demonstrate that these obligately anaerobic bacteria were able to grow well on 100% CO_2 (Hell et al., 2010) and were stimulated by the CO_2 produced by lactobacilli and other normal flora in the intestines (Hakalehto and Hänninen, 2012; Hakalehto 2015).

In case of dualistic balance between the two facultatively anaerobic groups of coliforms, namely A. mixed-acid fermenters, and B. 2,3-butanediol producing strains, the various groups seem to benefit from the metabolic products of the other one (also the gaseous ones) (Hakalehto et al., 2008; Hakalehto et al., 2010). This symbiosis seems to be advantageous particularly for *E. coli* and other acid producing strains since they are thus prevented from lowering their environmental pH to detrimental levels for their own growth. The klebsiellas, in turn, seem to exploit the volatile metabolic products of the *E. coli* (Hakalehto, 2010). This pattern of mutual cooperation is also emphasizing the fast "reactivity" of intestinal bacteria in their common intestinal habitat such as duodenum (Hakalehto, 2012). From the point of view of personalized medicine, it is important to know the status of the normal flora, and the dominant strains in it.

5. Strategies for Using the PMEU

When the PMEU concept was originally developed in the Finnoflag Oy's laboratory in late 1990'ies, the main idea was to bring the cultivation into places where the microbes were sampled in order to

1. facilitate improved recovery, and to give a better picture or the basis of more strains being viable, and
2. to shorten the incubation period prior to actual detection.

Due to economic limitations we had to develop a basic model of the PMEU to be a kind of "compromise" of the versions that would have been optimal for different fields of application, such as clinical, industrial or environmental monitoring.

During the further testing of the PMEU equipment it was realized that by simplifying the basic conditions in the microecosystems around the microbes we had been able to find the means to boost the cultures, if only knowing the specific requirements of any culture, either a monotonous or a mixed one (Hakalehto et al., 2007). If the environmental conditions in any microecosystem surrounding the cells were deduced correctly, we would be able to simulate the *in vivo* circumstances (Hakalehto et al., 2008; Hakalehto et al., 2010). Consequently it would be possible to monitor various samples using different gas modes in the enrichment (Figure 1). Then it turned out to be possible to study the signal effects of microbial cells to each other with the PMEU (Hakalehto, 2011b, 2013b; Hakalehto and Hänninen, 2012). With these means it has been possible to investigate both intraspecies and interspecies interactions. These activities were recorded with PMEU versions having either optical sensors for UV, visual light or IR, or sensors for the volatiles (Hakalehto and Heitto, 2012, Hakalehto et.al. 2013a).

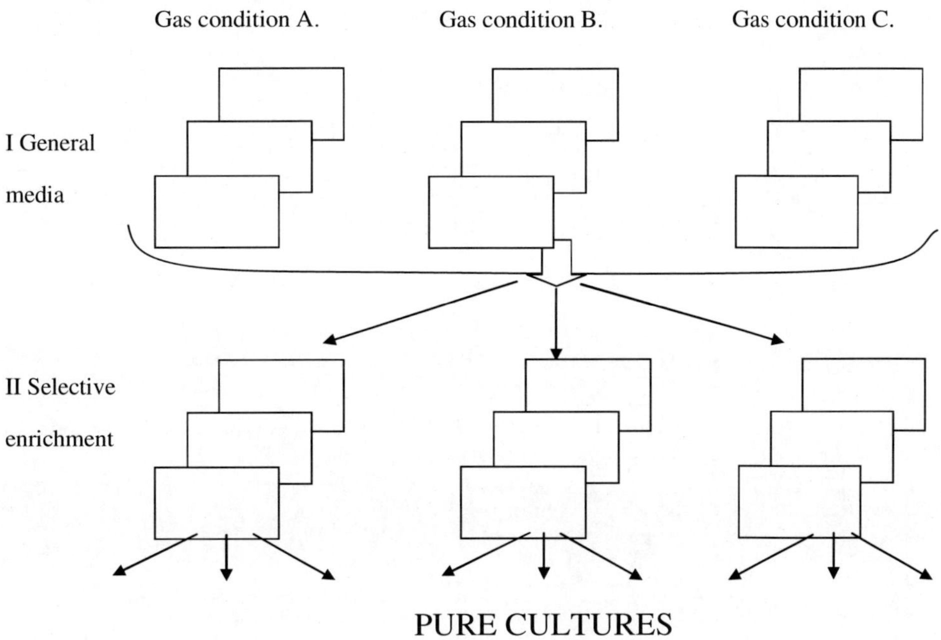

Figure 1. Strategy of sampling and enrichment/detection/identification using various gas modes in the PMEU (A. aerobic, B. microaerobic, C. anaerobic) at the same time. Further samples from the PMEU syringes after the initial enrichment in the generalized growth media (I). They will be then inoculated into various selective media (II) for wider characterization of the microflora.

The PMEU approach has been tested for the industrial hygiene control (Mentu et al., 2009; Hakalehto, 2012), for medical investigations (Pesola et al., 2009; Pesola and Hakalehto, 2011b; Hakalehto, 2012), for clinical hygiene control (Hakalehto, 2006, 2010; Hell et al., 2010), for detecting pathogens (Hakalehto et al., 2007; Pitkänen et al., 2009; Hakalehto, 2013b; Hakalehto et al., 2014), for water hygiene applications (Heitto et al., 2009; Wirtanen and Salo, 2010; Hakalehto et al., 2011a; Hakalehto et al., 2013a), as well as for hospital patient monitoring (Hakalehto et al., 2009; Pesola et al., 2011; Pesola et al., 2012; Laitiomäki et al., 2014), and for researching the microbes on human skin and in the wounds (Hakalehto and Hänninen, 2012). The PMEU can be effectively used for boosting the growth of many slowgrowing bacteria, such as Mycobacterium sp. (Hakalehto 2013, Hakalehto et al 2014b).

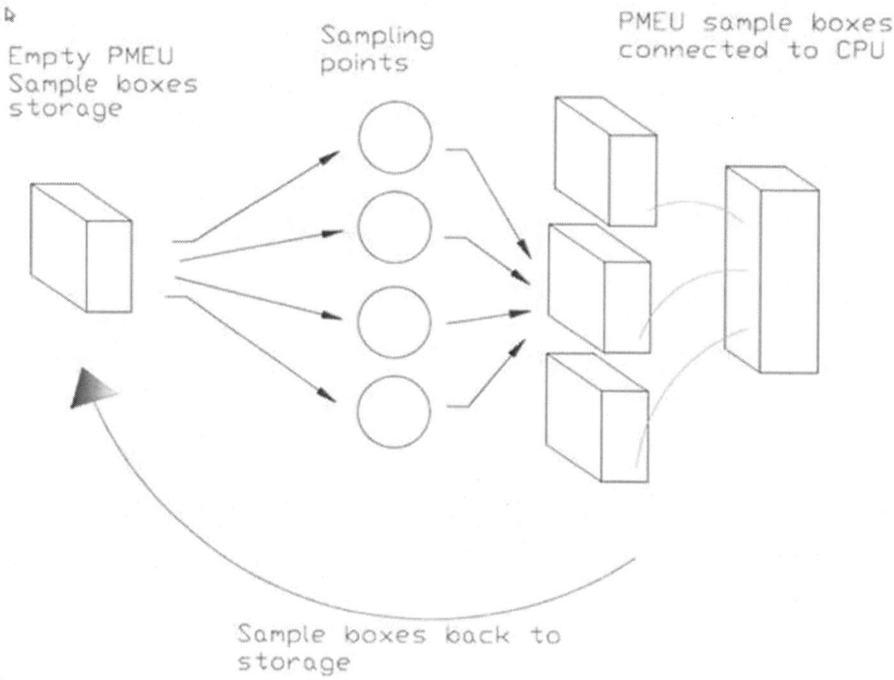

Figure 2. Schematic presentation of the modular PMEU system e.g., for hospital use. CPU = Central Processing Unit. Diagram by Juha Jokelainen, Samplion Oy.

The essential features of the PMEU technology are

1. temperature control with the precision of 0.1°C
2. selective, homogenous distribution of nutrients and growth factors
3. adjustable gas flow (aerobic, microaerobic, or anaerobic)

In an ordinary PMEU equipment these parameters are monitored and preset into desired values within a syringe container that acts as a sampler, cultivation chamber, and a sample applicator at the same time (Hakalehto, 1998). The internal conditions in the syringe are adjusted according to the purpose of the enrichment. In some cases as many strains as possible are recovered, and they could be detected before any domination or overgrowth by any single strain will occur. Alternatively, the PMEU culture could be used for more selective enrichment by carefully choosing and adjusting the key parameters. Some basic principles of PMEU cultivation have been presented in various articles and books regarding this matter (Hakalehto, 2010, 2011a, 2011b, 2012, 2013b, 2014, 2015). The PMEU concept has been successfully used also for investigating various aspects of microbial ecology (Hakalehto et al., 2008; Pesola et al., 2009; Hakalehto et al., 2010; Hakalehto & Hänninen, 2012). The PMEU approach has been used for detecting the influences of antibiotics or defensins or other anti-microbial substances on pure or mixed microbial cultures (Mentu et al., 2009; Pitkänen et al., 2009; Hakalehto et al., 2010; Hakalehto, 2011a; Samgina et al. 2012). Also the direct cultivation in a highly selective liquid medium has been attempted without enrichment in the case of salmonellas (Hakalehto et al., 2011a). The PMEU simulation of behavior of the bioprocess production organisms has been carried out in the PMEU environment successfully since the PMEU is effectively revealing the metabolic interactions on the cellular level (Hakalehto et al., 2013b; Hakalehto, 2015).

6. The Hospital Use of PMEU

At the present time, the hospital microbiology has been arranged into large central laboratories where the specimens are collected from different wards. Additionally, an increasing part of the microbiological analysis is carried out using POC (point-of-care) techniques. However, entire analysis or almost all of the POC is focused on finding specific microbes in the samples. Studies on microflora in general are mostly lacking, or inadequate ones.

Increase of hospital-acquired infections and their antibiotic resistance has become one of the most serious threats for the modern health care system. More and more bacterial strains invulnerable when facing any existing antibiotic treatments are found in the hospitals. Those threats have started spreading also outside the health care system (Hakalehto, 2006). However, development work for new antibiotics has not been producing as much results as was hoped (Spellberg and Geffen, 2012). In future, we need intensified diagnostics and antibiotic treatments which are well-targeted, thus preventing the undesired and unnecessary development of new resistant forms of pathogenic bacteria. We need to improve alternative infection treatments and ways to support the normal flora. PMEU is a suitable instrument for this kind of development work and also to figure out the ways how hospital infections are spreading (Hakalehto, 1998, 2001).

On the other hand, microbial ecosystems of the human body are in continuous interactions with the host (Hakalehto, 2012). Also different microbial strains interact with each other. Therefore, hospital microbiology should include more than just an on/off type of testing. Not only the pathogens should be screened or searched for but the normal flora and commensal microbes should be monitored as well. This kind of general follow up strategy would give an idea of the overall condition of the patient. It could also serve well in the case of environmental samples collected for investigating the status of microbes that are hygienically relevant ones. Thus the patients could be helped more effectively and the spread of harmful strains and increased microbiological risks detected and prevented early enough. PMEU versions could be used in hospitals as modular systems (Figure 2).

Since the microbes of human body are in continuous exchange of information with our humoral, neuronal and immunological functions and with our organs, it is of utmost importance to get a real-time picture on the microbiological activities of the body (Lyte, 2010). On the basis of this information, an idea of the health status as well as of the effectivity of various treatments could be deduced. Any sudden alteration could also serve as an indication of a trend or risky development in the patient condition.

The essential preconditions for a successful microbiological testing:

1. adequate and appropriate sample collection
2. instantaneous enrichment/culture phase

3. continuous follow up of the cultivation results during the enrichment
4. compatible methods for detection and identification

If the sampling is not carried out wisely, any further results could be misleading, and then the following detection chain and analytical procedures could be performed at least partially in vain. Alas, it is very important to get the cultivation step to begin immediately after sampling. As a thumb rule, after 24h only 1% of the original microbes are viable if cultivation is not started earlier. Of course, this is dependent on the species and the sample type. In hospital microbiology, the results are often obtained within hours instead of days, and in days instead of weeks, when the PMEU approach is used (Hakalehto, 2010, 2013a). It is then also possible to enrich many strains during the active growth phase in the same culture. The septic bacteria were detected in a few hours only using the PMEU Scentrion® (Hakalehto et al., 2009). The antibiotic resistance markers were also screened with in an equally short period of time (Hakalehto, 2011a).

In Summer 2008 we investigated bacteria isolated from the samples of blood culture from newborn babies intensive care unit of Kuopio University Hospital by using the PMEU enrichment culture system of Finnoflag Oy (Kuopio, Finland) and the ChemPro 100i® gas detector of Environics Oy (Mikkeli, Finland). At the start the bacteria concentration was approximately 1 x 10E6 cells per millilitre and we noticed growth of the bacteria after culturing them in the PMEU for two to four hours. Even in cultures whose bacterial concentration was very low at the beginning, only 0.5 to 600 cells per millilitre, we were able to detect the growth already after three to five hours of enrichment cultivation (Hakalehto et al., 2009).

The PMEU method has been tested also in indicating *Clostridium difficile* bacteria during a co-operative project with the doctors of the University Hospital of Salzburger Landesklinikum's (SALK) in Austria. The significance of *C. difficile* in causing antibiotic-associated diarrhea has been increasing worldwide. Additionally, exceptionally robust pathogenic populations have been observed. Therefore, we need more efficient methods to detect *C. difficile*. For example in England only, almost 7000 people died in year 2007 because of this bacterium.

PMEU has opened up new views also for the investigations on other pathogenic bacteria, such as salmonellas (Hakalehto et al., 2007) and campylobacteria (Pitkänen et al., 2009). The development of microbial flora in the intestines of the newborns has been investigated in children of 0-2 years old (Pesola et al., 2009; Pesola and Hakalehto, 2011). PMEU has been also successfully benefiting in the survey of the microbial flora in water systems (Heitto, 2006; Heitto et al., 2006; Hakalehto et al., 2011a, Heitto et al.,2012; Hakalehto et al., 2013a). An economical expense-profit comparison paying attention on the development of preventive diagnostics has been published in Finland (Jääskeläinen, 2007).

With respect to the actual detection and identication, it could be carried out with such methods as PCR (Polymerase Chain Reaction) (Yamamoto, 2002). However, the contaminating bacteria are not always detectable with this method in low concentrations as the sample matrix could interfere with the test. For example, various chemicals could inhibit the enzymes required for the multiplication of the selected DNA sequences. The PMEU pre-enrichment has improved the applicability of the PCR in several cases (Pitkänen et al., 2009). It is noteworthy, that any result from biochemical, genetic or immunological testing should be considered in the light of the growth result and metabolic indications. By combining different data at key points of analysis we can achieve time-dependent parameters. The changes in these parameters, in turn, could be handled with artificial intelligence. As the experiences accumulating, it is possible to develop algorithms for interpreting the results. Specific software could be developed for this purpose. In a lecture of Dr. Chia Feng Lu (BIOtech Japan 2014) it was indicated that the development of treatment option is correlating with the number of new medical device innovations implemented to the market. Therefore, Japanese government is strongly encouraging such developments, also with legislative measures.

7. Alertness Based on the PMEU Technology

According to a general approximation most microorganisms belong to our natural environment, where they are normally acting in a balanced way. For example, the microbiome of our gastrointestinal areas constitute such a balance, which is essential for our good health (Hakalehto, 2012). Although this is a common situation, comparable to a city which is functioning in an organized way on an ordinary day, still there is always a possibility of a disaster, a catastrophe, or at least that of an alarming situation. A tragic example of this kind occurred in New York City as an act of terrorism in 2001 (Giuliani and Kurson, 2002). During this incidence and some of similar type, although less catastrophic ones, several microbial hazards have to be taken into consideration. This is the case also on an individual level with respect to a pathogenic threat.

Several hazardous microbes, or pathogens, form a risk for our body system. They threaten our lives, and health, as well as the processes in our industrial production. They also undermine the value of our environment (Jääskeläinen, 2007). It has to be taken into account that a threat of a pathogen is influencing our behavior. Therefore, any microbiological monitoring has to be combined with purposeful action in order to minimize the risks. This is especially true for the zones surrounding the human inhabitation. By protecting the nature and our environment from the influences of our current activities, we actually are protecting ourselves.

The PMEU Spectrion® technology was validated for detecting hygiene indicating *Escherichia coli* and other coliforms (Wirtanen and Salo, 2010). The PMEU technology has been used for safeguarding the municipal water distribution system (Hakalehto et al., 2011a). It could be used in combination with such universal technologies as the PCR (Polymerase Chain Reaction) (Pitkänen et al., 2009), immunotechniques (Hakalehto et al., 2007), ATP (Adenosine Triphosphate) method (Mentu et al., 2009), and Colilert™ cultivation method (Hakalehto et al., 2013a). The Coliline™ PMEU automated water monitoring system has been tested in the Finnish Polaris project in the Savonia Technology University's pilot plant for municipal water distribution, as well as with several water departments of various cities (Hakalehto et al., 2011a; Hakalehto, 2014).

In hospitals the PMEU system could serve also as an overall hygiene control monitoring system (Hakalehto, 2006, 2010). It could give an early warning on the septic infections (Hakalehto et al., 2009; Pesola et al., 2011; Laitiomäki et al., 2014). Any life-threatening infectioncases could be under control by using such sensitive techniques as the PMEU Scentrion® (Pesola et al., 2012). The risks caused by a particular group of microbes, such as *E. coli* (Hakalehto, 2011a), or antibiotic resistant strains (Hakalehto, 2011b), or *Clostridium difficile* as an emerging pathogen (Hell et al., 2010; Hell et al., 2012) have been evaluated from the PMEU perspective. The use of the PMEU could open up new visions of hospital microbiology, where improved patient survival figures could be combined with improved economics (Hakalehto, 2011a). New areas of microbial influences on our health, such as gastric microbiology, could be considered on individual basis (Hakalehto et al., 2011b; Hakalehto, 2012; Hakalehto, 2013b).

In fact, the microbial gas generation could serve as a selective factor in many mixed populations, and ecosystems based on them. For example, it has been detected in anaerobic cultures that increasing H_2 and CO_2 content in gaseous outflow leads to decreasing CH_4 and H_2O contents, and vice versa. This could lead to an assumption on the importance of CO_2 as a regulator, as indicated before (Hakalehto and Hänninen, 2012). Interestingly, clostridia are able to continue fast growth in a 100% CO_2 atmosphere (Hell et al., 2010). Thus the methane production could be associated with more stagnant conditions with slower rates of bubbling and liquid movements.

Since the PMEU technique is giving continuous information during the enrichment cultivation, all the accumulated data can be used to:

1. detect different microorganisms and subcultures within the mixed populations of various samples
2. get an idea of the growth characteristics of these subpopulations, as well as figure out their interactions in specific conditions
3. follow the succession of different strains during the course of cultivation

It is possible to collect subsamples from the PMEU trial during the development of the broth cultures. They could then be studied with any technique, such as with the PCR, GC-MS (Gas Chromatography - Mass Spectrometry), and various immunotechniques. The latter ones are surveyed with respect to the bacterial cell surface (Hancock and Poxton, 1988). Additionally, the optically sensored PMEU Spectrion® and the gas sensing PMEU Scentrion® versions are monitoring the situation with respect to microbial growth and metabolic reactions.

Using PMEU technology benefits from understanding the differences between microbiological analysis and normal chemical reactions. Generally speaking, the former can be called as microbe detection process (Hakalehto, 2010). This usually starts from sample collection followed by various enrichment steps and detection/identification. In the PMEU, the characterization of the pure or mixed cultures can be carried out without interrupting them during the entire process. For example, this kind of survey was carried out when studying the microbial utilization of discarded car washing solution by the PMEU (Hakalehto et al., 2011b). When some microbial strains in a normal laboratory culture eventually dominate the "ecosystem" in a successive manner, in the PMEU various phases of microbiome development can be identified (Hakalehto, 2012).

The PMEU cultivation normally lasts for about 7-8h, one working day. During that period of time, we are able to continuously gather information on various parameters, such as:

1. nutrient exhaustion
2. gas generation

3. turbidity
4. metabolic activities (by e.g., color changes in the medium)

In a way, a well-equipped PMEU unit constitutes a stand-alone research station for microbiological studies. The samples of gaseous, liquid or solid phase can be applied to the unit. They can also be automatically collected by various ASCS devices (Automatic Sample Collection System) (Hakalehto, 2010, Lecture at "Veden vaarat", in Finnish. "Dangers in Water", Tampere, Finland).

As an overall consequence of using different PMEU's, any microbiological condition can be monitored, simulated, characterized and studied in a most profound way. Any information can be compared with the previous knowledge. In the hospital environment it is possible to carry out statistical investigation and classifying of many parameters. Then any abrupt change or more prolonged trend could serve as an alarming signal (Hakalehto, 2011a). The same approach could be applicable to many situation in the different industries (Hakalehto et al., 2007; Mentu et al., 2009; Hakalehto et al., 2013b; Hakalehto, 2015), and in the environmental monitoring (Heitto et al., 2009; Pitkänen et al., 2009; Hakalehto et al., 2011a; Heitto et al., 2012).

In the microbiological analysis, selective medium is one basic element in the microbial identification. In addition, comparative studies on different gas atmospheres as well as on the gas flow parameters could be performed. Moreover, single strains could be isolated for further characterization. The consequent pure cultures could then also be studied with the PMEU method. Thus it is possible to establish a structural pattern of microbiological analysis on any sample material. Then the vertical line is consisting of increasingly refined and elaborate studies on subpopulations or individual components of the microflora, and the horizontal axis of the analysis is referring to variable growth conditions and parameters. The microbiological samples can also be transported from one department or work station to another one, or to the laboratory. Also their culture characteristics can be measured also during this transportation. Any collected data is becoming beneficial in the individualized and holistic treatment strategies.

8. Relationship of Body Weight with the Gut Microflora

In recent studies with extensive material of globally collected intestinal samples, using the modern molecular biology methods, three principal types or classes of gut flora have been established (Wu et al., 2011). They are supposed to largely reflect the nutritional variations worldwide. Already in 1909 it was found that there was a clear difference between the gut microflora of those individuals that have consumed carbohydrate-based food with the ones having a protein-rich diet (Kendall, 1909). This basic distinction was also reflecting the way how the microflora, and consequently the human organism, reacted to alterations in food composition (and also to other environmental parameters). *Lactobacillus rhamnosus* strain GG was successfully used in case of provisional studies with small children in the sense of producing long-term positive development regarding maternal prenatal supplementation of the probiotics (Luoto et al., 2010).

It is also possible to influence the colonic flora by the diet (Walker et al., 2011). However, it is not clear whether this change in the colonic flora is reflecting previous events in the intestinal flow, or provoked mostly in the colon.

It has also been documented that obese persons have increased levels of strains belonging to Firmicutes, for example butyric acid bacteria, in their cecum (Ley et al., 2006, Backhed et al., 2007). This is probable an indication of and result from microbial activities in the upper intestines (Hakalehto et al., 2008). If 2,3-butanediol fermentation is dominating there over the acid fermentations this could lead to increased ethanol production. Ethanol, in turn, is readily assimilated by the host body. In practice we could demonstrate the generation of ethanol after the consumption of some soft drinks into the gases breathed out (results not shown here). The increased ethanol produced in the 2,3-butanediol fermentation is a way for the microbe cells to convert sugars rapidly into other substances and hence to lower the osmotic pressure in the small intestines (Hakalehto, 2012). The possibility to treat obesity by up-regulating the colonic fermentation has been suggested (Conterno et al., 2011). However, in the light of the above-mentioned influence of diet on the small intestinal microflora, it could be even more effective to focus on the upper small bowel in efforts for developing a more balanced intestinal flora (Hakalehto and Jaakkola, 2013).

The dualistic balance between the members of various groups of *Enterobacteriaceae* seems to be the foundation of the BIB (Bacterial Intestinal Balance) in duodenum and in entire small intestines (Hakalehto et al., 2008; Hakalehto et al., 2010). In the cecum and in the entire colonic region such strains as lactobacilli and clostridia dominate. They attach onto the epithelial walls using e.g., their slowly synthetized S-layer proteins (Schneitz et al., 1993). Enteric strains, on the contrary, are exploiting rapidly expressed fimbrial and adhesive structures (Hakalehto et al., 2000; Hakalehto et al., 2007). In the colon active normal flora could prevent overgrowth of putrefactive strains by CO_2 formation (Hakalehto and Hänninen, 2012). The latter study is an example of the usefulness of the PMEU in studying gaseous interactions. The effect of gas flow and its composition on *E. coli* has also been reported earlier (Hakalehto, 2011b).

9. Individualization of Oncological Care

In the light of above postulations, it is no wonder that some of the most effective cytostatic drugs were developed by Pharm-Italia in Milan in the beginning of the 80's from antibiotics. The trade name Adriamycin® became well known, and so were the effective substances, doxorubicin, and relative substances, such as epirubicin and idarubicin (Dr. Dagiel Dagan, personal communication). At 1990 this R&D was purchased by Swedish Pharmacia to be then sold soon to UpJohn.

In the 1950s the Italian Farmitalia Research Laboratories began an organized effort to find anticancer compounds from soil-based microbes. In a soil sample taken from the area surrounding the Castel del Monte, a 13th-century castle, a new strain of *Streptomyces peucetius*, was isolated. This species producing a red pigment was found to secrete antibiotic that was effective against tumors in mice. Since a group of French researchers discovered this compound at about the same time, the two teams named the compound daunorubicin, combining the name Dauni, a pre-Roman tribe that occupied the area of Italy where the compound was isolated, with the French word for ruby, rubies, describing the color. Clinical trials began in the 1960s, and the drug was successful in treating acute leukemia and lymphoma. However, by 1967, it was recognized that daunorubicin could produce fatal cardiac toxicity (Tan et al., 1967).

Researchers at Farmitalia soon discovered that changes in biological activity could be made by minor changes in the structure of the compound. A strain of *Streptomyces* was mutated using *N*-nitroso-*N*-methyl urethane, and this new strain produced a different, red-colored antibiotic. They named this new compound Adriamycin, after the Adriatic Sea, and the name was later changed to doxorubicin. The Doxorubicin showed better activity than daunorubicin against mouse tumors, and especially solid tumors. It also showed a higher therapeutic index, yet the cardiotoxicity remained (Di Marco et al., 1969).

Daunomycin or daunorubicin is a natural anthracyclin isolated originally from *Streptomyces peucetius.* Doxorubicin, epirubicin and idarubicin belong to anthracyclin antibiotics which are derived by chemical semisynthesis from a bacterial species. They work by intercalating DNA, with the most serious clinical adverse effect being life-threatening heart damage. These agents are commonly used in the treatment of a wide range of cancers, including hematological malignancies (blood cancers, like leukaemia and lymphoma), many types of carcinoma (solid tumours) and soft tissue sarcomas (Tacar et al., 2013).

Doxorubicin is photosensitive, and it should be protected from light from affecting it. It is also available in liposome-encapsulated forms, that is, pegylated forms.

Doxorubicin interacts with DNA by *intercalation* and inhibition of macromolecular biosynthesis (Momparler et al., 1976; Fornari et al., 1994; Tacar et al., 2013). This inhibits the progression of the enzyme topoisomerase II, which relaxes supercoils in DNA for transcription (Pommier et al., 2010). Doxorubicin stabilizes the topoisomerase II complex after it has broken the DNA chain for replication, preventing the DNA double helix from being resealed and thereby stopping the process of replication. It may also increase free radical production, hence contributing to its cytotoxicity (Rossi, 2013). Consequently, the antioxidant therapies could be important for optimizing the results from these cancer therapies.

The planar aromatic chromophore portion of the molecule intercalates between two base pairs of the DNA, while the six-membered daunosamine sugar sits in the minor groove and interacts with flanking base pairs immediately adjacent to the intercalation site, as evidenced by several crystal structures (Frederick et al., 1990).

By intercalation, doxorubicin can also induce histone eviction from chromatin. As a result, DNA damage response, epigenome and transcriptome are deregulated in doxorubicin-exposed cells (Pang et al., 2013).

Because of individual difference in metabolism also the treatments and dosing of medicines need to be adjusted in order to achieve effective anticancer treatment with tolerable side-effects. Fixed dosing may be good for one patient but too low or high for another one.

Personalized medicine should also be applied for the antibiotic treatments of cancer patients. During neutropenia a wide-spectrum antibiotic treatment should be used, but ideally the antibiotic load should be diminished by effective microbial diagnostics.

10. Contribution of Microflora Disturbances to Chronic Illnesses and Malfunctions

In the intestinal areas the leaky gut syndrome leading to bacterial penetration has been associated (Brown, 2012) with such illnesses as

- fibromyalgia
- chronic fatique syndrome
- autism
- depression
- asthma
- urticaria
- autoimmunity
- type 2 diabetes

The latest association with blood sugar level disturbances may be linked to the disturbed sugar metabolism as a consequence of invading bacteria, which produce their metabolites directly into the blood circulation.

In here, the probiotic strains have been shown to counteract the damage and they can reduce intestinal permeability at least in the case of *Lactobacillus rhamnosus GG* (Francavilla et al., 2010) and *Saccharomyces boulardii* (Ockenga et al., 2005).

The irritable bowel syndrome (IBS) has been recently reviewed by Dr. Mike Wakeman (2012). This syndrome could be a consequence of similar developments as the excessive growth of some bacteriological components of the intestinal balance (BIB) (Hakalehto, 2011a, 2012, 2013). It could also be treated with probiotics as demonstrated *in vitro* by Hakalehto and Jaakkola (2013). This IBS is associated with excessive carbohydrate malabsorption (Wakeman, 2012). This could lead the thoughts to excessive growth of freely trespassing small gut flora opportunistically overmetabolizing the available sugars. This kind of sequelae could then be attenuated by fiber-associated lactic acid bacteria (LAB) as described earlier (Hakalehto and Jaakkola, 2013). Fitting well into this picture, there has been reported a 9-fold decrease in the bifidobacterial number of the IBS-D (IBS with predominant diarrhea) patients (Carroll et al., 2001). It is noteworthy also that high-fibre diets were accepted as effective therapeutic measures to regularize bowel function (Wakeman, 2012). This is in line with our results with prebiotic flax, having a significant attenuation of excessive *E. coli*, *Klebsiella* sp. or *S. aureus* growth together with a selected probiotic mixture (Hakalehto and Jaakkola, 2013).

The mucosal surface where most pathogens enter the host are protected by the antibodies produced onto the mucosal associated tissues (Yamamoto et al., 1996). It has been shown that two Th2 cell-derived cytokines, for example, IL-5 and IL-6, are of particular importance for inducing surface IgA-positive ($sIgA^+$) B cells to differentiate into IgA plasma cells. It has been also shown that targeted disruption of the IL-6 gene resulted in a deficiency of IgA plasma cells in mucosa-associated tissues (Ramsay et al., 1994). This demonstrates the delicate mechanisms which protect the body specifically against invading pathogens.

Many toxic substances cause damage to the immunological system. Heavy metals, such as mercury, can cause anti-immune dysfunction (Klassen, 1990), many bodily malfunctions, and even the increase in the prevalence of antibiotic resistant bacteria (Summers et al., 1993). One possible mechanism of their adverse effects could be the inactivation of human defense proteins, such as human β-2 and other defensins (Hakalehto, 2011a). Several micro-organisms can also suppress immune pathways (Baxt et al., 2013). Many antioxidants, in turn, could detoxify the heavy metals. This could be carried out by selenium by binding of equimolar Hg-Se complex to a specific plasma protein (Yoneda and Suzuki, 1997).

Increased intestinal permeability in the IBS can be reversed with glutamine supplementation (Wakeman, 2012).

Conclusion

As the balanced and functional microbiological link of the human metabolism is an essential foundation for good health, it is logical to aim for analyzing the microflora of individual patients during the course of treatments. Whatever the basic illness is, the analysis of the changes in the normal flora could serve as a valuable source of information on:

1. patient general condition
2. course of disease
3. additional or chained disturbances in health
4. effectiveness of treatment
5. medicine side-effects
6. potential microbiological risks
7. individual nutritional levels
8. development of immune system and its basic protective capacity

Looking at the list above will reveal at one glimpse the key role and potential of personalized clinical microbiology (in health care development). Moreover, since we live in a modern society with such risk factors as industrially overprocessed or chemicalized food, extensive travel, environmental pollution, unhealthy buildings, mental and physiological stress, etc., the multiple syndromes and emerging infections have to be continuously monitored. Up to that alertness we need effective and straightforward evaluation of antibiotic resistance markers. These need to be investigated on individual level if the root causes of the current crisis in health care are to be eradicated. The microbes are related to many pathogenic, also cancerous, situations. Understanding their behavior may lead to remarkable breakthrough in the therapies of serious illnesses.

References

Baxt, L. A., Garza-Mayers, A. C., Goldberg, M. B. Bacterial subversion of host innate immune pathways. *Science*, 2013; 340, 697-701.Brown, B. Intestinal permeability getting to the guts of functional medicine. *CAM*, May 2012, 10-11.

Bäckhed, F., Manchester, J. K., Semenkovich, C. F., Gordon, J. I. Mechanisms underlyingthe resistance to diet-induced obesity in germ-free mice. *Proc. Natl. Acad. Sci. USA*, 2007; 104, 979–984.

Carroll et al. *Neurogastroenterol.*, 2001; 23, S1-13.

Conterno, L., Fava, F., Viola, R., Tuohy, K. M. Obesity and the gut microbiota: Does up-regulating colonic fermentation protect against obesity and metabolic disease? *Genes Nutr.*, 2011; 6, 241-260.

Di Marco, A., Gaetani, M., Scarpinato, B. Adriamycin (NSC-123, 127): a new antibiotic with antitumor activity. *Cancer Chemother. Rep.*, 1969; 53, 33–37.

Fornari, F. A., Randolph, J. K., Yalowich, J. C., Ritke, M. K., Gewirtz, D. A. Interference by doxorubicin with DNA unwinding in MCF-7 breast tumor cells. *Mol. Pharmacol.*, 1994; 45, 649–656.

Francavilla, R., Miniello, V., Magistà, A. M., de Canio, A., Bucci, N., Gagliardi, F., Lionetti, E., Castellaneta, S., Polimeno, L., Peccarisi, L., Indrio, F., Cavallo, L. A randomized controlled trial of *Lactobacillus GG* in children with functional abdominal pain. *Pediatrics*, 2010; 126, e1445-1452. Frederick, C. A., Williams, L. D., Ughetto, G., van der Marel, G. A., van Boom, J. H., Rich, A., Wang, A. H. Structural comparison of anticancer drug-DNA complexes: adriamycin and daunomycin. *Biochemistry,* 1990; 29, 2538–2549.

Frederick, C.A., Williams, L.D., Ughetto, G., van der Marel, G.A., van Boom, J.H., Rich, A., Wang, A.H.-J. Structural comparison of anticancer drug-DNA complexes: Adriamycin and daunomycin. *Biochemistry*, 1990; 29, 2538-2549.

Giuliani, R., Kurson, K. *Leadership*. Hypensi: New York City, USA. 2002.

Hakalehto, E. Syringe for collecting microbiological sweep samples. US Patent 5846209 A; 1998.

Hakalehto, E. Menetelmä ja laite mikrobiologisten näytteiden rikastamista ja tutkimista varten (Method for detecting microbes from an enrichment culture). Finnish Patent No. 106561; 2001.

Hakalehto, E. Semmelweis' present day follow-up: Updating bacterial sampling and enrichment in clinical hygiene. *Pathophysiology,* 2006; 13, 257-267.

Hakalehto, E. Hygiene monitoring with the Portable Microbe Enrichment Unit (PMEU). *41st R3 -Nordic Symposium. Cleanroom technology, contamination control and cleaning. VTT Publications 266.* Espoo, Finland: VTT (State Research Centre of Finland); 2010.

Hakalehto, E. Antibiotic resistant traits of facultative *Enterobacter cloacae* strain studied with the PMEU (Portable Microbe Enrichment Unit). In Press. In: Méndez-Vilas A, editor. *Science against microbial pathogens: communicating current research and technological advances. Microbiology book series Nr. 3.* Badajoz, Spain: Formatex Research Center; 2011a.

Hakalehto, E. Simulation of enhanced growth and metabolism of intestinal *Escherichia coli* in the Portable Microbe Enrichment Unit (PMEU). In: Rogers MC, Peterson ND, editors. *E. coli infections: causes, treatment and prevention.* New York, USA: Nova Publishers; 2011b; 159-175.

Hakalehto, E, editor. *Alimentary microbiome - a PMEU approach.* New York, US: Nova Science Publishers, Inc.; 2012, 263 p..

Hakalehto, E. Enhanced mycobacterial diagnostics in liquid medium by microaerobic bubble flow in Portable Microbe Enrichment Unit. *Pathophysiology*, 2013a 20, 177-180.

Hakalehto, E. Interactions of *Klebsiella* sp. with other intestinal flora. In: Pereira, L. A., Santos, A. editors. *Klebsiella infections: Epidemiology, pathogenesis and clinical outcomes*. New York, US: Nova Science Publishers, Inc.; 2013b.

Hakalehto, E. Bacteriological indications of human activities in the ecosystems. In: Armon, R; Hänninen, O, editors. *Environmental Indicators*. Germany: Springer Verlag; 2014. In print.

Hakalehto, E. Enhanced microbial process in the sustainable fuel production. In: Jinyue, Y, editor. *Handbook of Clean Energy Systems*. USA and UK: Wiley JR & Sons.; 2015. In print.

Hakalehto, E., Hänninen, O. Gaseous CO_2 signal initiate growth of butyric acid producing *Clostridium butyricum* both in pure culture and in mixed cultures with *Lactobacillus brevis*. *Can. J. Microbiol.,* 2012; 58, 928-931.

Hakalehto, E., Heitto, L. Minute microbial levels detection in water samples by Portable Microbe Enrichment Unit Technology. *Environment and Natural Resources Research,* 2012; 2, 80-88.

Hakalehto, E., Jaakkola, K. Synergistic effect of probiotics and prebiotic flax product on intestinal bacterial balance. *Clinical Nutrition,* 2013; 32, Suppl. 1, S200.

Hakalehto, E., Hujakka, H., Airaksinen, S., Ratilainen, J., Närvänen, A. Growth-phase limited expression and rapid detection of *Salmonella* type 1 fimbriae. In: Hakalehto, E., editor. *Characterization of Pectinatuscerevisiiphilus and P. frisingiensis surface components. Use of synthetic peptides in the detection of some Gram-negative bacteria.* Kuopio, Finland: Kuopio University Publications C. Natural and Environmental Sciences 112; 2000.

Hakalehto, E., Pesola, J., Heitto, L., Närvänen, A., Heitto, A. Aerobic and anaerobic growth modes and expression of type 1 fimbriae in Salmonella. *Pathophysiology,* 2007; 14, 61-69.

Hakalehto, E., Humppi, T., Paakkanen, H. Dualistic acidic and neutral glucose fermentation balance in small intestine: Simulation *in vitro*. *Pathophysiology*, 2008; 15, 211-220.

Hakalehto, E., Pesola, J., Heitto, A., BhanjDeo, B., Rissanen, K., Sankilampi, U., Humppi, T., Paakkanen, H. Fast detection of bacterial growth by using Portable Microbe Enrichment Unit (PMEU) and ChemPro100i® gas sensor. *Pathophysiology,* 2009; 16, 57-62.

Hakalehto, E; Hell, M; Bernhofer, C; Heitto, A; Pesola, J; Humppi, T; Paakkanen, H. Growth and gaseous emissions of pure and mixed small intestinal bacterial cultures: Effects of bile and vancomycin. *Pathophysiology,* 2010; 17, 45-53.

Hakalehto, E., Heitto, A., Heitto, L., Humppi, T., Rissanen, K., Jääskeläinen, A., Hänninen, O. Fast monitoring of water distribution system with portable enrichment unit: Measurement of volatile compounds of coliforms and *Salmonella* sp. in tap water. *Journal of Toxicology and Environmental Health Sciences,* 2011a; 3, 223-233.

Hakalehto, E; Vilpponen-Salmela, T; Kinnunen, K; von Wright, A. Lactic Acid bacteria enriched from human gastric biopsies. *ISRN Gastroenterol,* 2011b; 2011, 109183.

Hakalehto, E, Heitto, A. & Heitto, L.. Fast coliform detection in portable microbe enrichment unit (PMEU) with Colilert® medium and bubbling. *Pathophysiology*, 2013a; pii: S0928-4680(13)00025-4. doi: 10.1016/j.pathophys.2013.05.001. [Epub ahead of print]

Hakalehto, E., Jääskeläinen, A., Humppi, T., Heitto, L. Production of energy and chemicals from biomasses by microorganisms. In: Dahlquist, E, editor. *Biomass as Energy Source:*

Resources, Systems and Applications. London, UK: CRC Press, Taylor & Francis Group; 2013b.

Hakalehto E, Nyholm O, Kagambèga, A., Bonkoungou, I., Haukka K., Heitto A. Development of microbiological field methodology for water and food-chain hygiene analysis of *Campylobacter* sp. and *Yersinia* sp. in Burkina Faso. *Pathophysiology*, 2014a. In print.

Hakalehto, E., Heitto, A., Heitto, L., Rissanen, K., Pesola, I., Pesola, J. Enhanced recovery, enrichment and detection of *Mycobacterium marinum* with the Portable Microbe Enrichment Unit (PMEU). 2014 http://dx.doi.org/10.1016/j.pathophys.2014b.07.005.

Hancock, I. C., Poxton, I. R. Bacterial cell surface techniques. Chichester, USA: John Wiley&Sons.; 1988; 329p.

Heitto, L. Uusi bakteerimenetelmä paljastaa kuormituksen alkuperän. In Finnish. ("New bacterial detection method uncovers the origin of bacterial load."). *Aquarius*, 2006.

Heitto, L., Heitto, A., Hakalehto, E. Tracing wastewaters with faecal coliforms and enterococci (In Finnish, with English abstract). In: Simola H. (ed.), Seminar on Large Lakes 2006, University of Joensuu, Publications of the Karelian Institute No. 145 (2006) 101-106.

Heitto, L., Heitto, A., Hakalehto, E. Tracing waste waters with faecal enterococci. Poster in European Large Lakes Symposium, Norrtälje, Sweden; 2009.

Heitto, L., Heitto, A., Hakalehto, E. Environmental monitoring using the enrichment of hygienic indicators. In: Hakalehto, E, editor. *Alimentary microbiome - a PMEU approach.* New York, NY, USA: Nova Science Publishers, Inc.; 2012; pp. 215-231.

Hell, M., Bernhofer, C., Huhulescu, S., Indra, A., Allerberger, F., Maass, M., Hakalehto, E. How safe is colonoscope-reprocessing regarding *Clostridium difficile* spores*? The Journal of Hospital Infection* Vol. 76, Supplement 1: Abstracts, 8th International Congress of the Hospital Infection Society, 10-13 October 2010, Liverpool, UK, S21-22.

Hell, M., Sickau, K., Chmelizek, G., Kern, J. M., Maass, M., Huhulescu, S., Allerberger, F. Absence of *Clostridium difficile* in asymptomatic hospital staff. *Am. J. Infect. Control,*, 2012; 40, 1023-4.

Jääskeläinen, A. Talousveden riskienhallinnan kustannus-hyötyvertailu. (In Finnish) ("Cost-benefit analysis in risk management of household waters"). Kuopio, Finland: Savonia-ammattikorkeakoulu, Tekniikka; 2007.

Kendall, A. I. Some observations on the study of the intestinal bacteria. *J. Biol. Chem.*, 1909; 6, 499–507.

Klassen, C. D. Heavy metals and heavy-metal antagonists. In: Gilman, A. C., Rall, T. W., Niew, A. S., Taylor, P., editors. *The Pharmacological Basis of Therapeutics*. 8th edition. New York, USA: Pergamon Press; 1990, pp. 1598-1602.

Laitiomäki, E., Pesola, J., Hakalehto, E. *Projected improvement in the fast microbiological analysis of neonatal blood samples; 2014*. Submitted for publication.

Ley, R. E., Peterson, D. A., Gordon, J. I. Ecological and evolutionary forces shaping microbial diversity in the human intestine. *Cell*, 2006; 124, 837-848.

Luoto, R., Laitinen, K., Nermes, M., Isolauri, E. Impact of meternal probiotic-supplemented dietary connselling on pregnancy outcome and prenatal and postnatal growth: a douple-blind, placebo-controlled study. *Brit. J. Nutr.*, 2010; 103, 1792-1799.

Lyte, M. The microbial organ in the gut as a driver of homeostasis and disease. *Med. Hypotheses*, 2010; 74, 634-638.Mentu, J. V., Heitto, L., Keitel, H. V., Hakalehto, E.

Rapid microbiological control of paper machines with PMEU method. *PaperijaPuu/Paper and Timber*, 2009; *91*, 7-8 (90th Anniversary).

Momparler, R. L., Karon, M., Siegel, S. E., Avila, F. Effect of adriamycin on DNA, RNA, and protein synthesis in cell-free systems and intact cells. *Cancer Res.,* 1976; 36, 2891-2895.

Ockenga, J., Borchert, K., Stüber, E., Lochs, H., Manns, M. P., Bischoff, S. C. Glutamine-enriched total parenteral nutrition in patients with inflammatory bowel disease. *Eur. J. Clin. Nutr.,* 2005; 59, 1302-1309.

Pang, B., Qiao, X., Janssen, L., Velds, A., Groothuis, T., Kerkhoven, R., Nieuwland, M., Ovaa, H., Rottenberg, S., van Tellingen, O., Janssen, J., Huijgens, P., Zwart, W., Neefjes, J. Drug-induced histone eviction from open chromatin contributes to the chemotherapeutic effects of doxorubicin. *Nature Communications,* 2013; 4. 1908.

Pesola, J., Hakalehto, E. Enterobacterial microflora in infancy - a case study with enhanced enrichment. *Indian J. Pediatr.,* 2011; 78, 562-568.

Pesola, J., Heitto, A., Myöhänen, P., Laitiomäki, E., Sankilampi, U., Paakkanen, H., Riikonen, P., Hakalehto, E. Enhanced bacterial enrichment in the microbial diagnostics of pediatric neutropenic sepsis. (Poster abstract). In: Lähteenmäki, P., Grönroos, M., Salmi, T., editors. *NOPHO 29th Annual Meeting.* Turku, Finland: NOPHO; 2011; 59.

Pesola, J., Vaarala, O., Heitto, A., Hakalehto, E. Use of portable enrichment unit in rapid characterization of infantile intestinal enterobacterial microbiota. *Microb. Ecol. Health Dis.,* 2009; 21, 203-210.

Pesola, J., Paakkanen, H.., Hakalehto, E. Enhanced diagnostics of pyelonephritis – a case study. *Int. J Med. Med. Sci*, 2012; 2, 273-277.

Pitkänen, T., Miettinen, I. T., Heitto, A., Pesola, J., Hakalehto, E. Enhanced enrichment and detection of thermotolerant Campylobacter species from water using the Portable Microbe Enrichment Unit and real-time PCR. *Can. J. Microbiol.*, 2009; 55,849-58. doi: 10.1139/w09-040.

Pommier, Y., Leo, E., Zhang, H., Marchand, C.DNA topoisomerases and their poisoning by anticancer and antibacterial drugs. *Chemistry & Biology*, 2010; 17, 421-433.

Ramsay, A. J., Husband, A. J., Ramshaw, I. A., Bao, S., Matthaei, K. I., Kohler, G., Kopf, M. The role of interleukin-6 in mucosal IgA antibody responses *in vivo*. *Science*, 1994; 264, 561-563.

Randow, F., MacMicking, J. D., James, L. C. Cellular self-defence: how cell-autonomous immunity protects against pathogens. *Science*, 2013; 340, 701-706.

Rossi, S., editor. *Australian Medicines Handbook* (2013 ed.). Adelaide: The Australian Medicines Handbook Unit Trust; 2013.Samgina, T.; Vorontsov, E.; Gorshkov, V.; Hakalehto, E.; Hänninen, O.; Zubarev, R. ; Lebedev. Composition and antimicrobial activity of the skin peptidome of Russian brown frog *Rana temporaria*. *J Proteome Res*, 2012; 11, 6213-22.

Schneitz, C., Nuotio, L., Lounatma, K. Adhesion of *Lactobacillus acidophilus* to avian intestinal epithelial cells mediated by the crystalline bacterial cell surface layer (S-layer). *J. Appl.Bacteriol.*, 1993; 74, 290-294.

Spellberg, B., Geffen, D. New antibiotic development: barriers and opportunities in 2012. *APUA (Alliance for the Prudent Use of Antibiotics) Newsletter*, 2012; 30.

Summers, A. O., Wireman, J., Vimy, M. J., Lorscheider, F. L., Marshall, B., Levy, S. B., Bennett, S., Billard. L. Mercury released from dental silver filling provokes an increase in mercury and antibiotic bacteria in oral and intestinal floras of primates. *Antimicrob. Agents Chemother.*, 1993; 37, 825-834.

Tacar, O., Sriamornsak, P., Dass, C. R. Doxorubicin: an update on anticancer molecular action, toxicity and novel drug delivery systems. *The Journal of Pharmacy and Pharmacology*, 2013; 65, 157-170.

Tan, C., Tasaka, H., Yu, K. P., Murphy, M. L., Karnofsky, D. A. Daunomycin, an antitumor antibiotic, in the treatment of neoplastic disease. Clinical evaluation with special reference to childhood leukemia. *Cancer*, 1967; 20, 333-353.

Wakeman, M. Nutritional interventions and irritable bowel syndrome: a review. *CAM*, July 2012, 21-28.

Walker, A. W., Ince, J., Duncan, S. H., Webster, L. M., Holtrop, G., Ze, X., Brown, D., Stares, M. D., Scott, P., Bergerat, A., Louis, P., McIntosh, F., Johnstone, A. M., Lobley, G. E., Parkhill, J., Flint, H. J. Dominant and diet-responsive groups of bacteria within the human colonic microbiota. *ISME J.*, 2011; 5, 220-230.

Valley, G., Rettger, L. F. The influence of carbon dioxide on bacteria. *J. Bacteriol.*, 1927; 14, 101-137.

Williams, S. Hospital at home. In: Bond, C., editor. *Evidence-based Pharmacy*. London, UK: Pharmaceutical Press; 2000, pp. 131-153.

Wirtanen G, Salo S. PMEU-laitteen validointi koliformeilla (In Finnish) ("Validation of the PMEU equipment with coliforms").;Report VTT-S-01705-10, Statement VTT-S-02231-10; 2010.

Wu, G.D., Chen, J., Hoffmann, C., Bittinger, K., Chen, Y.Y., Keilbaugh, S.A., Bewtra, M., Knights, D., Walters, W.A., Knight, R., Sinha, R., Gilroy, E., Gupta, K., Baldassano, R., Nessel, L., Li, H., Bushman, F.D;.,Lewis, J.D. Linking long-term dietary patterns with gut microbial enterotypes. *Science,* 2011; 334, 105-108.

Yamamoto, Y. PCR in diagnosis of infection: detection of bacteria in cerebrospinal fluids. *Clin. Diagn. Lab. Immunol.*, 2002; 9, 508-514.

Yamamoto, M., Vancott, J. L., Okahashi, N., Marinaro, M., Kiyono, H., Fujihashi, K., Jackson, R. J., Chatfield, S. N., Bluethmann, H., McGhee, J. R. The role of Th1 and Th2 cells for mucosal IgA responses. In: Weiner, H. L., Mayer, L. F., editors. *Oral tolerance – mechanisms and applications.* New York, USA: The New York Academy of Sciences, Annals of The New York Academy of Sciences, 1996; 778, 64-71.

Yoneda, S., Suzuki, K. T. Detoxification of mercury by selenium by binding of equimolar Hg-Se complex to a specific plasma protein. *Toxicol. Appl. Pharmacol.*, 1997; 143, 274-280.

In: Microbiological Clinical Hygiene
Editor: Eino Elias Hakalehto

ISBN: 978-1-63463-428-1

Chapter 19

Antibiotic Resistance Essentials

***Elias Hakalehto*[1]*, Ilkka Pesola*[2]*, Jouni Pesola*[3] *and Markus Hell*[4]**
[1]Department of Environmental Sciences, University of Eastern Finland, Kuopio, Finland
[2]Dental Clinic, Kuopio, Finland
[3]Department of Pediatrics, Kuopio University Hospital, Kuopio, Finland
[4]Zentrum für Krankenhaushygiene und Infektionskontrolle der SALK, Universitätsklinikum Salzburg, Salzburg, Austria

Abstract

One type of so called emerging infections threatening our modern healthcare system are increasing antibiotic resistant forms of different pathogenic bacteria among the population. These strains carry various genetic markers encoding the resistance. Most worrisome cases are the multi-drug resistant (MDR) forms of various hazardous bacteria. In nature antimicrobial substances occur as "molecular weapons" in the struggles between different microbes for space and nutrients. In those "scattered" (on the basis of nutrient distribution) conditions, these means for the confrontations are a natural part of maintaining the balances in the microbial community. However, when those genetic traits are implemented into organisms belonging to the "enhanced" type of ecosystem, e.g., in the human intestines, their influence on the microflora can be a drastic one, and sometimes adversely contributing to the BIB (Bacteriological Intestinal Balance) during or after antibiotic medications. The substantial administration of antibiotics in human health care, as well as in animal husbandry, for example, has caused the rapid increase of the resistant strains in the environment, also in our "inner biosphere". In case of acute infection risks for a patient, rapid screening of the potential resistance factors of the causative microbial agents is of crucial importance.

1. Introduction

Microbes live in a world that is a much "larger" one than our own perception of the environment. Because they are essentially invisible to our naked eye, we have to use our imagination for conceiving the real proportions of their existence. Still, regardless of the small size of the micro-organisms, they contribute to our lives on everyday basis as friends, foes, threats and health potentials. We need instruments that assist our imagination in traversing into the depths of microbial microscale and the molecular nanoscales. “There is plenty of room at the bottom” said 1959 American Physicist Richard Feynman in his lecture referring to the miniatyrization of the technologies to the atomic scale. To some extent this saying is true also with respect to the world of microbes and biomolecules. In any case, in the microscopic world of the microbes the naturally occuring competition is often quite abundant. Therefore, soil bacteria and fungi produce antibiotics. They can also exhibit genetically inherited capabilities of withstanding specific antibiotics. This is called antibiotic resistance.

Mapping the exchange of genetic material between pathogens and other microbial strains gives us clues and opens up new perspectives for understanding and restricting the spread of drug-resistant strains. The treatment of antibiotic-resistant infections costs $ 35 billion annually in the US only. Some of the worst kinds of infections are the drug-resistant salmonellas and the MRSA. The strains possessing antibiotic resistant characteristics go on growing when sensitive strains fade away. When a remaining strain causes an infection, the resistance has to be taken into consideration in the cure procedures, like β-lactamase resistance developing during the infection following each other during childhood with a sequence of antibiotic treatments (Pesola and Hakalehto, unpublished data). Research on the PMEU studies regarding rapid characterization of *Escherichia coli* and other coliforms have been presented earlier (Hakalehto 2011a, Hakalehto et al. 2013)

The increasing problem of antibiotic resistance has provoked great concern on the ways, how to avoid catastrophes in the health care (Dantas and Sommer, 2014).

The most bile tolerant bacterial groups, such as coliforms and enterococci seem to colonize most often also the biliary tract (Hakalehto et al., 2010). Some intestinal bacteria carry out the deconjugation of bile acids. For example, all the enterococci could perform this function, whereas none of the *E. coli* or *Klebsiella mobilis* strains were able to carry it out (Shindo and Fukushima, 1976). They also transfer useful compounds into poisonous forms. In the intestinal sludge the conditions can allow rapid spread of genetic elements in a mixed population causing *e.g.,* distribution of antibiotic resistance plasmids (McKenna, 2011). This is increasing the risks of emerging new infections of previously known pathogens uncontrollable by the traditional antibiotic cure approach (Nordmann et al., 2011). That epidemiological development could worsen the capabilities of the healthcare system for controlling the communicable diseases, and it eventually produces carriers of the antibiotic resistant strains in the hospitals (Hakalehto, 2006). New effective tools and measures need to be invented or adopted for the fight against the spreading infective strains.

In case of intestinal microflora, bacterial strains are usually in better shape than in such generally more nutrient-deprived ecosystems, such as soil matrices (Hakalehto, 2012a, 2014). The alimentary tract microbiome is also directed towards fast and joint exploitation of the nutrient flow. There the microbes are also in movement along the digesting food.

Consequently, the antibiotic resistance markers could also get flushed and faded away within some time, whereas in the soil they could be more persistent in spores and other robust forms of microbial existence.

Naturally, the use of antibiotics will increase the potential for provoking resistance also in the intestines. Additionally, mixed microbial communities of the gut are protecting themselves and each other against antimicrobial effects with joint metabolic action. This is actually the true nature of well-functioning normal flora. In case of a newborn child, the effects of antibiotic medications were compensated in about 6 months, and the *status quo* was more or less returned (Pesola and Hakalehto, 2011).

However, it is important to keep in mind that developments in the GI tract are rather fast by nature. On the other hand, some commensal flora has rooted as a permanent normal flora in the early childhood.

Multidrug-resistance of the members of the *Enterobacteriaceae*, for example, is defined as sensitivity to one or less of the following antibiotic groups (lead substances of the groups listed here according to Mattner et al., 2012):

- piperacillin/tazobactam
- cefotaxime
- imipenem, meropenem or ertapenem
- ciprofloxacin

2. Short History of Antibiotic Resistance

In 1928, Alexander Fleming noticed that in a Petri dish bacteria were killed by a fungus of the genus *Penicillium*. Sulfonamide was the first commercially available antibacterial developed by a research team led by Nobel Prize -winner Gerhard Domagk in 1932 at the Bayer Laboratories of the IG Farben conglomerate in Germany (Bosch and Rosich, 2008).

In 1939 René Dubos reported the discovery of the first naturally derived antibiotic, tyrothricin, containing 20% gramicidin and 80% tyrocidine, from *Bacillus brevis*. It was one of the first commercially manufactured antibiotics universally and was very effective in treating wounds and ulcers during World War II (van Epps, 2006).

However, it could not be used systemically because of toxicity. Florey and Chain succeeded in purifying the first penicillin, penicillin G, in 1942 (Florey, 1946).

In 1952, Joshua and Esther Lederberg showed that there were some penicillin-resistant bacteria occuring before the onset of penicillin treatment.

Penicillin resistance of *Staphylococcus aureus* was found in 1947. Methicillin-resistant *Staphylococcus aureus* (MRSA) was first detected in Britain in 1961. The first identified case of vancomycin resistant *Staphylococcus aureus* was detected in Japan in 1996. The first documented strain with complete (>16 μg/ml) resistance to vancomycin, termed vancomycin-resistant *Staphylococcus aureus* (VRSA) appeared in the United States in 2002 (Bozdogan et al., 2003).

In order to prevent the antibiotic resistance against β-lactam antibiotics, the combination of amoxicillin and clavulanic acid was invented around 1977/78 by British scientists Crowley working at Beecham corporation. A US patent was granted in 1985 (US 4441609).

3. Alarming Distribution of Antibiotic Resistance

The antibiotic susceptibility monitoring of pathogens is of growing importance because of increasing tendency towards bacterial resistance development (Ariffin et al., 2000; Ayalew et al., 2003; Siu et al., 1999). The antibiotic resistance pressure is highest at hospital wards using long courses of broad-spectrum antibiotics. This is the case especially in neonatological, hematological and oncological units and also in the plastic surgery wards.

In cancer patients, for example, the increasing intensity of the chemotherapy is related to more prolonged neutropenias and more difficult infections (Crokaert, 2000). In the treatment of these patients the time for getting the results of antibiotic susceptibility monitoring should be reduced to minimum. Otherwise the proper treatment could be delayed and the outcome of the cure procedures endangered.

The clinical sector is facing an increasing and remarkable threat of antibiotic resistance strains causing incurable infections (Wellington et al., 2013). For example, in England there were 5 patient cases related to carbapenem, extremely wide-spectrum antibiotic, resistance in 2006, whereas the number of these cases was 600 in 2013 (Public Health England, 2014). Because of such developments, and together with more ambivalent and vague diseases resulting from emerging mixed infections, the hospital system has been referred to be in crisis (Figure 1).

In UK and Ireland the prevalence of multi-resistant ESBL-producing *E. coli* and *Klebsiella* increased between 2001 and 2006. Meanwhile, more ciprofloxacin resistance was detected among ESBL-non-producing *Enterobacteriaceae.*

MRSA prevalence among *S. aureus* strains was 40 - 42% from 2000 – 2005, but decreased to 31% in 2007. However, the prevalence of resistance in community-acquired respiratory infections was stable and relatively low during the same period (Reynolds, 2009).

Dissemination of various antibiotic resistant variants of different bacteria have been tracked globally (Figure 2a-c; Molton et al., 2013).

These illustrations give an idea of the microbiological side of globalization. In order to effectively prevail in the microbial communities of human origin these resistance markers need a continuous incubation in somewhat selective conditions.

This is a consequence of the type of microbial ecosystems e.g., in the digestive tract where these ecosystems are of the "enhanced" type. In them, any specific trait is easily diluted out, unless their continuous selection is provided within the microbial "biosphere" as a result of high human population density and use of antibiotics.

Prof. Tim Evans, of the RCP, said: "This evidence is very distressing. All hospital patients deserve to receive safe, high-quality sustainable care centred around their needs.

"Yet it is increasingly clear that our hospitals are struggling to cope with the challenge of an ageing population who increasingly present to our hospitals with multiple, complex diseases.

"We must act now to make the drastic changes required to provide the care they deserve."

The report said the solution lay in concentrating hospital services in fewer, larger sites that were able to provide excellent care round-the-clock, seven days a week.

But it also said this would require improvements in community services as there were many patients who ended up in hospital because of a lack of help close to home.

Jeremy Hughes, chief executive of the Alzheimer's Society, said: "These latest findings are alarming but, unfortunately, not surprising.

"It is painfully evident that the healthcare system stands on the brink of crisis.

"People with dementia are going into hospital unnecessarily, staying in too long coming out worse."

Figure 1. Excerpt from BBC News, "Hospitals 'on brink of collapse" (Nick Triggle, 13.9.2012).

This contradicts to the situation in soil, for example, where the microbial ecosystems are more "scattered ones" (Hakalehto, 2012a, 2014). In practice, this means abundant competition between the microbes in which the antibiotic substances are used as weaponry.

Therefore, it can be postulated that the corresponding markers could in fact better prevail in the environment than in the intestinal community. This naturally warrants more profound and wider research, but our results are in line with this assumption.

The extended-spectrum beta-lactamase (ESBL) –producing *Klebsiella pneumoniae* strains are important pathogens worldwide (Persichino et al., 2013).

Bacteremias caused by these strains are associated with higher mortality rates than the non-ESBL *K. pneumoniae* strains. The carbapenem antibiotics are useful against these strains.

New Delhi metallo-lactamase (NDM-1) is a growingly important antibiotic resistance causing enzymatic trait (Dortet et al., 2014). This compromises the efficacy of almost all lactam-antibiotics (except aztreonam).

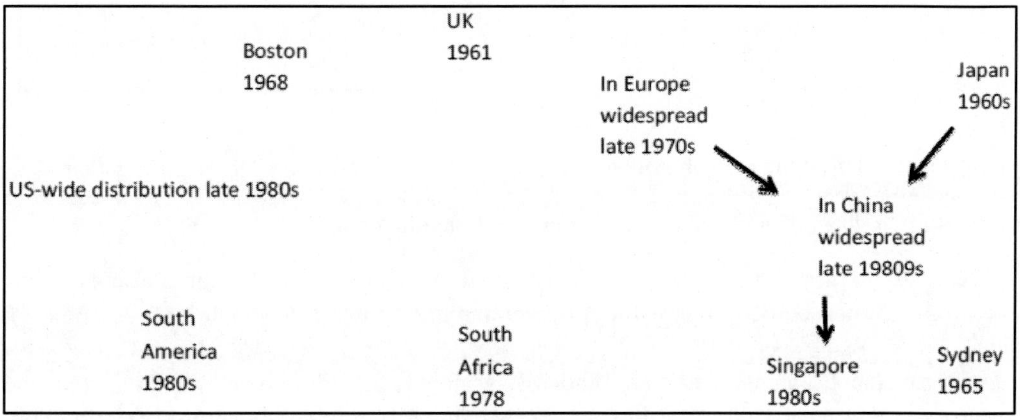

a

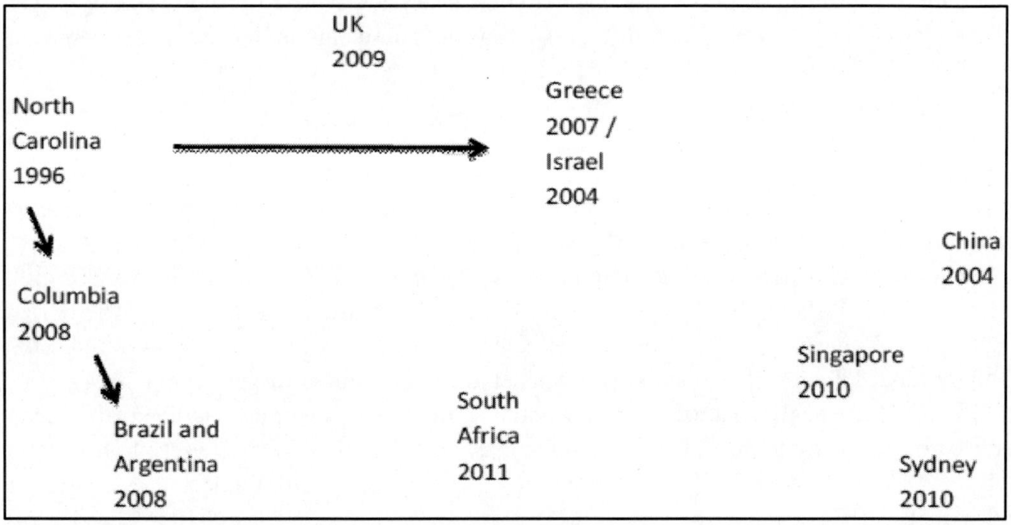

b

Figure 2. (Continued).

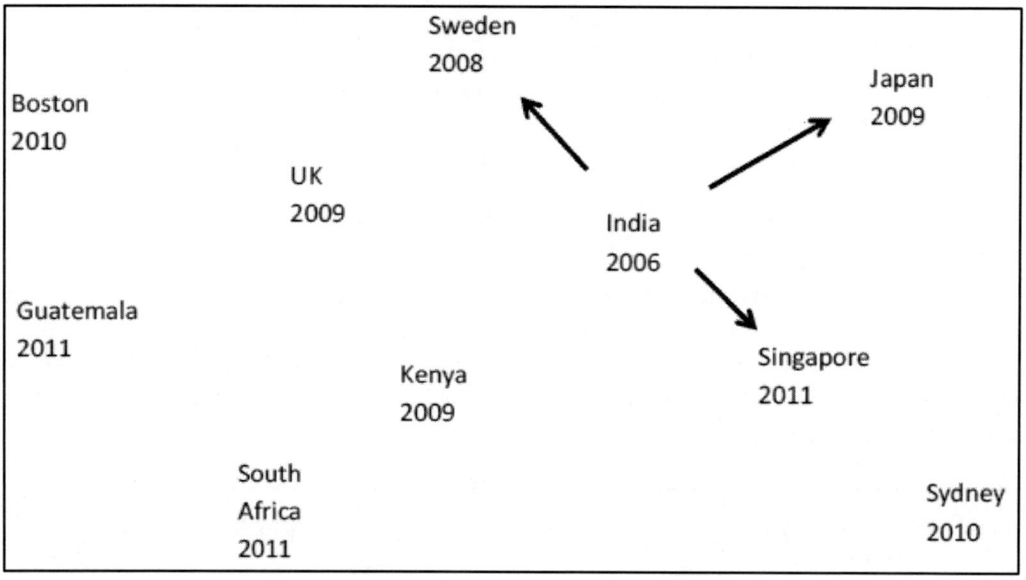

c

Figure 2. a) Global dissemination of healthcare-associated MRSA strains. b) Global dissemination of carbapenemase-resistant *Klebsiella pneumonia* (KPC). c) Global dissemination of New Delhi metallo-β-lactamase-1 producing *Enterobacteriaceae*. Modified from Molton et al., 2013.

These strains are also resistant to carbapenems that are often used as a final option. Remaining antimicrobials, like colistin and gentamicin are associated with high potential of toxicity.

Also resistance against these antibiotics has already been documented. To avoid the resistance development combination treatment by using different combinations of antibiotics, e.g., colistin and carbapenems or colistin-doripenem-ertapenem, has been suggested to treat the carbapenem-resistant *Klebsiella* (CRK) pathogens (Valachis and Kofteridis, 2013).

The main reservoir of NDM producers is Indian subcontinent, but the secondary reservoir seems to be Balkan regions and the Middle East. Recently a new regional reservoir of CRK has been detected also in Russia (Zubareva et al., 2013).

In addition to NDM-1 there is also in Europe a growing concern regarding *Klebsiella pneumoniae* carbapenemases (KPC) that has caused both national and international epidemics (Grundmann et al., 2010). Proportions of multidrug-resistant strains in European Intensive Care Units are presented in Figure 3 (Mattner et al., 2012).

Some established routes for the dissemination of antibiotic resistance are the meat or milk producing farms, where these medicines have often been used irresponsibly. There is a plentiful of references about this important issue, and many countries have now limited the use of antibiotics in animal husbandry (Liebana et al., 2013; Garcia-Migura et al., 2014).

Moreover, the negligence of the corresponding rules have been criminalized. In human health care increasingly careful consideration has been demanded for prescription criteria when the treatment of microbial infections as a whole (Piper and Kaplan, 2012; van der Velden et al., 2012).

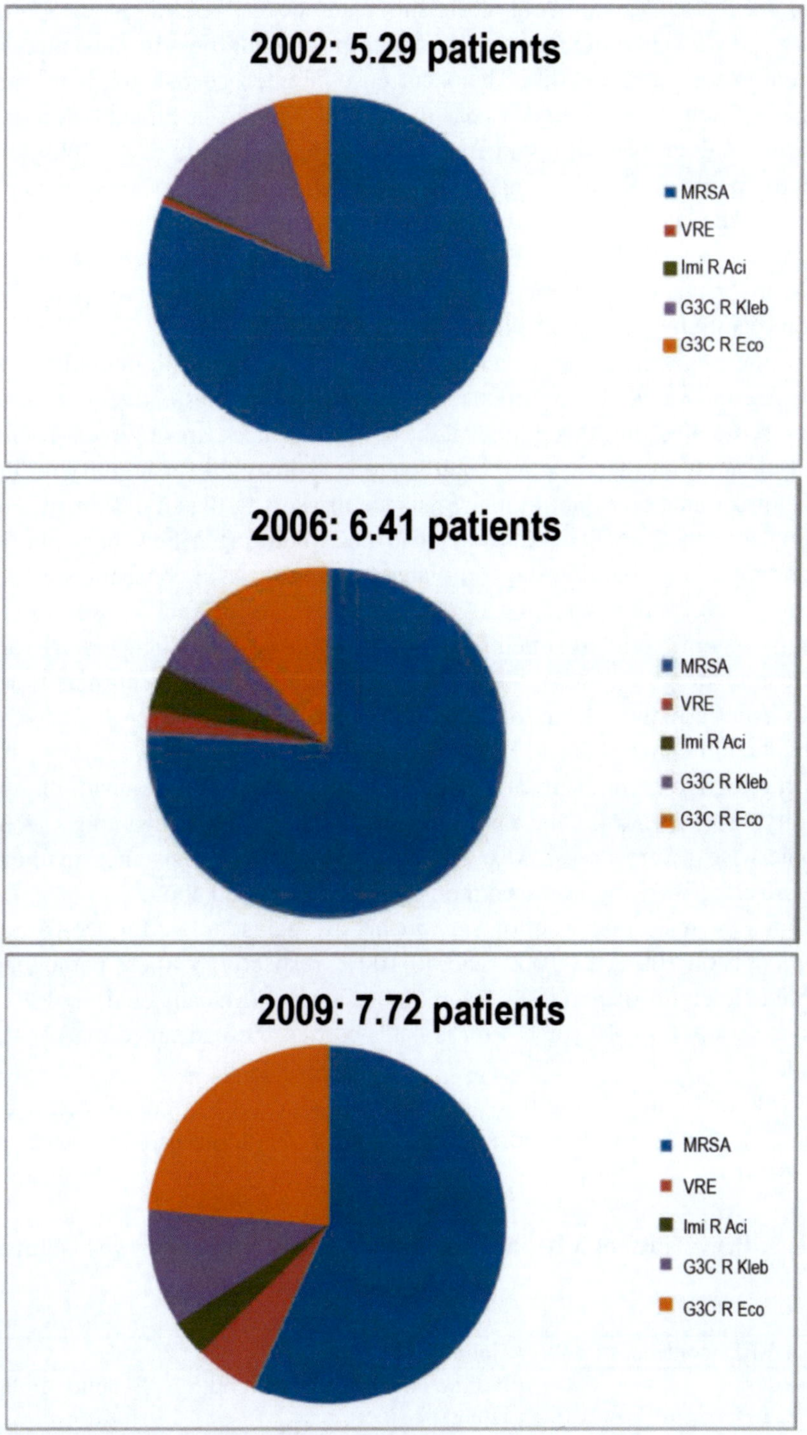

Modified from Mattner et al., 2012.

Imi R Aci = imipenem-resistant *Acinetobacter baumanii.* G3C R Kleb = Group 3 cephalosporin-resistant *Klebsiella pneumonia*. G3C R Eco = Group 3 cephalosporin-resistant *E. coli.*

Figure 3. Proportions of multidrug resistance (MDR) in European Intensive Care Units in 2002, 2006 and 2009 (patients with MDR per 1000 patient days are indicated for different years).

The incidence of vancomycin resistant enterococcal cases in proportion to all *Enterococcus faecalis* infections in various European countries is presented in Table 1 (modified from Werner et al., 2008). The occurrence of enterococcal strains in forest industry and municipal effluent outlet samples near the city of Kuopio in Finland were typed on the basis of known preferences of different enterococcal species (Heitto et al., 2009).

This study pointed out the important contribution of the nearest major source of contamination in the species distribution when the water samples were enriched. The use of the PMEU method revealed major oxygen tolerant strains which otherwise could have been omitted in the investigation. This piece of investigation also implied to the potential routes for dissemination of antibiotic resistance in the waste water.

In theory, the municipal wastewater treatment plants as well as circulation water system such as pulp factory could have enriched any specific strain effectively. Consequently, it could well be postulated that this strain might be a resistance carrying one. Therefore, more sophisticated research on the environmental bacteria is justified for identifying the potential routes for the dissemination of antibiotic resistance markers in the environment. For example, in one patient case the patient in question had been building a new boat platform on the lakeside spending whole working days in water for weeks. As a consequence he acquired a multi-resistant *E. coli* strain which was nearly fatal for him, and whose eradication took several months of antibiotic treatments. Fortunately, in case of such extensive periods of using antibacterial drugs we have shown that the recovery of the normal flora could be achievable in about 6 months from infecting strains belonging to *Enterobacteriaceae* at least in case of small children (Pesola and Hakalehto, 2011).

However, effective monitoring of these strains from the patients, inside the hospital, on the community level and from the environment could help in preventing the outcome of deadly or otherwise severe cases. Also the distribution of the resistance markers could be prevented more effectively by increased monitoring as described above.

Even though the resistance level of *Salmonella* sp. against ampicillin, co-trimoxazole and chloramphenicol is 68-100%, 38-100% and 40-100%, respectively, these pathogens are much more susceptible to ciprofloxacin (0-15%) in blood samples (Mshana et al., 2013).

In the same study only 1% of *E. coli* isolates carried the resistance markers against this ciprofloxacin.

In this light our finding of ciprofloxacin resistant strains of *E. coli* in bathing lake water samples near Stockholm, Sweden, during years 2005-2006 deserves some particular interest (Hakalehto, 2011b).

Table 1. Prevalence of VRE among clinical *Enterococcus faecalis* isolates in Europe in 2007

Proportion of VRE incidences (%)	Countries
< 1	Nordic countries, Baltic coutries, Benelux, Poland, Hungary
1-5	Spain, France, Austria, Switzerland, Croatia, Slovenia
5-10	Czech Republic
10-20	Germany, Italy, Portugal
20-30	United Kingdom
> 30	Ireland, Greece

According to Werner et al., 2008.

It could be postulated that these strains originated from abroad since the corresponding beach is in the active use of immigrated citizens.

This is an implication to the movements of antibiotic resistance pools across the international borderlines. We could also speculate on some enrichment of specific markers among these incomers in their new homeland, in remote and distinct conditions when compared with the countries of their origin.

Clostridium difficile is considered to be a leading cause of hospital-acquired diarrhea. Treatment with wide-spectrum antibiotics, chemotherapy and prolonged hospitalization are risk factors for *C. difficile* infections (CDI). In Austria the clinical CDI was related to 8.45% lethality, and cluster of CDI were detected in hospitals (Indra et al., 2008). High age as well as ribotypes 018 and 056 are associated with complicated disease outcome (Bauer et al., 2011). CDI shows a high rate of recurrence.

It seems to be predominantly of monoclonal origin, but occasionally it can also be polyclonal (Hell et al., 2011). The eradication of *C. difficile* has been extremely challenging.

In treatment of diarrhea related to the CDI the avoidance of additional antibiotic treatments is important. Also successful results have been achieved by using the multistrain probiotic products (Hell et al., 2013).

4. Transfer of Resistance

Basic mechanisms for the transfer of the antibiotic resistance traits are genetic ones. In a murine model, neonatal antibiotic treatment also altered the developmental gene expression of the gastrointestinal tract and the development of gut barrier function (Schumann et al., 2005). The distribution of the genetic material with antibiotic resistance genes can facilitate intraspecies, and sometimes also interspecies “contagion” of new cells with the capability of undermining the antimicrobial effects.

These mechanisms can include plasmid transmission, conjugation and transduction (with bacterial viruses). The genes coding antibiotic resistance characteristics can be changed as transposable elements from one place to another within the chromosomal material or bacterial plasmids (Cuypers et al., 1988).

On the other hand, the antibiotic resistance is sometimes caused by inactivating enzymes (Leslie et al., 1988). The mechanisms of antibiotic resistance presented in the preceding references give an impact on the abilities of microbes to change their environment in order to inactivate the antibiotics or to dilute their effect on the bacteria.

This is not necessarily directly based on genetic characteristics. Accordingly, microbial ecosystem, biofilm, etc., may increase the antibiotic tolerance of the microbial strains.

It has been shown that the resistance can also be transferred between different farm animals (Liebana et al., 2006). In order to prevent this, it is of utmost importance to maintain a high standard of hygiene in the farm environment, as well. Sometimes the species in microbial communities may together protect the members against antibiosis. This effect may base on metabolic function, inactivation of antimicrobials, physical barriers and / or other phenomena. The microbes may also alter the environmental conditions into direction which adds protection.

5. Microbial Community Impacts on Antibiotic Effect

In case of the intestinal microbial ecosystems, the antibiotics do not normally play any significant role, but their outcome is most likely provoked by the medical use of these substances (Hakalehto, 2012a). Even though they are often considered as "weapons" used by various micro-organisms in the interspecies competition, they are mostly needed in the so called "scattered" ecosystems which as such include occasional prevalence of adequate nutritive factors. There microbes mostly live under continuous lack of resources. This type of microbial ecosystem is common in soils, for example. The intestinal microbiome is, on the contrary, based on BIB (Bacterial Intestinal Balance) (Hakalehto, 2011a, b). This feature is ruling out any excessive use of antibiotics for struggling for the space in the intestines. In this "enhanced" ecosystem, the balance is based on diversity. This, in turn, is benefitting all members of the microflora, and most importantly the human host. This delicate balance is important for our health, and changing it will ultimately lead to illnesses and imbalances (Jaakkola and Hakalehto, 2012).

6. Essence of Antibiotic Resistance

Naturally occurring antibiotic resistance amongst bacteria and other microbes is traditionally associated with soil ecosystems (Popowska et al., 2012). These ecosystems as such are mostly "scattered" type, the term describing the scarce and uneven location of nutrients and growth factors in this environment (Hakalehto, 2012a). These circumstances are favorable for competition between microbial strains and for the prerequisite of life.

Unlike the soil ecosystems, our digestive system contains areas and niches where under prolonged periods of time prevail nearly optimal conditions for microbial growth. Such environment can be found in the duodenum after meals, for example (Hakalehto et al., 2008). When prehydrolyzed stomach contents are sprayed into the starting point of the small intestines, pancreatic bicarbonates are neutralizing the HCl-derived acidity. These basic substances are directed into the gut through one and same port, called *papilla vateri*. After these substances are mixed into the degrading food, the outcoming viscous fluid, chyme, starts its movement along the small bowel. This downward transfer during which 80 % of our nutritive uptake is taking place, is the onset of a column or gradients of intestinal joint metabolic continuum (Kendall, 1909; Hakalehto, 2012a, b; Hakalehto et al., 2012). The time period between the food arrival to the duodenum and its relocation to the starting point of the large intestines, through ileo-caecal valve into caecum, takes 6-7 hours which is the time period identical to the life cycle of such enteric bacteria as *Escherichia coli* and *Klebsiella* sp. in the PMEU unit (Hakalehto et al., 2008).

It can be stated that the inoculation of the chyme into the duodenum is in a way the foundation for the BIB (Hakalehto, 2011a, 2012b, 2013, Hakalehto et al. 2013).

During the digestive process natural antibiotic resistance is not as common as in the poorer soil conditions, for example. In fact, the BIB is inherently favoring the versatile flora in the gut. This versatility has also been found to be one of the prerequisites of the (human) host health. It was shown by Hakalehto et al. (2010) that a dualistic (or symbiotic) culture of acid-producing *E. coli* and neutral substances producing *Klebsiella mobilis* was able to maintain its balance and function also in the presence of newcoming other strains (*Bacillus cereus* and *Staphylococcus aureus*).

Because of the need for rapid nutrient uptake in the small intestines, the surface epithelium of the gut wall is consisting of one cell layer only. This causes some risks to the general health, too. With respect to potential immunodeficiency caused by e.g., chemical intoxication, our working hypothesis has been stated regarding one potential sequence of events:

1 a toxic substance is causing a leaky gut and temporarily weakening the defenses.
2 bacterial strain, e.g., *Staphylococcus* sp. is invading the body and encapsulates into the adipose tissue / intracellularly
3 the nutrient drainage caused by inflammation etc. is replaced by storage lipids, and staphylococci are liberated into lymphatic tissues, rooting in there
4 the bacterium is distributed to the entire body system, where it is exhausting and breaking down various tissues enzymatically
5 the lipid capsules around the bacterial cells provoke the cholecystokinin secretion of human cells in the digestive tract, and the intestines are acidified e.g., due to increased bile secretion (in one particular patient case the duodenal pH was around 1)
6 osmotic pressure in the lymphatic tissues is increasing, causing swelling and thirstiness
7 as the bacterium is attacking basically defenseless (with respect to innate immunity) tissues, B cells are increased, but B plasma cells are then dying as the situation is calming down. However, B memory cells are all the time increasing causing superantigen formation.
8 IgG production of the B cells is based on T helper cells, and their growth factors. T cells require for their action a contact with the bacterial cells, which is not formed through the lipophilic capsule (consisting possibly of host own lipids).
9 Antibiotic treatments and high hygiene standards are limitating the direct contacts of the T helper cells with the bacterial cells, which could be lowering the IgG level slightly, but not IgM which acts independently.

In our experiments with a symbiotic enterobacterial culture between klebsiellas and *E. coli* we found out that the numbers of the viable cells of the latter strain rose up to the level of 10 000 000 cells per ml in the presence of the antibiotic netilmicin compared with some hundreds of recovered cells in the *E. coli* pure culture (results not shown here).

Reasons behind this kind of big difference in between the ability to survive of *E. coli* cells alone and with the related *Klebsiella* sp. could be a faster distribution of the resistance plasmid in the mixed culture, but this seems rather unlikely. In previous experiments we have shown that these two genera of enterobacterial groups regularly grow equally well together in a mixed culture than separately in pure cultures with nearly identical yields in cell numbers in both cases (Hakalehto et al., 2008). This implies to metabolic cooperation between the species, which also has been documented (Hakalehto et al., 2010). This cooperation could thus include also the inactivation of the antibiotic by klebsiellas, for the benefit of *E. coli* strains as well.

The poor ability of *E. coli* culture to grow alone in presence of an antibiotic substance could then be a result of the lack of some specific, individual or general, activity of the klebsiellas. Consequently, it can be deduced that *in vivo* the changes of one strain could be improved by some metabolic activity of the other. This effect could hypothetically include enzymatic action directed toward the antibiotic activity, or some physiological functions modifying the environment by the klebsiellas in this case. Also the gas conditions could have an influence to growth parameters (Hakalehto, 2011a, 2013; Hakalehto and Hänninen, 2012).

The Coliline PMEU™ device (Berner Oy, Helsinki, Finland) has been tested in several water departments during the Finnish nationwide Polaris project. It proved out effective tool for automatic sample collection and screening of indicator bacteria and pathogens (Hakalehto and Heitto, 2012; Hakalehto et al. 2013). In case of coliform testing Colilert™ by Idexx Inc. (Ohio, US) was used as standardized growth medium. Besides coliformic growth, also total bacterial load, and members of *Pseudomonas* sp. (Hakalehto et al., 2011; Hakalehto, 2012b) and fecal enterococci (Heitto et al., 2012) were effectively studied with the PMEU technology. The detection of a single *E. coli* cell with the PMEU in less than 10 hours was verified in a validation study conducted by the VTT, State Research Centre of Finland, using the bubble flow in the PMEU Spectrion® (Wirtanen and Salo, 2010).

The importance of built–in gas bubble flow in the PMEU was verified in several studies with the PMEU (Hakalehto et al., 2013). Also in case of *Campylobacter* sp. the PMEU enrichment method alone or in conjunction with the real-time PCR was found to be more effective method for the detection of pathogens in water than the corresponding ISO standard method (ISO 17995:2005) (Pitkänen et al., 2009).

In order to further exploit the use of PMEU technology for pathogen screening, we performed a field study in Burkina Faso in Western Africa for identifying contaminating *Campylobacter* sp. and *Yersinia* sp. in municipal waste water used for irrigation and in the chicken offered for sale in the local market in Ouagadougou (Hakalehto et al., 2014).

Besides the microaerobic bacteria, or facultative anaerobes, the PMEU method has been used for detecting obligate anaerobic pathogens, such as *Clostridium difficile* (Hell et al., 2010), and aerobes, such as *Bacillus cereus* (Mentu et al., 2009). In case of *Salmonella* sp. it was proved out that the anaerobic metabolism was equally effective than the aerobic one in maintaining cell growth (Hakalehto et al., 2007). However, the cell surface antigens varied depending on the mode of gas flow. In case enterococci in the forest factory waste water treatment pools, the PMEU turned out to favor somewhat different subpopulations than the traditional laboratory methods if oxygen was regulated in the gas flow (results not shown here). In general, it could thus be stated that any variation in the method of enrichment can cause qualitative variation, if not quantitative alterations, in the composition of the microflora. This has to be taken into account in the source-tracking studies (Heitto et al., 2009). In the hospital setting it can be stated that the more heterogenous the flora is, the better the hygienic situation generally is (Hakalehto, 2006; Manzoni et al., 2013). In case of facultative dualistic balance between species, it was shown to persist even if new foreign bacterial strains (*Staphylococcus aureus* and *Bacillus cereus*) were introduced to the mixed culture (Hakalehto et al., 2010). This demonstrating the principle of "enhanced ecosystem" on BIB (Hakalehto, 2011a, 2012a, b, 2013) reflects the duodenal tract as the origins of the small intestine movement of chyme. The antibiotic resistance in the chyme populations was studied with the PMEU Spectrion® (Hakalehto, 2011b; Laitiomäki et al., 2014).

It is noteworthy that even though these strains are exhibiting culture growth during the chyme movements, some cells always manage to remain on the duodenal walls constituting as a seed culture for future inoculation of the chyme. This makes it theoretically possible to have the antibiotic resistance preserved and maintained on these epithelial walls.

The *Enterobacterium cloacae* was infected via clinical devices as neonatal blood contaminant that was carrying antibiotic resistance according to PMEU studies (Hakalehto, 2011b).

Both the antibiotic resistance and viral epidemics may spread during the same outbreaks of hospital infections of such bacteria as *C. difficile* (see the Chapter 15 of this book). These combined infections of viral origin and disseminating harmful antibiotic resistant bacteria lead to dysbiosis, where the inner space of the body, epithelial surfaces, tissues, or host intracellular fluids are contaminated with persistent bacterial strains. Such phenomenon was demonstrated in case of intestinal staphylococci which were shown to exercise their detrimental effects on the neonatal host by two mechanisms in recent study by the University College of London (Edwards et al., 2012):

1 direct epithelial cytopathy
2 superantigen-mediated T cell activation

In our earlier mentioned patient case, peritoneal isolates of hemolytic *Staphylococcus epidermidis* where partially encapsulated as "minicells" into lipophilic microcolonies.

The individual cells were about 1/10 of the size of the corresponding laboratory strains (Hakalehto, unpublished results). According to our hypothesis, this type of contaminant was hiding in the lymphatic tissues during continuous doxycyclin medication (results not shown here). Their colonies were dissociated with some surface active substances and cell size increased after some cycles of cultivation, in the PMEU, or in the laboratory.

This implied also to intracellular forms of pathogens, or to robust resting forms of these bacteria. This mode of hiding, persistent illness is somewhat parallel to the borreliosis, for example. A special polysaccharide capsule has been reported on *Staphylococcus haemolyticus* (Flahaut et al., 2008). Consequently, the contaminating bacteria could have means for escaping out of the reach of any antibiotic influence.

7. Combined Hospital Infections

In the present situation with many factors influencing the etiology of many diseases, novel preparedness and planning action is required for keeping the healthcare standing on its foot. In 2012 there was an article published by the BBC about the hospital system collapsing because of the new diseases (Triggle, 2012).

Some important tools for avoiding catastrophic direction include:

- early warnings on emerging infections
- mapping of the microbiological risks in buildings
- food and nutrition safeguarding, development of food hygiene protocols and technologies

- sophisticated environmental control, source-tracking and definition of sources and routes of contamination
- understanding microbial metabolism and interactions in microbial communities
- new materials for anti-microbial building works
- innovative diagnostics, translational medicine for transferring the results from research laboratories into the use of the patient work quickly
- personalized medicine, bed-side diagnostics
- travel medicine
- understanding microflora development,
- microbes and digestion link studies
- intracellular pathogens and parasites monitored
- improved control of immunodeficiencies

In the core of any hygiene maintenance operation is the availability of pure water. It has to be safeguarded by modern methods even if the conditions are otherwise difficult and the infrastructure not existing (Hakalehto et al., 2014). This is a prerequisite for all efforts in promoting human health. Portable Microbe Enrichment Unit technology (PMEU) has been developed for water department hygiene monitoring with ASCS (Automated Sample Collection System) (Hakalehto, 2011a; Hakalehto et al., 2013).

This approach has been tested in water departments (Hakalehto et al., 2011) and for pathogen monitoring (Hakalehto and Heitto, 2012; Hakalehto, 2014).

Similarly, clean water is needed for food production, and its qualities in irrigation needs to be screened with such methods as the PMEU (Hakalehto et al., 2014).

Most sensitive bacterial monitoring was achieved in water (Hakalehto et al., 2011), food (Hakalehto et al., 2014), and in hospital hygiene monitoring (Laitiomäki et al., 2014) by using the PMEU Scentrion® version measuring emitted gaseous subtrates (VOC's, volatile organic substrates).

8. Studying Antibiotic Resistance

Physical factors often confine the target cells and prevent the antibiotic influences directed against them. These include slime layers, capsules, intracellular pathogenesis, spores and other persistent forms.

Tests for antibiotic resistance monitoring have to be continuously developed taking into account these factors. Preferably, also more point-of-care methods should be developed.

In order to test quickly the effect of various antimicrobial compounds on the bacterial strains, the PMEU broth could be loaded with e.g., different antibiotics or other bacteriostatic or bacteriosidic substances. The impacts of vancomycin and bile substance oxgall were studied on pure and mixed cultures of intestinal bacteria (Hakalehto et al., 2010).

Some bacteria are naturally resistant to some antibiotics, which means that some mechanisms of antibiotic action are not as effective to some of the strains or species as to the other. For example, vancomycin is hampering the cell wall peptidoglycan layer build up. The peptidoglycan is generally more accessible in the Gram-positive bacteria than in the Gram-negatives. Therefore, it has to be taken into account that not all shortages in the antibiotic susceptibilities are due to acquired resistance factors such as extrachromosomal genetic elements.

Microbial growth can be detected by on site by optical, thermal or gas sensing equipment, and the information is transferred via the internet or other data transfer solutions to the user or controller of the PMEU system. The bacterial growth, for instance, could be illustrated by growth curves based on the attenuation of IR radiation in the cultivation broth (Wirtanen and Salo, 2010). Simultaneous screening with UV light makes it possible to select and identify *E. coli* amongst the coliformic cultures which could also be detected by optically sensing the yellow color formed in Colilert™, for example.

It is important to be conscious of the fact that antibiotic resistant strains are not always selected in the clinical setting only.

Potential other sources or routes of antibiotics in the environment have been listed as modified from Shahid et al. (2010):

1 Sewage
- unprocessed drug will pass into environment along with feces and urine
- waste treatment plants may enrich resistant strains
- also the metabolites of various drugs accumulate

2 Animal production and veterinary practice
- antibiotics often used as growth promoting ingredients in animal feeds
- also added to fishery waters
- these practices forbidden or restricted in many countries
- standard veterinary treatments

3 Medical waste
- various utensils, consumables etc. have got in contact with antibiotics, and inevitably end up into mixed waste

4 Household products
- many antibacterial substances are added into household products, such as toothpastes, paints, anti-mold materials etc.

5 Crop-sprays
- if plant diseases are prevented or treated with anti-microbials, they spread into environment

9. Antimicrobial Influences Studied by the PMEU

In a profound study on the development of the fecal microflora during the first 32 months of a boy child gives an idea of the recovery of the microbiome after antibiotic treatments (Pesola and Hakalehto, 2011). The establishment of the enterobacterial flora was delayed by several courses of antibiotics right after birth, and the recovery of the flora took about half a year. Later one the recovery of the microflora after courses of antibiotics was achieved in about three months according to these PMEU studies where the isolated strains were also typed biochemically. The medications increased the resistance for β-lactam antibiotics among the microbiota, but the corresponding genetic traces vanished in rather short period of time. Therefore, it could be justified to require repetition of tests concerning the antibiotic resistant strains and their prevalence within the intestines or other body fluids or surfaces of any particular individual. The well designed system for determining the distribution and storage of antibiotic resistance, and the routes of its spreading from individual to individual, are highly needed for improving the healthcare security (Hakalehto, 2006, 2011b).

The PMEU equipment has been used for determining the influence of bile substances and vancomycin on some bacterial strains (Hakalehto et al., 2010). When some neonatal septic isolates were studied with the PMEU Spectrion®, a multi-resistant *Enterobacter cloacae* strain was found indicating the risk of spreading antibiotic resistance by the hospital equipment (Hakalehto, 2011b).

The cleaning effectivity of the colonoscopic equipment was found to be adequate in a study with a PMEU monitoring *Clostridium difficile* (Hell et al., 2010).

Even though the *C. difficile* contamination was verified in some patients from the untreated coclonoscopes, no presence of the endospore-forming anaerobes was detected after the cleaning procedures.

Traditional microbiological approach for investigating the bacterial behaviour includes culture methods. However, these studies are often carried out by maintaining growth conditions which are very restrictive for the microbes on the cellular level. The nutrients may be available but the individual cells are hampered at the same time, as their speed of metabolism is limited by several factors inside the culture broth or on the plate. These factors do not necessarily play a major role in the natural conditions, such as on the surfaces of the human epithelial membranes, especially in the small intestines. Where the human uptake of nutrients is the most rapid one the individual cells are acting differently from the manner in which they grow and metabolise in the laboratory cultures in general.

The PMEU acts as a simulator for the intestinal conditions in the microscopic-scale. Reaction speed of the energy-generating machineries of the bacterial cells is enhanced by creating a uniform environment of submerged growth including proper exchange of gaseous substances and nutrient diffusion.

These beneficial and close to natural conditions surrounding the cells make it possible to find answers to questions regarding the molecular communication between different bacterial cells or strains, or between them and their host organism.

E. coli is a typical intestinal bacterium. It is participating both in the normal flora, as well as in some infections. The circumstances behind its opportunistic pathogenesis should be understood on the basis of its normal appearance as a member of the human microbiota. *E. coli* has been shown to maintain symbiotic or commensalistic relationships with other members of the microbial community in the intestines.

These interactions could also be researched by using the PMEU.

The speed of detection of *E. coli* in water and in foods is demonstrated (Wirtanen and Salo, 2010; Hakalehto et al., 2013). Then the entry to the human alimentary tract by an intruding strain is simulated in the PMEU, where the established role of the balanced normal flora could also be studied in terms of ecological succession, biofilm formation, competition and cooperation with the host body.

Different bacterial structures take also part in the interactions. Flagellar and fimbrial molecules, endotoxins and quarum sensing molecules, as well as antibiotic functions could be investigated in the PMEU. The enrichment units provide means for detecting the metabolic cooperation between various bacterial strains.

Gas Flow Follow-Up

The initial validation of the combination of PMEU and ChemPro100i® gas monitoring for pure and mixed bacterial cultures has been published earlier (Hakalehto et al., 2008; Hakalehto et al., 2009). Gas flow from the PMEU culture was studied by gas sensor technology (ChemPro100i® Chemical Detector) with a delay line to record the cell signals from evaporating substances. Together these combined equipment form the PMEU Scentrion® device prototype (Samplion Oy, Siilinjärvi, Finland). The detector intake air was taken through a NBC filter to ensure a clean background air. During the measurements, the outlet air from each cultivation point was mixed into the detector's intake flow producing a dilution factor around 22.

Samples were taken through a delay line to maintain the relative humidity constant during the measurement. The individual sampling time was about 3 seconds from the exhaust of each culture and the sampling period varied between 2 and 3 hours. Measurements were recorded into a PC with a special ChemPro UIP –program (Environics Oy, Mikkeli, Finland) and written out with a LogInspector –Program (Environics Oy). The responses of different sensors were compared to the first measurement (kept as a zero reference).

The Matter of Antibiotic Resistant Strains and Research on Them Using the PMEU System

The PMEU technologies have been developed in order to

1 begin the microbial cultivation immediately after sampling,
2 speed up the enrichment of the desired strains,
3 investigate the events on cellular level in a liquid bacterial culture, and
4 monitor the interaction between various microbes, as well as microbes and their hosts.

Any droplet of the culture broth inside the PMEU is identical to the other ones in the same PMEU enrichment syringe illustrating the bacterial behaviour in specific temperature and growth medium, and with respect to gas composition and flow bubbling through the culture. The improved diffusion of gaseous compounds, nutrients and waste materials promote the microbial metabolism.

In the PMEU studies we have been able to find out and document symbiotic relationships between different bacteria. These interactions could take place *in vivo* in the midst of several host body functions. For example, there exists a BIB maintaining the pH and other conditions in the small intestines, and consequently in the entire intestinal tract (Hakalehto, 2011a). In these studies it was demonstrated by the PMEU method that the so called mixed-acid producing *E. coli* strains could cooperate with the more neutral substances producing *Klebsiella/Enterobacter* group of strains, which produce 2,3-butanediol besides ethanol, some organic acids, and hydrogen and carbon dioxide gases (Hakalehto et al., 2008). The cooperation of these facultative anaerobic bacteria is maintaining a dualistic balance which could be the foundation of the BIB, this balance being capable of sustaining other incoming species, which could not alter the proportions between the two facultative groups (Hakalehto et al., 2010).

Another example related to the bacterial interactions is the growth promoting signal effect of lactobacilli on the clostridial strains in the PMEU which is mediated by the CO_2 in the intestinal environment (Hakalehto and Hänninen, 2012).

In these cases the bacterial species are together formulating their surroundings for the common benefit of the microbial communities. This interaction is vital for all participants, and is also maintaining healthy conditions in the host body (Wopereis et al., 2014).

The microbes in nature are often prepared for less peaceful confrontations, which could also be seen as like efforts of returning the balance in the microenvironments. The antibiotic substances are generally speaking the "molecular weapons" which are used by bacterial and mould and other microbial strains for conquering and maintaining space in the populated microbial communities (Duquesne et al., 2007).

They are directed toward the competing other strains in soil, for example. In medicine, these molecules of microbial origin have been converted into healing agents since the discovery of penicillin by Sir Alexander Fleming in London, England, year 1929 (Fleming, 1929). This finding of a mould strain preventing the staphylococcal growth on a Petri dish has consequently contributed to the saving of millions of lives, and it has facilitated the eradication of many devastating communicable diseases from our societies.

However, if a particular pathogenic bacterium could produce resistant forms against such antibiotic medicines, they again constitute an increased health risk (Hakalehto, 2006). The bacterial strains in the small intestines carrying the antibiotic resistance genes have been shown to transfer the corresponding genetic material and traits to other strains and species. This enrichment of antibiotic resistance markers is increasing the risk of multiresistant strains which could form a severe threat to the entire healthcare system.

In Figure 4 the recent developments of Gram-negative facultative (ESBL) and Gram-positive staphylococcal multiresistant (MRSA) infections in Finland are illustrated.

In the present study we wanted to investigate the antibiotic resistance among the facultative, or coliformic, bacterial strains isolated from neonatal patients at the Kuopio University Hospital (KUH) wards in Kuopio, Finland (Figure 5). In such studies we monitored the outgoing gas flow which carries information about the bacterial existence in the samples or their behaviour in the cultures with PMEU Scentrion® (Hakalehto et al., 2009; Hakalehto, 2011a), or exploited also optical, IR or UV radiation for the bacterial monitoring in various real-life or laboratory samples using the PMEU Spectrion® (Hakalehto, 2010, 2011b). In recent studies we were able to demonstrate also the usability of the PMEU method for screening neonatal faecal strains (Pesola and Hakalehto, 2011), and for screening the lactobacilli on the gastric surfaces (Hakalehto et al., 2011).

In the former study it was demonstrated that an individual child with numerous heavy antibiotic treatments during his first years.

In the experimentation with the PMEU Spectrion® at 37°C it was shown that relatively low human beta-defensin-2 (HBD-2) concentrations compared to the clinically used antibiotic doses were able to hamper the growth of *E. coli* (Figure 6) (Hakalehto, 2011a). This effect is comparable with the antibiotic function on the same bacterial strain but with even a 1000-fold magnitude.

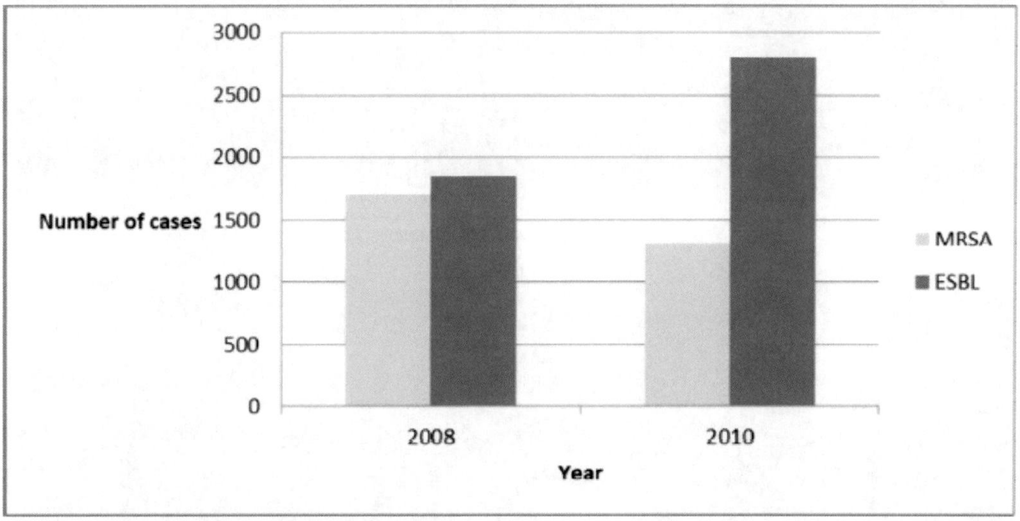

Source: Infectious Disease Register, Finland.

Figure 4. Recent trends of Gram-negative facultative (ESBL) and Gram-positive staphylococcal multiresistant (MRSA) infections in Finland (modified from Hakalehto 2011b). These developments reflect in the former case the increased dissemination rate of the resistant strains, whereas the decrease in the latter could be resulting from improved hand and other hospital hygiene.

Similarly the mucosal antibodies influence on keeping the small intestinal membranes clear enough of bacterial intruders (or prevailing strains) and thus prevent the formation of colony or slime on the intestinal walls. Actually, the effective distribution of the IgY type of anti-bacterial antibody was in the mouth and throat membranes was demonstrated using immunotechniques (Hakalehto and Kuronen, 1998). Thus it could be deduced that in the mucosal surfaces there are many regulating factors which from the limit from the host part for the microbial growth. One of the most important ones is undoubtedly the bile function. Amongst the intestinal bacteria the most bile tolerant ones, such as facultative coliforms and the enterococci, tend to occupy the upper small intestines (Hakalehto et al., 2010).

Less well-known effects are the host hormonal and neurological regulation which could also have an effect on the gut microbiota (Lyte, 2010). The picture of the BIB would then be completed according to the hypothesis by the selection according to bile tolerance and possibly also by the allowance of the immune system for certain inherited or from early childhood originating strains to occupy the uppermost gut areas, and simultaneously either supporting each other or possibly sometimes competing with each other by the antibiotic function.

Besides the regulation of gas flow into the cultures it has been possible to monitor the outgoing gas flow which carries information about the bacterial existence in the samples or their behaviour in the cultures (Hakalehto et al., 2009).

Similarly, the PMEU principles are possible to be applied for the bacterial detection in various real-life samples using also optical, IR or UV radiation.

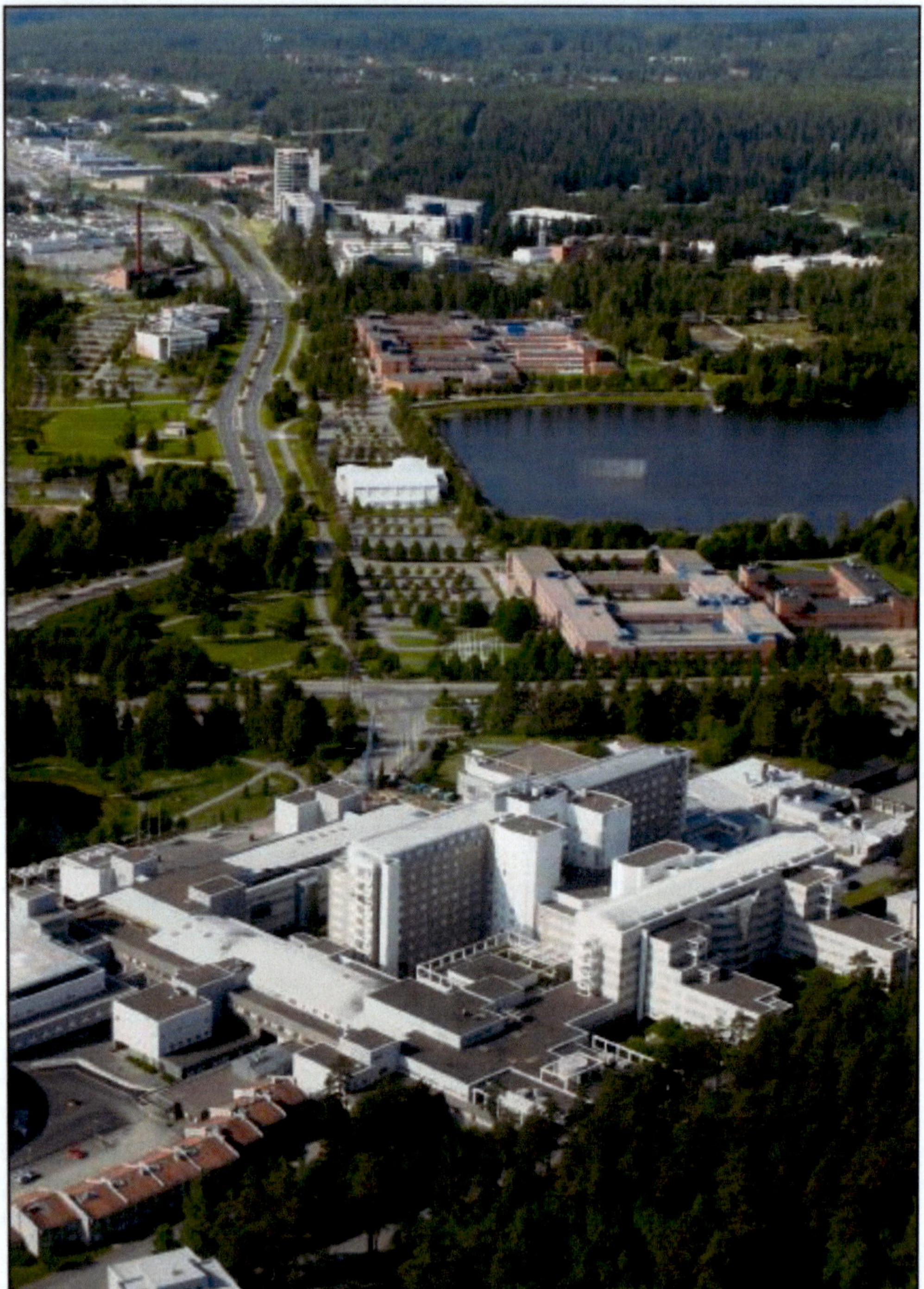

Figure 5. Aerial photograph of Kuopio University Hospital. In Finland a big governmental rearrangement of healthcare administration was recently agreed between political decision makers (23.3.2014). Hygiene control in hospitals is in key position in avoiding deteriorating of the level of European healthcare.

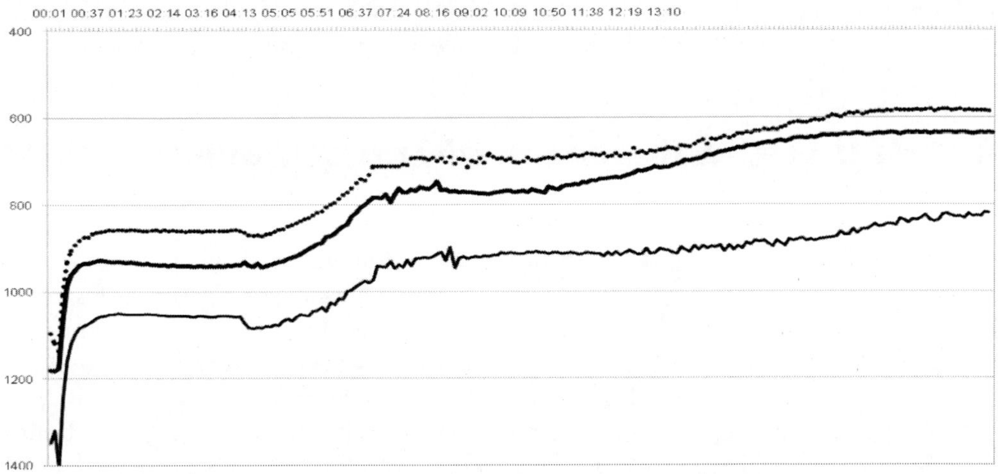

Figure 6. The *Escherichia coli* patient strain isolated from the Neonatal Intensive Care Unit of the Kuopio University Hospital, Finland, was cultivated at 37 °C in TYG broth in the PMEU Spectrion® (Hakalehto, 2011a). This cultivation was carried out in constant anaerobic N_2 flow without any addition (the uppermost curve), and with concentrations of 4ng/ml (middle curve) or 50ng/ml (lowermost curve) of human beta-defensin-2 (HBD-2). Interestingly, the initiation of growth was not delayed by the defensins, but the growth was somewhat attenuated by these small additions. The final cell content after 21 hours of the PMEU culture was about 1.7 x 10E9 per ml of medium in the control culture and with the lower defensin concentration, whereas with the higher addition the final cell concentration was 1.1 x 10E9 per ml of medium. The final pH´s were 6.90, 6.87 and 6.79, respectively, the original pH of the pure medium being 6.95.

These parameters give information not only regarding the bacteria numbers but also on the growth phase, well-being and interactions of the strains.

In the PMEU all the strains in a coculture grow in a logarithmic fashion after the lag-phase, provided that the conditions are favorable for them. Thus the simultaneous follow up of several strains could be made possible, if less selection is used in the cultivation. Regardless of the method of sensing, the growth information is transferred via the internet or other data transfer solutions to the user or controller of the PMEU system. This makes it possible for a medical doctor, for instance, to get information about the results from the microbiological analysis in real-time (Hakalehto, 2010).

Plate Culture

In the hygiene analysis, the research with PMEU enrichment broths could be accompanied with more traditional methods, such as plate culture. In the beginning, in order to obtain the correct dilution, the strains are often diluted with distilled water or buffer solution. The strains are then plated before enrichment or after enrichment, 100 μl per plate, on CHROMagar™ plates prepared from the powder obtained from CHROMAgar Microbiology (Paris, France), and onto XLD (Difco laboratories, Detroit MI, US) plates (for the salmonellas), for example. Two parallel plate cultivations should normally be made out of for each dilution. All plates are incubated at 37 °C in case of intestinal isolates. The plates can be studied after two days of cultivation. In the water distribution network studies THG plates,

Chromagar plates (see above) as well as Total Plate Count and Coli/Coliform Dry Cult™ media slips (Orion Diagnostica Oy, Espoo, Finland) were used for colony enumeration.

10. PMEU in the Research of Intestinal Microbiota

In a way, it could be said that human health is for a big part getting along with one's own microbes. Therefore, researching the microbial presence on epithelial surfaces, in the body fluids and within the tissues is an increasingly important valuable perspective for inspecting and understanding the human health. In any case, these studies are mostly limited to demonstrating the bacterial or other microbial occupation without being able to investigate the *in vivo* metabolic functions or interactions of the microbes. Consequently, we have developed the PMEU device for simulating, simplifying and further researching the intestinal microbial ecosystems (Hakalehto, 2010).

How to Use the PMEU?

The three principal sets of functions of the PMEU comprise of:

1 creating the environmental conditions resembling the natural setting
2 by using various real-time measurements confining the bacterial growth and function inside the PMEU syringes, or equivalent, and together with further microbiological cultivations ----->
3 detecting the cell growth and function (together with identification)

This approach is offering simple but effective means for screening up the influences of the composition of microflora, temperature, pH, atmosphere, on the defined part or section of e.g., intestinal ecosystem. The perspective could also be broadened to the PMEU equipment used for *in vitro* studies or treatments (Hell et al., 2010). Cultivation systems resembling the PMEU have also been used for example in the Pasteur Institute in Paris, mainly for genetic studies of micro-organisms (Frachon et al., 2006). This type of devise allows the fast follow up of the changes in the microbial culture. In the PMEU number of parameters has been limited to the most essential ones, and the microbial growth is being monitored, by using the infrared (IR), ultra violet (UV) or optical sensors (Wirtanen and Salo, 2010; Hakalehto and Heitto, 2012).

Also separate microscopic or spectroscopic measurements (Mentu et al., 2009), immunoassays (Hakalehto et al., 2007), and real-time PCR (Pitkänen et al., 2009) have been used successfully for detecting bacteria in the PMEU cultures.

The PMEU could be directly exploited in the detection of coliformic and *E. coli* growth in the Colilert™ media (IDEXX Laboratories, Inc., Maine, US) medium which is used for detecting fecal contamination in waters (Figure 7a-b) (Fricker et al., 2008; Pitkänen et al., 2009). PMEU method has also been validated for the verification of coliforms in water samples by the State Research Centre of Finland (VTT) (Wirtanen and Salo, 2010).

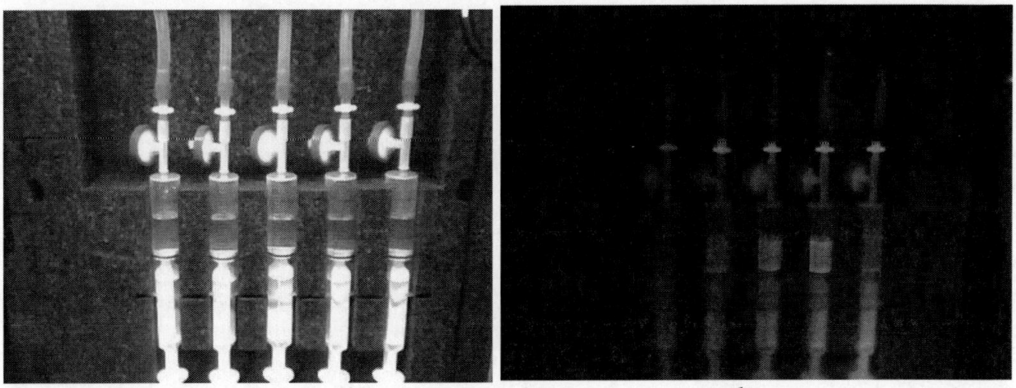

a b

Figure 7. (a-b) The PMEU method has been exploited in the detection of coliformic and *E. coli* growth in the Colilert™ media (IDEXX Laboratories, Inc., Maine, US) (Hakalehto, 2011a). This medium is used for detecting fecal contamination in waters.

Indirect means for verifying the growth and activity of microbes according to their metabolic functions in the PMEU include the measurement of metabolic functions, such as ATP concentration (Mentu et al., 2009), or the emission of volatile organic compounds (the voc's) (Hakalehto et al., 2009; Hakalehto and Hänninen, 2012, Laitiomäki et al., 2014). The latter method is one of the most sensitive ways for acquiring real-time information on the microbe populations.

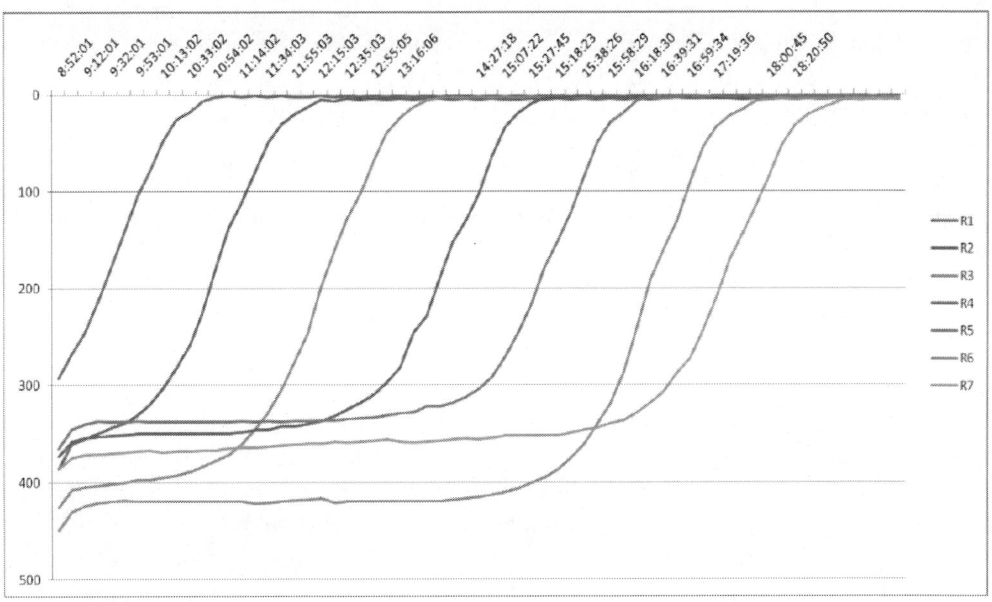

Figure 8. The quantification of the bacteria by "extrapolating" the growth curves obtained from PMEU cultivations. In the case of *E. coli* this means about one hour shortening in the onset of growth (in the PMEU graph) per 10-fold increase of the initial cell concentration (Hakalehto, 2011a).

It is also possible to quantify the bacteria by "extrapolating" the growth curves obtained from PMEU cultivations. In the case of *E. coli* this means about one hour shortening in the onset of growth (in the PMEU graph) per 10-fold increase of the initial cell concentration (Figure 8). In principle, the PMEU method has been able to help more microbe cells to recover in from the samples compared with other cultivation means (Heitto et al., 2009; Pesola and Hakalehto, 2011).

Escherichia coli, and other coliformic strains form a group of facultative anaerobic bacteria which is typical for the human intestinal tract, although it is often not associated with the small intestines (Levinson, 2006).

In fact, even though *E. coli* is less numerous in the duodenum, jejunum or ileum, than in the colon, it may possess some important functions in the regulation of the conditions in these areas important for human nutrition (Hakalehto et al., 2008; Hakalehto, 2011a). This bacterium, together with the other so-called coliformic bacteria and fecal enterococci, represents around 60% of the microflora in the bile duct and most likely also on the duodenal epithelial surfaces (Hakalehto et al., 2010). Sampling from the bile duct of 249 patients produced 973 aseptically collected microbial isolates in an Austrian hospital during three years. More than ten percent of the strains (12.6%) was identified as *E. coli.* It can tolerate relatively high levels of bile substances which makes it possible for it to survive also in the upper small intestines. There the *E. coli* strains are able to regulate and maintain the intestinal conditions in symbiosis with the human host body and the strains of *Klebsiella/Enterobacter* group (Hakalehto et al., 2008). Together with these neutral end-products producing facultative coliforms the acid-producing *E. coli* strains contribute to making up the foundation of the BIB. Therefore, *E. coli* and other coliforms have also emerged amongst all the intestinal microbes as the most important hygiene indicating bacteria in water, food, cosmetics etc., indicating fecal contamination (Edberg et al., 2000, Hakalehto et al., 2010).

Moreover, the *E. coli* bacterium has been used for decades as a model organism in the studies of bacterial cell structure, function and genetics as well as hygiene indicator (Rompré et al., 2002).

In the human body system the *E. coli* strains also offer a model system for investigating the molecular communication between different microbes and man. The interactions of various microbial subpopulations as members of the microbiota can also be studied on the basis of considering *E. coli* as "one of the major bacteriological building blocks" of the intestinal flora and an important factor in its development (Hakalehto et al., 2008; Pesola et al., 2009; Hakalehto, 2011a; Pesola et al., 2012). The PMEU technology offers a tool for these kinds of evaluations.

For example, in a neonatal patient the occupation of the small intestines was shown to be delayed by several months after antibiosis following the birth (Pesola and Hakalehto, 2011).

In this kind of example, the vulnerability of the microbiota could be observed. In fact, the unbalanced microbial composition and function could also explain many diseases, disturbances and malfunctions of the alimentary tract, and it has been postulated that human body and its microbiota form a kind of "superorganism" (Lederberg, 2000). The malfunctioning of this symbiotic system is likely to include for instance the small intestinal bacterial overgrowth (SIBO) and irritable bowel syndrome (IRS) (Ford et al., 2009), and most likely also endocolitis (Ishikawa et al., 2003) and Crohn´s disease (Lodes et al., 2004).

These diseases contribute to the general health status of an individual by many ways. For example, the SIBO is increasing the occurrence of rosacea significantly (Parodi et al., 2008), and is treated with an antibiotic, rifaximin which is not penetrating the intestinal membranes (Pimentel, 2009). This example demonstrates the need for understanding the molecular communication on the mucosal membranes, and between different bacteria on them.

When using the PMEU one is actually observing the multiplied picture on the cellular microcosm on the membraneous surfaces.

Function of Antibiotics and Peptides on the Microflora Variations

In order to test quickly the effect of various antimicrobial compounds on the bacterial strains, the PMEU broth could be loaded with e.g., different antibiotics or other bacteriostatic or bacteriosidic substances. The impacts of vancomycin and bile substance oxgall were studied on pure and mixed cultures of intestinal bacteria (Hakalehto et al., 2010). We have also studied the influences of some synthetic peptides, in which case it was possible to detect the inhibiting influences of very low peptide concentrations on the growth curves in the PMEU cultivation (results not shown here). The frog skin peptides, and their effect on *S. aureus* and the salmonellas has been studied with the PMEU (Samgina et al., 2012). Similarly we were able to monitor the growth inhibition of human beta-defensin-2 (HBD-2) on the *E. coli* patient strain. This defensin (HBD-2) is a cysteine-rich cationic low molecular weight antimicrobial peptide, which is produced by a number of epithelial cells and exhibits potent antimicrobial activity against Gram-negative bacteria (Schröder and Harder, 1999).

In Figure 9 there is a growth curve from aerobic *E. coli* culture grown without any antibiotic addition in the TYG broth (a), and with 50IU/ml of penicillin G (b), 0.25mg/ml cefuroxin (c), and 0.025 mg/ml netilmicin. The cultivation took place in the PMEU Spectrion® at 37 °C in aerobic conditions (with continuous sterile air flow). Bacterial growth was observed only when no antibiotic was used in the cultivation indicating the sensitivities of the studied bacterial strain to the used medications.

11. Future Perspectives

The development of new antimicrobial agents has faced remarkable difficulties. The race against the increasing antibiotic resistance of the microbes is in a very challenging phase.

Careful monitoring of microbiota and effective diagnostics of infecting pathogens are crucial for more directed antimicrobial treatment.

However, until rapid and accurate tests for infective agents like *Streptococcus pneumoniae* are available, the initial treatment will remain empirical (Jones et al., 2010).

Likewise in case of Fleming finding of the antibacterial action of *Penicillium,* also in future more attention should be paid to the detection of antibiotic substances of different microbes. There are interesting data on substances possessing antibiotic activities against various pathogens.

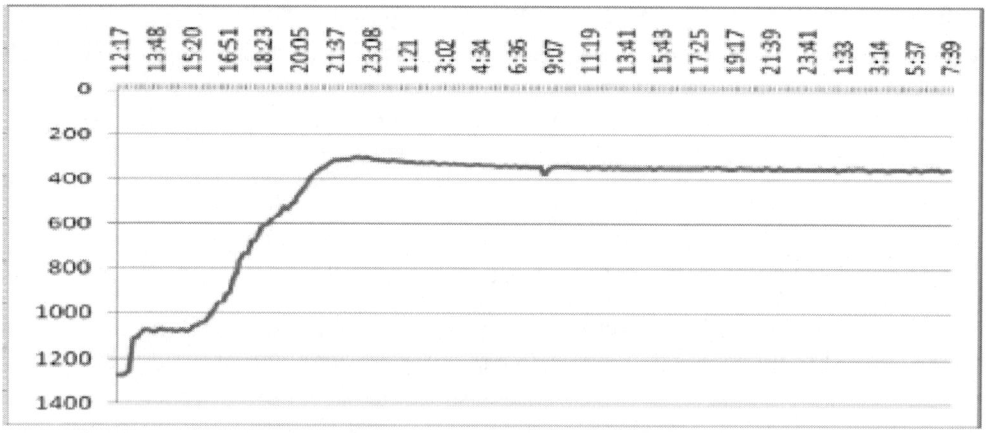

a

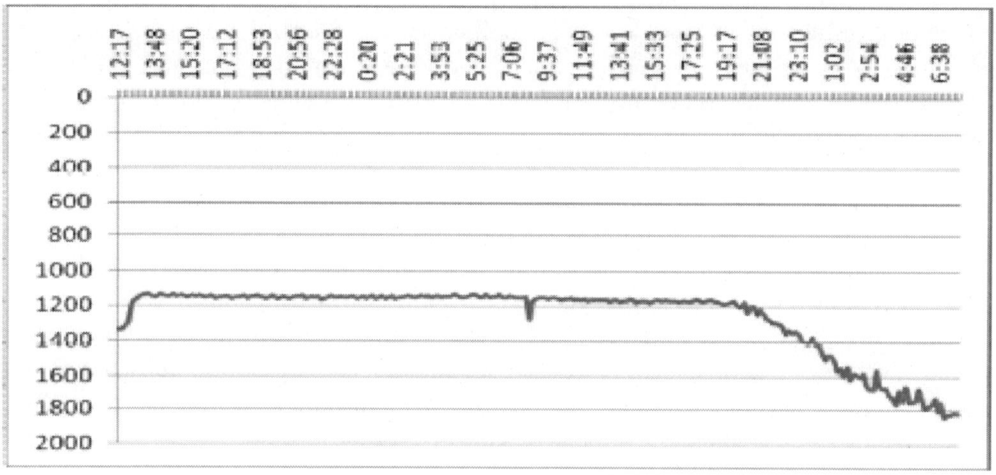

b

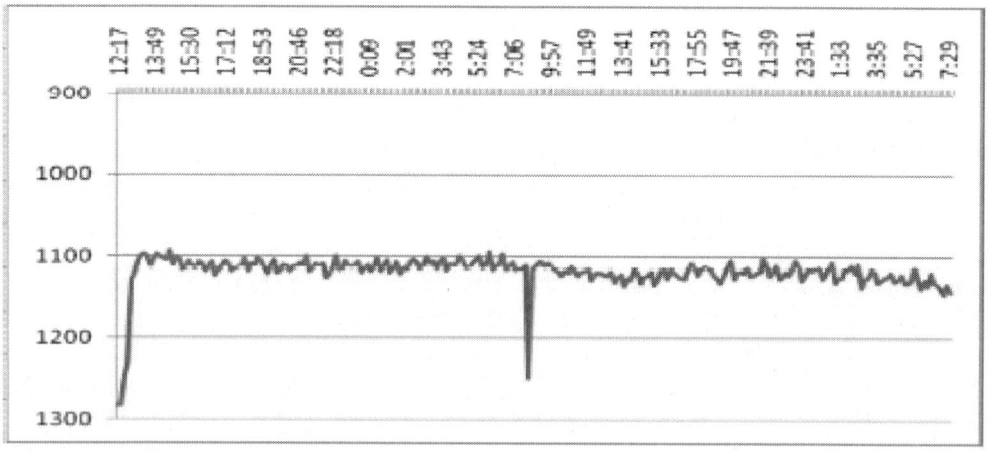

c

Figure 9. (Continued).

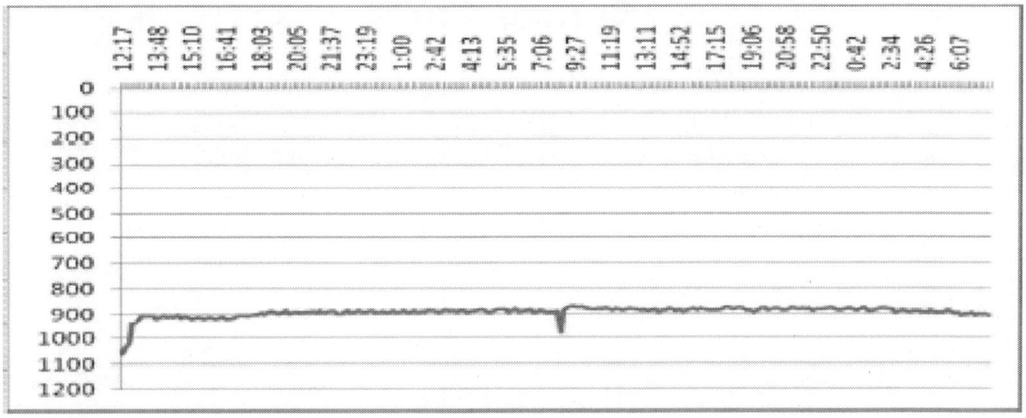

d

Figure 9. The growth curves of different *E. coli* cultures in the PMEU in aerobic conditions. In the curve (a) no antibiotics were added to the TYG medium, whereas the other syringes contained benzylpenicillin (b), cefuroxime (c), and netilmicin (d) (Hakalehto, 2011a).

In nature there are tremendous resources of microbes yet unknown. For example, it has been stated that termites have several hundred species of gut microbes unique to them capable to utilize dead plant materials effectively (Hongoh, 2010). The growing understanding of the capabilities of these microbes could provide new tools also for the search of new antibiotic compounds.

Both *Aspergillus* sp. strain FKI-2136 and *Streptomyces* sp. K04-0144 have shown imipenem potentiating effects against MRSA (Koyama et al., 2005; Fukumoto et al., 2008). *Rhodococcus* sp. K01-B0171 produces produces two types of antimycobacterial agents, lariatin A and B (Iwatsuki et al., 2006). Also calpinactam produced by fungal strain *Mortiella alpina* FKI-4905 is active against mycobacterial strains (Koyama et al., 2010a), but also against other bacteria and fungi (Koyama et al., 2010b). On the other hand, some interesting antibacterial metabolites of *Actinomyces* sp. have been found (Koyama et al., 2013).

Citridone A that has originally been isolated from the culture broth of *Penicillium* sp. FKI-1938 can both potentiate antifungal miconazole against *Candida albicans* and inhibit the MRSA (Fukuda et al., 2014). Antibiotic treatments may have relatively long-lasting harmful effects on the intestinal microbiota. It has been suggested that in addition to probiotic lactobacilli, that have been used for balancing the gut during and after the antibiotic treatments, also yeasts could be used in order to buffer the lactic acidosis resulting from a mixed antibiotic therapy with numerous substances in short small bowel patients (Bongaerts et al., 2005).

The effectivity of the older antibiotic agents towards bacteria could also be enhanced by overcoming the barriers of natural resistance.

This could be achieved, e.g., through investigating the antibiotic-sensitive strains of the species being normally resistant towards the antibiotic in question (Rida et al., 1996).

Conclusion

The global distribution of antibiotic resistant strains has been followed up widely by international organizations. In the worsening situation, however, new measures are required for the monitoring of the resistance both in global scale and on the individual level.

Proper understanding is warranted on the structure and function of the pathogens, as well as the transmission of the antibiotic resistance traits between various species and strains. Also the penetration of the medicinal molecules into the tissues, and into microbial biofilms, needs to be further investigated.

References

Ariffin, H., Navaratnam, P., Mohamed, M., Arasu, A., Abdullah, W. A., Lee, C. L., Peng, L. H. Ceftazidime-resistant *Klebsiella pneumoniae* bloodstream infection in children with febrile neutropenia. *Int. J. Infect. Dis.,* 2000; 4, 21-25.

Ayalew, K., Nambiar, S., Yasinskaya, Y., Jantausch, B. A. Carbapenems in pediatrics. *Ther. Drug Monit.,* 2003; 25, 593-599.

Bauer, M. P., Notermans, D. W., van Benthem, B. H., Brazier, J. S., Wilcox, M. H., Rupnik, M., Monnet, D. L., van Dissel, J. T., Kuijper, E. J. ECDIS Study Group. *Clostridium difficile* infection in Europe: a hospital-based survey. *Lancet,* 2011; 1, 377, 63-73.

Bongaerts, G., Severijnen, R., Skladal, D., Bakkeren, J., Sperl, W. Yeast mediates lactic acidosis suppression after antibiotic cocktail treatment in short small bowel? *Scand. J. Gastroenterol.*, 2005; 40, 1246-1250.

Bosch, F., Rosich, L. The contributions of Paul Ehrlich to pharmacology: a tribute on the occasion of the centenary of his Nobel Prize. *Pharmacology*, 2008; 82, 171-179.

Bozdogan, B., Esel, D., Whitener, C., Browne, F. A., Appelbaum, P. C. Antibacterial susceptibility of vancomycin – resistant *Staphylococcus aureus* strain isolated at the Hershey Medical Center. *JAC*, 2003; 52, 864-868.

Crokaert, F. Febrile neutropenia in children. *Int. J. Antimicrob. Agents,* 2000; 16, 173-176.

Cuypers, H., Dash, S., Peterson, P. A., Saedler, H., Gierl, A. The defective En-I102 element encodes a product reducing the mutability of the En/Spm transposable element system of Zea mays. *EMBO J.*, 1988; , 7, 2953-2960.

Dantas, G., Sommer, M. O. A. How to fight back against antibiotic resistance. *American Scientist*, 2014; 102, 42-51.

Dortet, L., Poirel, L., Nordmann, P. Worldwide dissemination of the NDM-type carbapenemases in Gram-negative bacteria. *Biomed. Res. Int.*, 2014; 2014, 249856. doi: 10.1155/2014/249856. Epub. 2014 Mar. 26.

Duquesne, S., Petit, V., Peduzzi, J., Rebuffat, S. Structural and functional diversity of microcins, gene-encoded antibacterial peptides from enterobacteria. *J. Mol. Microbiol. Biotechnol.,* 2007; 13, 200-209.Edberg, S. C., Rice, E. W., Karlin, R. J., Allen, M. J. *Escherichia coli*: the best biological drinking water indicator for public health protection. *Symp. Ser. Soc. Appl. Microbiol.,* 2000; 29, 106S-116S.

Edwards, L. A., O'Neill, C., Furman, M. A., Hicks, S., Torrente, F., Pérez-Machado, M., Wellington, E. M., Phillips, A. D., Murch, S. H. Enterotoxin-producing staphylococci cause intestinal inflammation by a combination of direct epithelial cytopathy and superantigen-mediated T-cell activation. *Inflamm. Bowel Dis.*, 2012; 18, 624-640.

Flahaut, S., Vinogradov, E., Kelley, K. A., Brennan, S., Hiramatsu, K., Lee, J. C. Structural and Biological Characterization of a Capsular Polysacchatide Produced by *Staphylococcus haemolyticus*. *J. Bacteriol.*, 2008; 190, 1649-1657.

Fleming, A. On the antibacterial action of cultures of a *Penicillium*, with special reference to their use in the isolation of B. Influenzae. *British Journal of Experimental Pathology,* 1929; 10, 226-236.

Florey, H. W. The use of micro-organisms for therapeutic purposes. *Yale J. Biol. Med.*, 1946; 19, 101-117.Ford, A. C., Spiegel, B. M., Talley, N. J., Moayyedi, P. Small intestinal bacterial overgrowth in irritable bowel syndrome: systematic review and meta-analysis. *Clin. Gastroenterol. Hepatol.,* 2009; 7, 1279-1286.

Frachon. E., Bondet, V., Munier-Lehmann, H., Bellalou, J. Multiple microfermentor battery: a versatile tool for use with automated parallel cultures of microorganisms producing recombinant proteins and for optimization of cultivation protocols. *Appl. Environ. Microbiol.*, 2006; 72, 5225-5231.Fricker, C. R., Bullock, S., Murrin, K., Niemelä, S. I. Use of the ISO 9308-1 procedure for the detection of *E. coli* in water utilizing two incubation temperatures and two confirmation procedures and comparison with defined substrate technology. *J. Water Health*, 2008; 6, 389-397.

Fukuda, T., Shimoyama, K., Nagamitsu, T., Tomoda, H. Synthesis and biological activity of Citridone A and its derivatives. *The Journal of Antibiotics,* 2014; 1-6.

Fukumoto, A., Kim, Y. P., Hanaki, H., Shiomi, K., Tomoda, H., Õmura, S. Cyslabdan, a new potentiator of imipenem activity against methicillin-resistant *Staphylococcus aureus*, produced by *Streotomyces* sp. K04-0144. *J. Antibiot.,* 2008; 61, 7-10.

Garcia-Migura, L., Hendriksen, R. S., Fraile, L., Aarestrup, F. M. Antimicrobial resistance of zoonotic and commensal bacteria in Europe: the missing link between consumption and resistance in veterinary medicine. *Vet. Microbiol.*, 2014; 170, 1-9.

Grundmann, H., Livermore, D. M., Giske, C. G., Canton, R., Rossolini, G. M., Campos, J., Vatopoulos, A., Gniadkowski, M., Toth, A., Pfeifer, Y., Jarlier, V., Carmeli, Y. The CNSE Working Group. Carbapenem-non-susceptible Enterobacteriaceae in Europe: conclusions from a meeting of national experts. *Euro Surveill.*, 2010; 15, pii=19711.

Hakalehto, E. Semmelweis' present day follow-up: Updating bacterial sampling and enrichment in clinical hygiene. *Pathophysiology,* 2006; 13, 257-267.

Hakalehto, E. Hygiene monitoring with the Portable Microbe Enrichment Unit (PMEU). *41st R3 -Nordic Symposium. Cleanroom Technology, Contamination Control and Cleaning. VTT Publications 266.* Espoo, Finland: VTT (State Research Centre of Finland); 2010; pp. 164-176.

Hakalehto, E. Simulation of enhanced growth and metabolism of intestinal *Escherichia coli* in the Portable Microbe Enrichment Unit (PMEU). In: Rogers, M. C., Peterson, N. D. editors. *E. coli infections: causes, treatment and prevention.* New York, US: Nova Publishers; 2011a.

Hakalehto, E. Antibiotic resistant traits of facultative *Enterobacter cloacae* strain studied with the PMEU (Portable Microbe Enrichment Unit). In Press. In: Méndez-Vilas, A., editor. *Science against microbial pathogens: communicating current research and technological advances. Microbiology book series Nr. 3.* Badajoz, Spain: Formatex Research Center; 2011b.

Hakalehto, E. Development of microbial ecosystems. In: Hakalehto, E., editor. *Alimentary microbiome - a PMEU approach.* Nova Science Publishers, Inc., New York, NY, US; 2012a; pp. 95-125.

Hakalehto, E., editor. *Alimentary microbiome - a PMEU approach.* New York, NY, US: Nova Science Publishers, Inc.; 2012b.

Hakalehto, E. Interactions of *Klebsiella* sp. with other intestinal flora. In: Pereira, L. A., Santos, A., editors. *Klebsiella Infections: Epidemiology, Pathogenesis and Clinical Outcomes.* New York, US: Nova Science Publishers, Inc.; 2013; pp. 1-33.

Hakalehto, E. Bacteriological indications of human activities in the ecosystems. In: Armon, R., Hänninen, O., editors. *Environmental Indicators.* Germany: Springer Verlag; 2014. In Print.

Hakalehto, E., Hänninen, O. Gaseous CO_2 signal initiate growth of butyric acid producing *Clostridium butyricum* both in pure culture and in mixed cultures with *Lactobacillus brevis. Can. J. Microbiol.,* 2012; 58, 928-931.

Hakalehto, E., Heitto, L. Minute microbial levels detection in water samples by Portable Microbe Enrichment Unit Technology. *Environment and Natural Resources Research,* 2012; 2, 80-88.

Hakalehto, E., Kuronen, I. A method for producing jelly sweets, which contain antibodies. WIPO Patent Application WO/1998/043610; 1998.

Hakalehto, E., Pesola, J., Heitto, L., Närvänen, A., and Heitto, A. Aerobic and anaerobic growth modes and expression of type 1 fimbriae in *Salmonella. Pathophysiology,* 2007;14, 61-69.

Hakalehto, E., Humppi, T., Paakkanen, H. Dualistic acidic and neutral glucose fermentation balance in small intestine: Simulation *in vitro. Pathophysiology,* 2008; 15, 211-220.

Hakalehto, E., Pesola, J., Heitto, A., Bhanj Deo, B., Rissanen, K., Sankilampi, U., Humppi, T., Paakkanen, H. Fast detection of bacterial growth by using Portable Microbe Enrichment Unit (PMEU) and ChemPro100i® gas sensor. *Pathophysiology,* 2009; 16, 57-62.

Hakalehto, E., Hell, M., Bernhofer, C., Heitto, A., Pesola, J., Humppi, T., Paakkanen, H. Growth and gaseous emissions of pure and mixed small intestinal bacterial cultures: Effects of bile and vancomycin. *Pathophysiology,* 2010; 17, 45-53.

Hakalehto, E., Heitto, L., Heitto, A., Humppi, T., Rissanen, K., Jääskeläinen, A., Paakkanen, H., Hänninen, O. Fast monitoring of water distribution system with portable enrichment unit – Measurement of volatile compounds of coliforms and *Salmonella* sp. in tap water. *Journal of Toxicology and Environmental Health Sciences,* 2011; 3, 223-233.

Hakalehto, E., Pesola, J., del Amo, E. M., Hänninen, O. Bacterial interactions in the small intestine and their contribution to host nutrient uptake. In: Hakalehto, E., editor. *Alimentary microbiome - a PMEU approach.* Nova Science Publishers, Inc., New York, NY, US; 2012 pp. 61-94.

Hakalehto, E., Heitto, A., Heitto, L. Fast coliform detection in portable microbe enrichment unit (PMEU) with Colilert® medium and bubbling. *Pathophysiology*, 2013; 20, 257-262.Hakalehto, E., Nyholm, O., Bonkoungou, I. J., Kagambega, A., Rissanen, K., Heitto, A., Barro, N., Haukka, K. Development of microbiological field methodology for water and food-chain hygiene analysis of *Campylobacter* spp. and *Yersinia* spp. in Burkina Faso, West Africa. *Pathophysiology*, 2014 Aug 4. pii: S0928-4680(14)00043-1. doi: 10.1016/j.pathophys.2014.07.004. [Epub ahead of print]

Heitto, L., Heitto, A., Hakalehto, E. Tracing wastewaters with faecal enterococci. Poster presentation in 2nd European Large Lakes Symposium, Norrtälje, Sweden, 10.-14. August, 2009.

Heitto, L., Heitto, A., Hakalehto, E. Environmental monitoring using the enrichment of hygienic indicators. In: Hakalehto, E. (Ed.): *Alimentary microbiome - a PMEU approach.* Nova Science Publishers, Inc., New York, NY, USA; 2012, pp. 215-231.

Hell, M., Bernhofer, C., Huhulescu, S., Indra, A., Allerberger, F., Maass, M., and Hakalehto, E. (2010). How safe is colonoscope-reprocessing regarding *Clostridium difficile* spores? *The Journal of Hospital Infection* Vol. 76, Supplement 1: Abstracts, 8th International Congress of the Hospital Infection Society, 10-13 October 2010, Liverpool, UK, S21-22.

Hell, M., Permoser, M., Chmelizek, G., Kern, J. M., Maass, M., Huhulescu, S., Indra, A., Allerberger, F. Clostridium difficile infection: monoclonal or polyclonal genesis? *Infection,* 2011; 39 , 461-465.

Hell, M., Bernhofer, C., Stalzer, P., Kern, J. M., Claassen, E. Probiotics in *Clostridium difficile* infection: reviewing the need for a multistrain probiotic. *Benef. Microbes,* 2013; 4, 39-51.

Hongoh, Y. Diversity and genomes of uncultured microbial symbionts in the termite gut. *Biosci. Biotechnol. Biochem.,* 2010; 74, 1145-1151.

Indra, A., Schmid, D., Huhulescu, S., Hell, M., Gattringer, R., Hasenberger, P., Fiedler, A., Wewalka, G., Allerberger, F. Characterization of clinical *Clostridium difficile* isolates by PCR ribotyping and detection of toxin genes in Austria, 2006-2007. *J. Med. Microbiol.,* 2008; 57, (Pt 6), 702-708.Ishikawa, H., Akedo, I., Umesaki, Y., Tanaka, R., Imaoka, A., Otani, T. Randomized controlled trial of the effect of bifidobacteria-fermented milk on ulcerative colitis. *J. Am. Coll. Nutr.*, 2003; 22, 56-63.

Iwatsuki, M., Tomoda, H., Uchida, R., Gouda, H., Hirono, S., Õmura, S. Lariatins, antimycobacterial peptides produced by *Rhodococcus* sp. K01-B0171, have a lasso structure. *J. Am. Chem. Soc.,* 2006; 128, 7486-7491.

Jaakkola, K., Hakalehto, E. Intestinal imbalances and diseases of the digestive tract. In: Hakalehto, E., editor. *Alimentary microbiome - a PMEU approach.* New York, NY, US: Nova Science Publishers, Inc.; 2012; pp. 127-160.

Jones, R. N., Jacobs, M. R., Sader, H. S. Evolving trends in *Streptococcus pneumonia* resistance: implications for therapy of community-acquired bacterial pneumonia. *Int. J. Antimicrobial Agents*, 2010; 136, 197-204.

Kendall A. I. Some observations on the study of the intestinal bacteria. *J. Biol. Chem.*, 1909; 6, 499–507.

Koyama, N., Nagahiro, T., Yamaguchi, Y., Masuma, R., Tomoda, H., Õmura, S. Stemphones, novel potentiators of imipenem activity against methicillin-resistant *Staphylococcus aureus*, produced by *Aspergillus* sp. FKI-2136. *J. Antibiot.,* 2005; 58, 695-703.

Koyama, N., Shigenobu, K., Fukuda, T., Nagamitsu, T., Yasuhara, T., Omura, S., Tomoda, H. Structure and total synthesis of fungal calpinactam, a new antimycobacterial agent. *Org. Lett.*, 2010a; 12, 432-435.

Koyama, N., Shigenobu, K., Nonaka, K., Masuma, R., Matsumoto, M., Omura, S., Tomoda, H. Calpinactam, a new anti-mycobacterial agent, produced by *Mortierella alpina* FKI-4905. *J. Antibiot.*, 2010b; 63, 183-186.

Koyama, N., Tokura, Y., Takahashi, Y., Tomoda, H. Discovery of nosokophic acid, a predicted intermediate of moenomycins, from nosokomycin-producing *Streptomyces* sp. K04-0144. *Bioorg. Med. Chem. Lett.*, 2013; 23, 860-863.

Laitiomäki, E., Pesola, J., Hakalehto, E. Projected improvement in the fast microbiological analysis of neonatal blood samples. Submitted for publication. 2014.

Lederberg, J. Infectious history. *Science*, 2000; 288, 287-293.

Leslie, A. G., Moody, P. C., Shaw, W. V. Structure of chloramphenicol acetyltransferase at 1.75-A resolution. *Proc. Natl. Acad. Sci. US.*, 1988; 854133-7.

Levinson, W. E. *Review of Medical Microbiology and Immunology* (9. ed.). McGraw-Hill Medical Publishing Division. p. 30. ISBN 978-0-07-146031-6; 2006.

Liebana, E., Batchelor, M., Hopkins, K. L., Clifton-Hadley, F. A., Teale, C. J., Foster, A., Barker, L., Threlfall, E. J., Davies, R. H. Longitudinal farm study of extended-spectrum β-lactamase-mediated resistance. *J. Clin. Microbiol.*, 2006; 44, 1630-1634.

Liebana, E., Carattoli, A., Coque, T. M., Hasman, H., Magiorakos, A. P., Mevius, D., Peixe, L., Poirel, L., Schuepbach-Regula, G., Torneke, K., Torren-Edo, J., Torres, C., Threlfall, J. Public health risks of enterobacterial isolates producing extended-spectrum β-lactamases or AmpC β-lactamases in food and food-producing animals: an EU perspective of epidemiology, analytical methods, risk factors, and control options. *Clin. Infect. Dis.*, 2013; 56, 1030-1037.

Lodes, M. J., Cong, Y., Elson, C. O., Mohamath, R., Landers, C. J., Targan, S. R., Fort, M., Hershberg, R. M. Bacterial flagellin is a dominant antigen in Crohn disease. *J. Clin. Invest.*, 2004; 113, 1296-1306.

Lyte, M. The microbial organ in the gut as a driver of homeostasis and disease. *Med. Hypotheses.*, 2010; 74, 634-638.

Manzoni, P., De Luca, D., Stronati, M., Jacqz-Aigrain, E., Ruffinazzi, G., Luparia, M., Tavella, E., Boano, E., Castagnola, E., Mostert, M., Farina D. Prevention of nosocomial infections in neonatal intensive care units. *Am. J. Perinatol.*, 2013;, 30, 81-88.

Mattner, F., Bange, F.-C., Meyer, E., Seifert, H., Wichelhaus, T. A., Chaberny, I. F. Preventing the spread of multidrug-resistant gram-negative pathogens. *Dtsch. Arztebl. Int.*, 2012; 109, 39-45.

McKenna, M. The enemy within. *Sci. Am.*, 2011; 304, 46-53.

Mentu, J. V., Heitto, L., Keitel, H. V., Hakalehto, E. Rapid microbiological control of paper machines with PMEU method. *Paperi ja Puu / Paper and Timber*, 2009; 91, 7-8 (90th Anniversary).

Molton, J. S., Tambyah, P. A., Ang, B. S. P., Ling, M. L., Fisher, D. A. The global spread of healthcare-associated multidrug-resistant bacteria: a perspective from Asia. *CID*, 2013; 56, 1310-1318.

Mshana, S. E., Matee, M., Rweyemamu, M. Antimicrobial resistance in human and animal pathogens in Zambia, Democratic Republic of Congo, Mozambique and Tanzania: an urgent need of a sustainable surveillance system. *Annals of Clinical Microbiology and Antimicrobials,* 2013; 12, 28-37.

Nordmann, P., Poirel, L., Toleman, M. A., Walsh, T. R. Does broad-spectrum beta-lactam resistance due to NDM-1 herald the end of the antibiotic era for treatment of infections caused by Gram-negative bacteria? *J. Antimicrob. Chemother.,* 2011; 66 , 689-692.Parodi, A., Paolino, S., Greco, A., Drago, F., Mansi, C., Rebora, A., Parodi, A.,

Savarino, V. Small intestinal bacterial overgrowth in rosacea: clinical effectiveness of its eradication. *Clin. Gastroenterol. Hepatol.*, 2008; 6, 759-764.

Persichino, J., Sutjina, M., Kim, D. *Klebsiella pneumoniae*: epidemiology, microbiology, pathogenesis and clinical management. In: Pereira, L. A., Santos, A., editors. *Klebsiella Infections: Epidemiology, Pathogenesis and Clinical Outcomes*. New York, US: Nova Science Publishers, Inc.; 2013; pp. 35-66.

Pesola, J., Hakalehto, E. Enterobacterial microflora in infancy - a case study with enhanced enrichment. *Indian. J. Pediatr.,* 2011; 78, 562-568.

Pesola, J., Vaarala, O., Heitto, A., Hakalehto, E. Use of portable enrichment unit in rapid characterization of infantile intestinal enterobacterial microbiota. *Microb. Ecol. Health Dis.,* 2009; 21, 203-210.Pimentel, M. Review of rifaximin as treatment for SIBO and IBS. *Expert Opin. Investig. Drugs,* 2009; 18, 349-358.

Piper, G. L., Kaplan, L. J. Antibiotic heterogeneity optimizes antimicrobial prescription and enables resistant pathogen control in the intensive care unit. *Surg. Infect. (Larchmt).*, 2012; , 13,194-202.

Pitkänen, T., Bräcker, J., Miettinen, I., Heitto, A., Pesola, J., and Hakalehto, E. Enhanced enrichment and detection of thermotolerant *Campylobacter* species from water using the Portable Microbe Enrichment Unit (PMEU) and realtime PCR. *Can. J. Microbiol.,* 2009; 55, 849-858.

Popowska, M., Rzeczycka, M., Miernik, A., Krawczyk-Balska, A., Walsh, F., Duffy, B. Influence of soil use on prevalence of Tetracycline, Streptomycin, and Erythromycin Resistance and Associated Resistance Genes. *Antimicrob. Agents Chemother.,* 2012; 56 , 1434-1443.

Public Health England. PHE launches toolkit to manage hospital infections caused by antibiotic-resistant bacteria. 2014-03-06. www.gov.uk/government/news/phe-launches-toolkit-to-manage-hospital-infections-caused-by-antibiotic-resistant-bacteria. 2014.

Reynolds, R. Antimicrobial resistance in the UK and Ireland. *J. Antimicrob. Chemother.*, 2009; 64, S1, i19-i23.

Rida, S., Caillet, J., Alix, J.-H. Amplification of a novel gene, *sanA*, abolishes a vancomycin-sensitive defect in *Escherichia coli. J. Bacteriol.,* 1996; 178, 94-102.Rompré, A., Servais, P., Baudart, J., de-Roubin, M. R., Laurent, P. Detection and enumeration of coliforms in drinking water: current methods and emerging approaches. *J. Microbiol. Methods*, 2002; 49, 31-54.

Samgina, T., Vorontsov, E., Gorshkov, V., Hakalehto, E., Hänninen, O., Zubarev, R., Lebedev, A. Composition and antimicrobial activity of the skin peptidome of Russian brown frog *Rana temporaria. J. Proteome Res.,* 2012; 11, 6213-6222.

Schröder, J. M.; Harder, J. Human beta-defensin-2. *Int. J. Biochem. Cell Biol.,* 1999; 31, 645-651.

Schumann, A., Nutten, S., Donnicola, D., Comelli, E. M., Mansourian, R., Cherbut, C., Corthesy-Theulaz, I., Garcia-Rodenas, C. Neonatal antibiotic treatment alters gastrointestinal tract developmental gene expression and intestinal barrier transcriptome. *Physiol. Genomics,* 2005; 23, 235-245.

Shahid, M., Khardodi, N., Tripathi, T., Bergman, S. Pharmaco-EcoMicrobiology: A newer component of medical sciences bridging pharmacovigilance, ecology, and environmental microbiology. *Journal of Infection and Public Health,* 2010; 3, 1-4.

Shindo, K., Fukushima, K. Deconjugation of bile acids by human intestinal bacteria. *Gastroenterol. Jpn.*, 1976; 11, 167-174.

Siu, L. K., Lu, P L., Hsueh, P. R., Lin, F. M., Chang, S. C., Luh, K. T., Ho, M., Lee, C. Y. Bacteremia due to extended-spectrum beta-lactamase-producing *Escherichia coli* and *Klebsiella pneumoniae* in a pediatric oncology ward: clinical features and identification of different plasmids carrying both SHV-5 and TEM-1 genes. *J. Clin. Microbiol.,* 1999; 37, 4020-4027.

Triggle, N. Hospitals 'on brink of collapse. *BBC News*, 13.9.2012.

Valachis, A., Kofteridis, D. P. Treatment strategies for infections caused by carbapenem resistant and pandrug resistant *Klebsiella* isolates. In: Pereira, L. A., Santos, A. editors. *Klebsiella Infections: Epidemiology, Pathogenesis and Clinical Outcomes*. New York, US: Nova Science Publishers, Inc.; 2013; pp. 107-131.

Van der Velden, A. W., Pijpers, E. J., Kuyvenhoven, M. M., Tonkin-Crine, S. K., Little, P., Verheij, T. J. Effectiveness of physician-targeted interventions to improve antibiotic use for respiratory tract infections. *Br. J. Gen. Pract.*, 2012; 62, e801-807.

Van Epps, H. L. René Dubos: unearthing antibiotics. *J. Exp. Med.,* 2006; 203, 259.

Wellington, E. M., Boxall, A. B., Cross, P., Feil, E. J., Gaze, W. H., Hawkey, P. M., Johnson-Rollings, A. S., Jones, D. L., Lee, N. M., Otten, W., Thomas, C. M., Williams, A. P. The role of the natural environment in the emergence of antibiotic resistance in gram-negative bacteria. *Lancet Infect. Dis.,* 2013; 13, 155-165.

Werner, G., Coque, T. M., Hammerum, A. M., Hope, R., Hryniewicz, W., Johnson, A., Klare, I., Kristinsson, K. G., Leclercq, R., Lester, C. H., Lillie, M., Novais, C., Olsson-Liljequist, B;., Peixe, L. V., Sadowy, E., Simonsen, G. S., Top, J., Vuopio-Varkila, J., Willems, R. J., Witte, W., Woodford, N. Emergence and spread of vancomycin resistance among enterococci in Europe. *Eurosurveillance*, 2008; 13: 1-11.

Wirtanen, G., Salo, S. PMEU-laitteen validointi koliformeilla (Validation of the PMEU equipment with coliforms). *Report VTT-S-01705-10, Statement VTT-S-02231-10; 2010.*

Wopereis, H., Oozeer, R., Knipping, K., Belzer, C., Knol, J. The first thousand days - intestinal microbiology of early life: establishing a symbiosis. *Pediatr. Allergy Immunol.,* 2014; Jun. 5. doi: 10.1111/pai.12232. [Epub. ahead of print].

Zubareva, N., Goncharov, A., Solomennyi, A. Multi-drug resistant *Klebsiella pneumoniae* and *Klebsiella oxytoca* strains in Russian hospital. In: Pereira, L. A., Santos, A. editors. *Klebsiella Infections: Epidemiology, Pathogenesis and Clinical Outcomes*. New York, US: Nova Science Publishers, Inc.; 2013; pp. 209-220.

In: Microbiological Clinical Hygiene
Editor: Eino Elias Hakalehto
ISBN: 978-1-63463-428-1

Appendices

Appendix 1

POSTULATES FROM AIRBORNE CONTAGION (Wells, 1955):

FIRST POSTULATE

The Castleman-Rayleigh theory of atomization defines the size of the droplets expelled by violent expiratory processes; the diameter of most of these droplets will not greatly exceed 10 microns.

SECOND POSTULATE

Raoult's law of molecular exchange at the surface of a liquid dictates that most droplets expelled by violent expiratory processes evaporate before reaching the ground. Raoult's law also defines the condensation of vapour upon a droplet; the concentration of glycol in a droplet depends more upon the humidity of the atmosphere than upon the amount of glycol added to the air.

THIRD POSTULATE

Stoke's law dictates that the nuclei of most droplets atomized indoors shall remain in atmosphere suspension until they are breathed or vented or until they die. Settling velocity becomes the aerodynamic dimension, which governs the retention of droplet nuclei in the atmosphere.

FOURTH POSTULATE

Conversely, Stoke's law governs the removal of droplet nuclei from the air by attraction or momentum. Generally, the product of settling velocity by an aerodynamic constant, fixed by conditions of collection, gives the negative natural logarithm of the uncollected fraction of particles. The aerodynamic constant of upper respiratory tract permits droplet nuclei to pass to the lung, where the aerodynamic constant insures their deposition.

FIFTH POSTULATE

Many parasites in the nuclei of droplets atomized indoors live until breathed or vented.

PHYSICAL SYNTHESIS

The dominant part, which the aerodynamics of droplet nuclei plays in the dynamic spread or airborne contagion, within and between population groups, is the theme of second part of this book. Let it suffice to say here that this role fits the dynamic pattern suggested by a statistical analysis of epidemics of contagious diseases. The ode of generation, their buoyance in air, their dispersion through indoor atmospheres, and their implantation in the lung when breathed – all adapt droplet nuclei for a leading part in the great drama of airborne contagion.

SIXTH POSTULATE

The vulnerability of parasites in droplet nuclei to lethal radiation may be expressed quantitatively, in terms of the Bunse-Roscoe reciprocity law, by the law of mass action: the number of parasites killed is proportional to the lethal radiation intercepted by the living organisms. These are more vulnerable in dry than in humid air, in aqueous suspension, or on moist agar surfaces.

SEVENTH POSTULATE

By Raoult's water evaporates from, and glycol vapour condenses upon, droplet nuclei (or vice versa) until the mole percentage of glycol in solution equals the relative pressure of the vapour at saturation. Humidity therefore dominates the equilibrium concentration of certain hydroxyl derivatives of certain hydrocarbons to which certain parasites in droplet nuclei suspended in atmospheres saturated with the vapours are vulnerable at mid-humidity ranges.

BIOLOGICAL SYNTHESIS

Quite irrespective of all theoretical considerations of the viability, longevity, and vulnerability of airborne parasites, the practical results of experiments conducted over a score of years demonstrate conclusively that many parasites in the nuclei of droplets expelled in indoor atmosphere can live until breathed or vented and during this period can be destroyed by lethal agents innocuous to the human occupants. The use of such agents constitutes the sanitary equivalent of ventilation.

EIGHT POSTULATE

The infectivity of certain airborne parasites against certain hosts depends as much upon the aerodynamic dimension of inhaled particles as upon the virulence of included parasites or the innate resistance of their hosts, for the tissue upon which a parasite is planted also governs the response of the host.

NINTH POSTULATE

The response to inhaled droplet nuclei contagium is quantal; the Poisson equation expresses reasonably well the relation between dosage and initial response, a quantum infection 63,2 per cent of homogeneously exposed hosts by definition. The manifestation of infection depends both upon the number of the parasites breathed and upon their rate of inhalation, for the response to subsequent infection may be modified by the reaction of the host to initial infection. Pulmonary disease has been induced quantitatively in experimental animals breathing parasites in droplet nuclei.

PARASITOLOGICAL SYNTHESIS

Animal studies conducted over a dozen years enabled us, first, to develop special techniques for the quantitative study of the pathogenesis of droplet infections and, second, to demonstrate quantitative that airborne parasites breathed in droplet nuclei may penetrate to the lungs and so induce respiratory disease. The infectivity of inhaled particles depended as much upon their aerodynamic dimension as upon the virulence of included parasites or the resistance of the host. However, this response was modified by prior experience with the same or other parasites. If, the, infectivity defines response and change in response defines reaction, we conclude that in experimental airborne tuberculosis quantal initial response was homogeneous even though reaction was heterogeneous.

TENTH POSTULATE

The mean discharge of airborne contagium per contagious carries is statistically determinate for a specific host-parasite relationship.

REVELATION 22:1-2

And he shewed me a pure river of water of life, clear as crystal…and on either side of the river, was there the tree of life, which bore twelve manner of fruits, and yielded her fruit every month; and the leaves of the tree were for the healing of the nations.

From: Wells, WF. Airborne contagion and air hygiene: an ecological study of droplet infection. Cambridge, MA: Harvard University Press; 1955.

Appendix II: Preoperative Skin-Antisepsis

Bernhofer, C. and Hell, M.
Zentrum für Krankenhaushygiene und Infektionskontrolle der SALK
ESCMID Collaborative Centre for Infection Control (ECC)
Universitätsklinikum der Paracelsus Medizinischen Privatuniversität (PMU) – Salzburg
Müllner Hauptstr.48
A-5020 Salzburg
Austria

OR routine procedures in Austria... a very practical approach – best practice model:

Patient, before going to the OR:	Bath or shower, including nail cleaning, hair washing and shaving, preferably in the evening before the surgery. Before minimal invasive surgery, give the belly button a second look – some people forget to clean it.
Skin-Antisepsis: When:	Before every breach of skin or mucous membranes
What:	In Austria, antiseptics are legally considered drugs. Therefore, only registered products may be used. Do never mix alcohol-based and water-based antiseptics or add other ingredients to antiseptic solutions.
Skin:	Alcohol: Isopropanol, n-propanol; we don't recommend ethanol 'cause we had already problems with skin reactions
Mucous membranes:	Octenidindihydrochloride or iodophores; chlorhexidine-based agents are not commonly used in German speaking hospitals
Who:	Trained surgeon or OR-nurse
When:	Immediately before surgery, after all other preparations are made.
Where:	In an operating room or a defined room in an outpatient department.
How:	Prepare sterile gauze swabs (fixed in an appropriate forceps) thoroughly drenched with antiseptic solution. Wipe skin/mucous membranes carefully and thoroughly at least four times. Change the swabs every time. Do not touch the disinfected area again. Take care that the disinfectant can't form a puddle underneath the Patient or accumulate in skinfolds.
Exceptions:	If there are pre-existing wounds or skin defects, don't use alcohol! Take care that alcohols can't get into eyes, mouth, nose or ear if you are working at the face of a patient. For infants, it might be better to use an iodophore or octenidindihydrochloride. Skin reactions to alcohols were observed at our pediatric surgery department. For surgeries regarding bones or joints, the disinfection of the limb has to be done circularly. This requires necessarily at least one assisting person.

A) General Recommendations

Before all invasive techniques and in particular before surgery, a skin and/or a mucous membrane disinfection is necessary. On healthy skin, alcohol should always be preferred. For wounds, mucous membranes and infants, water-based disinfectants are recommended; do consider allergies and contraindications, e. g. iodine allergy/thyroid illnesses.

Before surgery:

If possible, the patient takes a bath or shower, otherways is washed in bed. Disinfecting detergents are not necessary. To avoid skin reactions or enhance shedding of skin flora due to dry skin, its recommended in some guidelines to do this the evening before.

Before surgery at the face, head or neck wash the hair also, because this might not be possible afterwards for some time. In preparation of abdominal surgery, in particular minimal invasive techniques, special attention should be directed toward the thorough cleaning of the navel.

Before surgery at hands or feet the nails should be included into the preparation. Nail lacquer, hair clips, false teeth and private underwear as well as all kinds of jewellery need to be removed.

Experts in infection control agree on the fact, that preoperative shaving increases the risk of a surgical site infection. So, avoid shaving, shortening the hair is sufficient. If the surgeon insists on a complete hair removal, only clipping should be done, as close to the scheduled time of surgery as possible. A preoperative skin disinfection at the ward, with or without sterilized cover, is useless, more important and more effective would be a change of bedding and linens before the patienten is sent to the OR.

The preoperative skin antisepsis takes place in the OR, after all necessary lines are inserted and other preparations made. The disinfection itself can be done by a surgeon as well as an OR-nurse, after a surgical hand disinfection, with sterile gloves and a sterile forceps. In order to avoid contamination, it is better to done the sterile gown afterwards. The gloves have to be changed before further preparations.

Take care that no disinfectants accumulate under the patient, and/or in skinfolds. This could cause skin-irritation or burns, if cauterization is used. Furthermore, make suret hat alcohols can't get into the eyes, mouth, nose, into open wounds or on genital organs.

Don't use hand antiseptics for preoperative skin disinfection. They contain emollients, perfums and these may cause irritation or allergy. Besides, the emollients prevent tapes and drapes from adhering properly!

B) Procedure

1. Aseptic Surgery

The disinfection is done with fully soaked (but not dripping) swabs and strong wipes, in order to achieve an additional mechanical cleaning. Whenever possible, the disinfected area should be in every direction at least fifteen centimeters more than the intended incision site.

2. Surgery at Contaminated/Inflammed Areas, Preexisting Wounds or Colostomata

Use a mucous membrane disinfectant (e. g. an iodophore).

Exception: If the aim of the surgery is to eliminate the stoma, alcohol can and should be used, because of its higher efficacy.

3. Surgery at the Face

Alcohol-based disinfectants may not get into the eyes, the nose or the ears. If covering these areas is possible, the disinfection can oand should be done with alcohol.

4. Surgery at the Groin, in the Mouth or Nose

Use a water-based mucous membrane disinfectant.

Note that alcohol-based disinfectants can cause skin irritations and lingering pain on mucous membranes and sometimes on shaved skin areas e. g. the male groin lingering after the surgery for hours. Hence, prefer a water-based disinfectant for the male groin and in particular for children.

5. Surgery on Arms and Legs

In order to exclude confusion, marking of the extremity concerned by the surgeon before the patient is brought to the OR is strongly recommended! The disinfection itself is done with an alcohol-based disinfectant - exceptions see above. If the operating technique needs moving the Limb during surgery, a circular disinfection is required. Therefore, the assistance of a second person is always necessary, maybe even a third - with sterile gloves – is required.

If a disinfection of fingers or toes (or e.g., the male genital organ) is necessary, then a usual disinfection with forceps is difficult. The use of soaked gauze compresses (and of course change of the sterile gloves afterwards) is an easier alternative. A preoperative bath facilitates the disinfection in the OR.

An assistant keeps the extremity outstretched, standing as far as possible distant from the patient. The surgeon or OR nurse (preferably without sterile gown) disinfects first circularly the area of the intended incision, then likewise circularly toward fingers or toes and in direction to the groin or arm pit. If a disinfection of the complete arm or leg is required or the patient has a fracture, the assistance of a third person with sterile gloves is required, who holds the already disinfected area, while the first one finishes the disinfection proximally and distally. The extremity may be put down only after positioning of a sterile drape and if necessary after the attachment of sterile stockings.

6. Surgery on Children

For surgery on children, especially infants, regardless the localization, a mucous membrane disinfectant is recommended, since alcohol can cause adverse skin reactions. In addition, the cooling effect by the evaporation of alcohol needs to be considered in small infants.

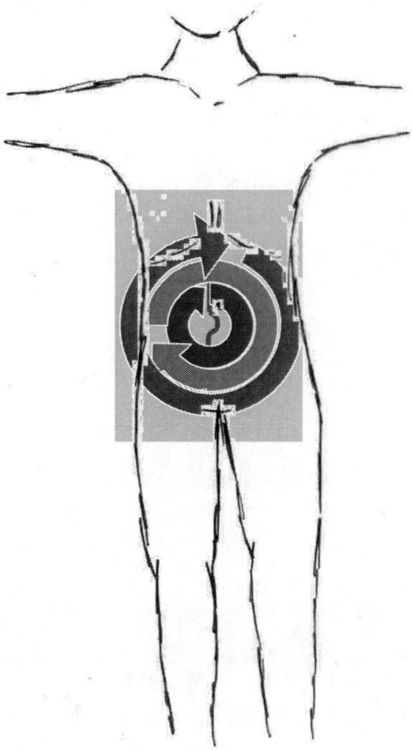

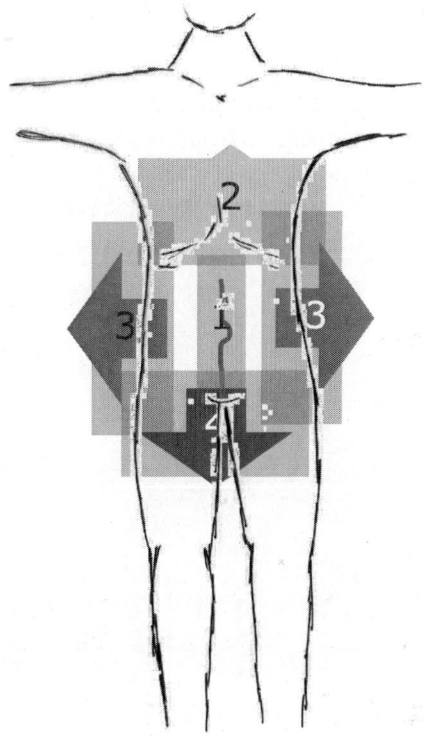

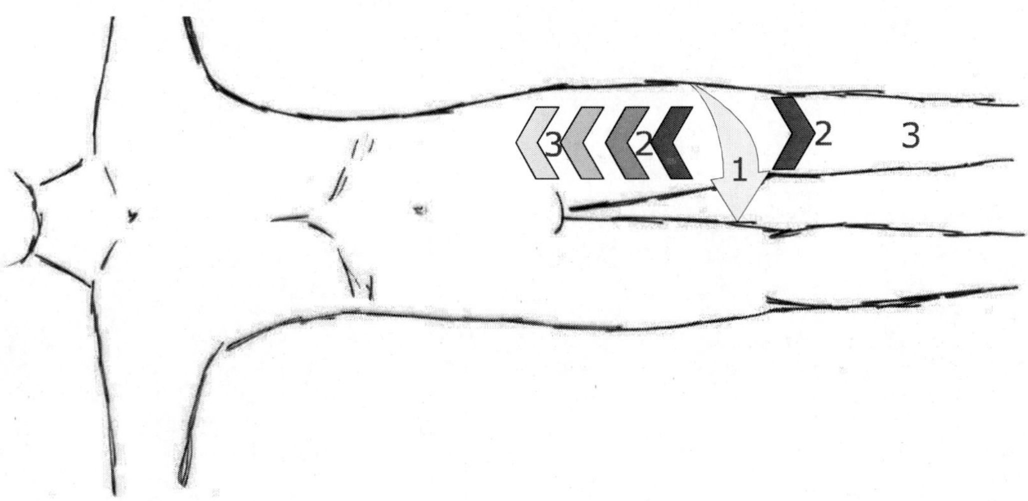

References

Austrian Standards plus GmbH. Chemical disinfectants and antiseptics — Surgical hand disinfection — Test method and requirements (phase 2, step 2). ICS 11.080.20. Identical (IDT) with prEN 12791:2013-07. Responsible Committee 215. Sterilization and disinfection of medical devices. Austrian Standards Institute/Österreichisches Normungsinstitut, Wien, Austria, 2013.

Goroncy-Bermes, P. Hand disinfection according to the European Standard EN 1500 (hygienic handrub): a study with Gram-negative and Gram-positive test organisms. *Int. J. Hyg. Environ. Health*, 2001; 204, 123-126.

Rotter, ML. European norms in hand hygiene. *J. Hosp. Inf.*, 2004; 56, S6–S9.

Suchomel, M; Gnant, G; Weinlich, M; Rotter, M. Surgical hand disinfection using alcohol: the effects of alcohol type, mode and duration of application. *J. Hosp. Inf.*, 2009; 71, 228-233.

Index

A

B

C

D

E

F

G

H

I

J

K

L

M

N

O

P

Q

R

S

T

U

V

W

X

Y